ENDOSONOGRAPHY

SERIES IN RADIOLOGY

Volume 17

For a list of the volumes in this series see final page of the volume.

Endosonography

edited by

BRUNO D. FORNAGE, M.D.

Associate Professor of Radiology
Chief, Section of Ultrasound,
The University of Texas M. D. Anderson Cancer Center,
Houston, Texas,

Director, Department of Radiology
Institut Jean Godinot, Reims, France

KLUWER ACADEMIC PUBLISHERS
DORDRECHT / BOSTON / LONDON

Library of Congress Cataloging-in-Publication Data

Endosonography.

    Includes index.
    1. Endoscopic ultrasonography. I. Fornage, Bruno.
[DNLM: 1. Endoscopy. 2. Ultrasonic Diagnosis.
WB 289 E56]
RC78.7.E48E53 1989   616.07'543   88-27379

ISBN-13: 978-94-010-6886-4   e-ISBN-13: 978-94-009-0885-7
DOI: 10.1007/978-94-009-0885-7

Published by Kluwer Academic Publishers,
P.O. Box 17, 3300 AA Dordrecht, The Netherlands.

Kluwer Academic Publishers incorporates the publishing programmes of
D. Reidel, Martinus Nijhoff, Dr W. Junk and MTP Press.

Sold and distributed in the U.S.A. and Canada
by Kluwer Academic Publishers,
101 Philip Drive, Norwell, MA 02061, U.S.A.

In all other countries, sold and distributed
by Kluwer Academic Publishers Group,
P.O. Box 322, 3300 AH Dordrecht, The Netherlands.

Preface

Following the development of gray-scale imaging, real-time scanning, Doppler examination, and high-frequency sonography, endosonography is one of the latest major breakthroughs in the history of diagnostic ultrasound. Although early attempts at inserting ultrasound transducers in natural cavities of the body can be traced back more than two decades, only in the past few years has technology allowed the development and commercialization of effective, easy-to-use endosonoscopic probes. Because the transducer can be placed in direct contact with or close to lesions, high frequencies (up to 12 MHz) can be used, yielding cross-sectional images of unsurpassed resolution. The availability of specially designed intracorporeal probes for specific natural cavities that are routinely explored by conventional (optical) endoscopy or palpation has significantly expanded the diagnostic applications of sonography. Transrectal and transvaginal examinations are now performed routinely in many institutions, and virtually all sonographic equipment manufacturers have in their line of products at least one endorectal and one endovaginal transducer. Most endosonoscopic probes connect to existing scanners, and for radiology departments, the investment for transrectal or transvaginal scanning will usually be limited to the purchase of the specific probe.

In this book, clinical applications of endosonography (excluding transesophageal echocardiography) are covered by European and North American experts. Current equipment and techniques of examination are described in detail to help newcomers get started in the field of endosonography. However, because endosonography is more operator dependent than regular ultrasound studies are, both adequate training and sufficient clinical practice are prerequisites for optimal results.

Bruno D. Fornage, M.D.
Associate Professor of Radiology
Chief, Section of Ultrasound
The University of Texas M. D. Anderson Cancer Center
Houston, Texas, U.S.A.

Contents

Contributors

Luigi Barbara, MD
Professor of Medicine
First Department of Internal Medicine
University of Bologna, Italy

Jacques L. Beco, MD
Department of Gynecology and Obstetrics
Hôpital de la Citadelle
University of Liège, Belgium

Luigi Bolondi, MD
Chief, Ultrasound Division
First Department of Internal Medicine
University of Bologna, Italy

Jörg A. Bönhof, MD
Department of Ultrasound
Deutsche Klinik für Diagnostik
Wiesbaden, F.R.G.

Patrice M. Bret, MD
Associate Professor of Radiology
McGill University;
Radiologist in Chief
Montreal General Hospital, Montreal, Canada

Gian Carlo Caletti, MD
Chief, Endoscopy
First Department of Internal Medicine
University of Bologna, Italy

Giulio Di Candio, MD
Assistant Professor of Surgery
Chief, Section of Ultrasound
Istituto di Patologia Chirurgica II
University of Pisa, Italy

Bruno D. Fornage, MD
Associate Professor of Radiology
Chief, Section of Ultrasound
The University of Texas MD
Anderson Cancer Center
Houston, Texas, U.S.A.
Director, Department of Radiology
Institut Jean Godinot, Reims, France

Hans H. Holm, MD, PhD
Professor of Urology
University of Copenhagen

Director, Department of Ultrasound
Herlev Hospital, Herlev, Denmark

Niels Juul, MD
Department of Ultrasound
Herlev Hospital, Herlev, Denmark

Peter Linhart, MD
Department of Gastroenterology
Deutsche Klinik für Diagnostik
Wiesbaden, F.R.G.

Nabil F. Maklad, MD, PhD
Professor of Radiology and Obstetrics,
Gynecology, and Reproductive Sciences
University of Texas Medical School at Houston;
Director of Ultrasound
Herman Hospital, Houston, Texas, U.S.A.

Franco Mosca, MD
Professor of Surgery
Director, Istituto de Patologia Chirurgica II
University of Pisa, Italy

Léandre G. Pourcelot, MD
Professor of Biophysics
Chairman, Department of Nuclear Medicine and
Ultrasound
University Hospital, Tours, France

Matthew D. Rifkin, MD
Professor of Radiology and Urology
Division of Diagnostic Imaging
Thomas Jefferson University Hospital
Philadelphia, Pennsylvania, U.S.A.

Jean-Pierre J. Schaaps, MD
Department of Gynecology and Obstetrics
Hôpital de la Citadelle
University of Liège, Belgium

Maseb S. Sulu, MD
Department of Gynecology and Obstetrics
Hôpital de la Citadelle
University of Liège, Belgium

Soren T. Torp-Pedersen, MD
Department of Ultrasound
Herlev Hospital, Herlev, Denmark

Acknowledgments

The editor wishes to express his gratitude to Rose Salazar and Véronique Dupuis for their secretarial assistance, and to Art Wimberly from the Department of Medical Graphics and Illustration, The University of Texas at Houston. He is also indebted to Suzanne Simpson, from the Department of Scientific Publications, The University of Texas at Houston, and to Dr James Lorigan for their editorial contribution in the preparation of this book.

1. General considerations on endosonographic equipment

LÉANDRE G. POURCELOT

Ultrasound imaging provides the physician with a great deal of information without risk to the patient. Conventional ultrasound is well established in the assessment of diseases of the heart, abdominal and pelvic organs, and soft tissues. However, visualization with this approach is limited in some areas of the abdomen and pelvis and in most of the mediastinum by obstacles to sound wave propagation. Bone and gas in the lungs and alimentary canal are each responsible for extreme variations in acoustic impedance, so that virtually all the acoustic energy of the incident beam is reflected rather than transmitted. Further, since the attenuation α of the beam is related to its frequency F as $\alpha = \alpha_0 F^\beta (\alpha_0 =$ attenuation coefficient at 1 MHz; $\beta \approx 1$), the transcutaneous visualization of deep structures requires the use of low frequencies, which limits image resolution and, consequently, the diagnostic capabilities. Frequencies greater than 3.5 MHz cannot usually be employed for transcutaneous examination of the abdominal and pelvic organs in adults.

Endoscopic ultrasound (or endosonography) circumvents these limitations. Without the obstacles of gas and bone, areas not accessible by conventional ultrasound can be imaged. Since the transducer is close to the region of interest, high frequencies can be used, improving spatial resolution and increasing diagnostic capabilities over external ultrasonography. Further, endoscopic ultrasound can be used in conjunction with fiberoptic endoscopy: the techniques are complementary, providing, respectively, in-depth visualization and a surface view.

Intracavitary ultrasound has only recently become popular. The esophageal route has been used to study the aortic arch and left carotid artery, the heart, esophagus, stomach, left lobe of the liver, biliary tree, and pancreas [1—5]. The rectal approach has been used for endoscopic sonography of the prostate, seminal vesicles, lower portion of the bladder, bladder neck, and more lately the urethra and rectum [6—14]. Transvaginal sonography has recently been used in the evaluation of the uterus and adnexa [15—17]. Transurethral scanning was specifically developed for the examination of the bladder [18, 19]. Evaluation of the uterus using intrauterine transducers has also been reported [20].

Technological requirements

Equipment design reflects the several requirements demanded by the special conditions of use. These requirements are:
1. Safety rules must be strictly observed, particularly as regards the protection of mechanically activated parts and electrical insulation. The endosonoscope must be waterproof, and it must also be easily sterilized.
2. The transducer must be miniature, notably so in a transesophageal or transurethral probe.
3. Adequate evaluation of an organ requires views made in at least two planes perpendicular to one another.
4. Ultrasound-guided biopsy, fiberoptic examination, or Doppler study should be possible during the endosonoscopic examination.
5. The stiff portion of a transesophageal endosonoscope should be as small as possible.

Bruno D. Fornage (ed.), *Endosonography*, pp. 1—7.
© 1989 *Kluwer Academic Publishers*.

Scanning modes

The basic ultrasound scanning techniques developed in conventional, external sonography are used in endosonography.

Mechanical sector scanning

Mechanical scanning with a single transducer results in a sector field of view that is usually perpendicular to the axis of the probe. The transducer mounted on the rotating axis (Fig. 1.1) can either oscillate, to scan a limited sector, or rotate a full 360°, generating a complete plane. The fixed transducer placed at the extremity of the probe can also operate in conjunction with a rotating 45° mirror used to reflect the beam perpendicularly to the probe axis (Fig. 1.2). This latter technique allows electronic focusing when an annular-array transducer is used. The major advantage of radial mechanical scanning is its simplicity and the availability of a wide range of transducers, from 3 to 12 MHz. Miniature radial transducers are available for transurethral and intrauterine scanning. Radial mechanical scanning has been widely applied to transrectal scanning [6—8]; it is also used in flexible esophageal endosonoscopes [3, 4]. In the latter case, however, rotation speed is limited by the risk of vibration.

A special mention must be made of the mechanical 'panoramic' (or 'end-firing') trans-

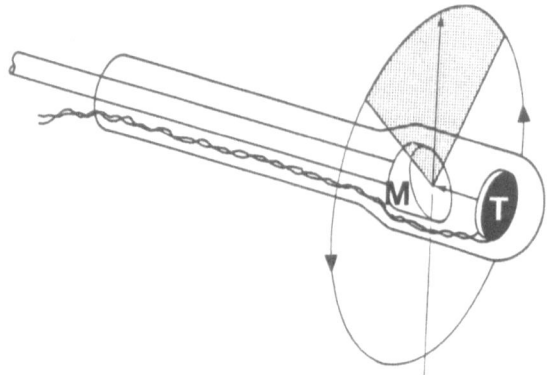

Figure 1.2. The axial rotation of the mirror (M), which reflects the beam emitted by the transducer (T), results in a scan plane perpendicular to the probe axis. Dynamic electronic focusing is available with an annular-array transducer.

vaginal transducers. An oscillating or rotating crystal scans a sector that is oriented forward along the axis of the probe. The resulting front view may exceed 180°.

Phased-array sector scanning

The transducer used in phased-array sector scanning consists of a small bar of several adjacent crystals, each less than 1 mm wide (Fig. 1.3). The image is obtained by electronic deflection of the beam; the ultrasound pulses from adjacent crystals are slightly delayed so that the wave front is propagated in an oblique direction

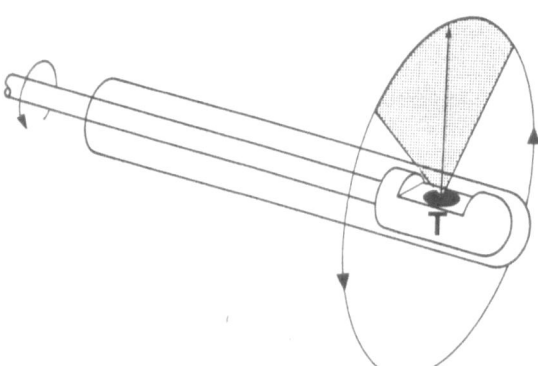

Figure 1.1. The radial mechanical scan is obtained by the oscillation or the complete rotation of the transducer (T) around the axis of the probe. The scanning plane is perpendicular to the probe axis.

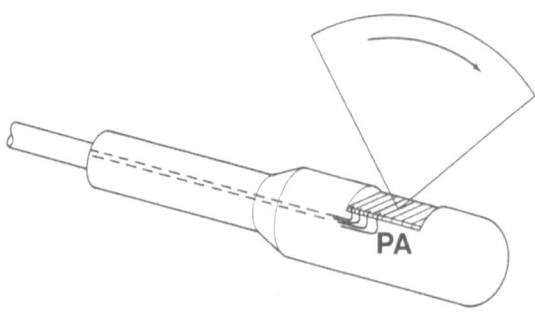

Figure 1.3. Phased-array sector scanning. The sector field of view is obtained through the dephasing of the beam emitted and received by each elementary crystal of the small linear transducer (PA). On this view, a longitudinally oriented sector scan is obtained since the phased-array transducer is placed along the probe axis.

determined by the value of the phase delay. This technique allows a maximum sector angle of 90°.

The advantages of this technique are that all mechanical movement is eliminated and that the transducer can be small. However, the electronic processing entailed is complex and therefore costly. This type of probe has been used in the transesophageal evaluation of the heart [1, 21]. More recently, transrectal and transvaginal phased-array sector probes have been developed.

Linear-array scanning

In linear-array intracavitary probes, the conformation is that of a bar of several centimeters consisting of many small contiguous crystals (Fig. 1.4). Groups of 4—20 adjacent crystals are fired simultaneously. After one group of crystals has completed its sound reception, the firing process is translated in 1-crystal increments so that one line of exploration is assigned to each crystal. The rapid electronic commutation of the various crystals provides up to 100 frames per second. There are no mechanically activated parts, and transducers of high frequencies, up to 10 MHz, have been successfully developed. The advantage of these transducers is that a homogeneous field is afforded by the parallel beam scanning. Also, variable electronic focusing is available. Linear-array scanning is ideal for evaluating superficial structures close to the transducer. Because the linear-array transducer is aligned along the probe axis, the probe is side-viewing. Linear-array probes are mainly used in transrectal scanning [9—13].

Convex-array sector scanning

Linear electronic scanning along a convex array of crystals (Fig. 1.5) provides a sector-type field of view whose angle depends on the curvature of the transducer. This recently developed scanning technique has the advantages both of linear-array electronic scanning, including a well-mastered electronic technology and the availability of high frequencies, and of sector scanning, including a reduced contact surface and widening of the ultrasound field of view at depth. Convex sector endoscopic transducers are now available for transvaginal and transesophageal examinations.

Comparison of sector and linear-array scanning

Linear-array scanning provides a homogeneous field of view, enabling adequate visualization of structures located in the near-field of the transducer. Nonhomogeneity of the image is sector scanning's major drawback: the near-field is poor because information is compressed into a limited surface, whereas the excessive spacing between each line in the far-field results in insufficient sampling. On the other hand, sector scanners are characterized by a small entry surface and an 'oblique' view in depth, allowing imaging of deep structures that might not be visualized by linear-array transducers. Currently,

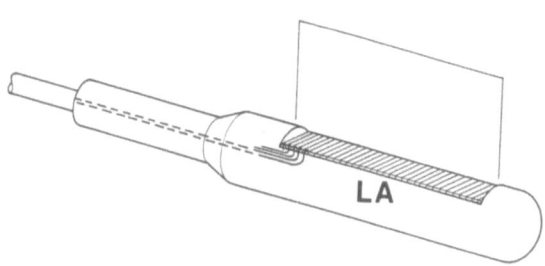

Figure 1.4. Linear-array electronic transducer operating by the sequential activation of the elementary crystals of the linear-array transducer (LA). The beams are parallel to one another.

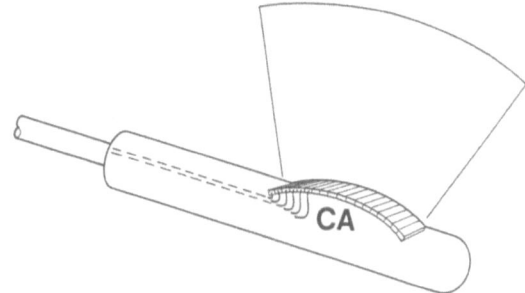

Figure 1.5. Electronic sector scanning obtained with a convex array (CA) of elementary crystals. The electronic processing of the signals is similar to that of the linear-array transducer described in Figure 1.4.

4

convex sector transducers are considered to provide the best compromise.

Bi- or multiplanar scanning

Until recently, ultrasound examination with commercially available intracavitary probes was limited to a single, fixed scanning plane, usually perpendicular or parallel to the axis of the probe. Three-dimensional evaluation required the consecutive use of two separate intracavitary transducers oriented 90° from each other. To overcome this shortcoming, various combined probes have been designed to provide biplanar

imaging, with transverse and sagittal scans, or even multiplanar imaging [11, 21, 22].

Biplane probes consist of either two separate fixed transducers or a single steerable transducer. Combinations include the following:

1. One transducer (or reflecting mirror) with two mechanical sector scanning movements. The transducer (or the mirror) can rotate (or oscillate) around the probe axis and around an axis perpendicular to that of the probe (Fig. 1.6).
2. Another configuration utilizes two separate single-crystal transducers (Fig. 1.7). The axial rotation of one transducer provides the transverse scanning plane, and the oscillation

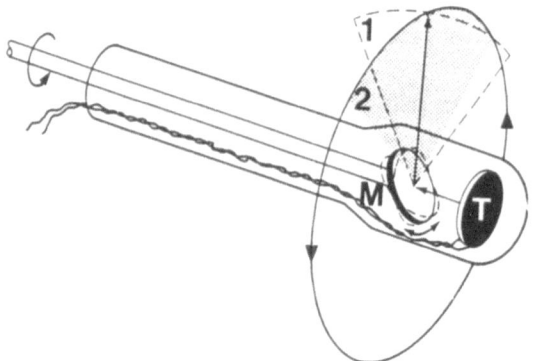

Figure 1.6. Example of biplane probe characterized by mechanical sector scanning in two orthogonal planes. The sagittal sector plane (1) is obtained through the oscillation in the sagittal plane of the mirror (M) facing the transducer (T). The transversely oriented radial scan (2) is obtained by the axial rotation of the mirror (M).

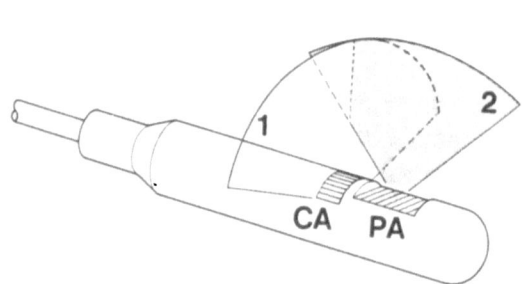

Figure 1.8. Biplane intracavitary probe combining a transversely placed convex-array transducer (CA), which provides the transverse sector scan (1), and a longitudinally oriented phased-array transducer (PA), which provides the sagittal sector plane (2).

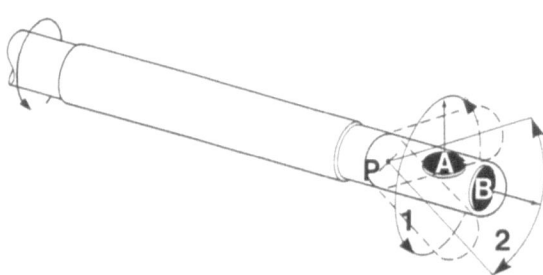

Figure 1.7. Biplane intracavitary probe associating two mechanically activated transducers. The axial rotation of transducer A provides the transverse scan plane (1). The oscillation of the mobile tip of the probe around a transverse axis in P allows the transducer B to scan the front-viewing sector (2).

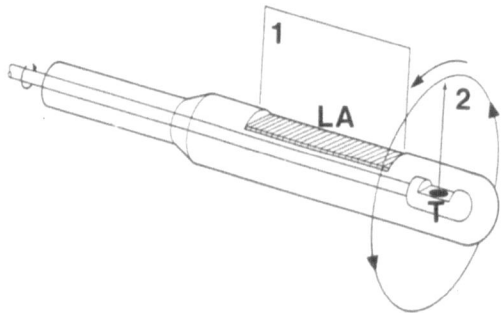

Figure 1.9. Biplane intracavitary probe combining a linear-array transducer (LA), which provides the longitudinally oriented scan plane (1), with rotating transducer (T), which provides the transversely oriented scan plane (2).

of a second transducer placed at the tip of the probe and facing frontward provides a front-viewing sector scan.

3. Two adjacent phased-array or convex sector transducers (in any combination) perpendicular to each other (Fig. 1.8).

4. A linear-array transducer associated with a mechanical radial scanner that is located at the end of the probe (Fig. 1.9).

Multiplane probes developed thus far use a mechanically activated single-crystal transducer that swivels around its ultrasound axis so that the operator can select the transverse, the sagittal, or any oblique scanning plane.

The goal of all these arrangements is to provide at least two perpendicular scanning planes. The outlook for rapid improvement in biplane and multiplane intracavitary probes is excellent given recent technological developments in the industry and thanks to feedback about new clinical applications.

Focusing and resolution

Two different types of spatial resolution have to be considered in ultrasound tomography: axial and lateral. Axial resolution is the smallest distance that can be resolved axially. It depends on the duration of the ultrasound pulse emitted by the transducer, which is a function of the ultrasound wavelength (or frequency) and the damping of the transducer. It also depends on the electronic processing of the signal. The axial resolution of currently available ultrasound units is better than 1 mm. Lateral resolution is the smallest distance that can be resolved transversely. It can be improved by any means that reduces the beam width — that is, by focusing techniques. In probes using a single, mechanically activated crystal, focusing is achieved by using a concave transducer or by affixing an additional acoustic lens to the front surface of the plane transducer. The beam is thus focused at a fixed depth. With electronic multielement transducers, focusing is achieved by the electronic emulation of an acoustic lens through the introduction of delays at the emission and recep-

tion of the signals. This electronically controlled system lets the operator adjust the focal zone to the region of interest.

Examination techniques

Examination techniques in endosonography comprise direct apposition of the transducer and the cavity wall, direct instillation of water or saline solution into the lumen, and the use of a water-distended balloon surrounding the transducer. The first technique can be used in endosonography of the alimentary canal and transvaginal scanning. Direct instillation of saline solution is used in transurethral scanning of the bladder; it is also an alternative in endosonography of the upper gastrointestinal tract. The balloon technique is used when the cavity in which the probe is inserted is fairly large (e.g., in transrectal scanning of the prostate); the water-distended balloon has the advantage of moving the transducer away from the cavity wall, which can be clearly visualized.

Needle biopsy guidance

Endosonography can be used to guide needle biopsies of small abnormalities. Optimal visualization of the biopsy needle requires that the distal portion of the needle be entirely contained in the scan plane and perpendicular (or at least markedly oblique) to the ultrasound beam [11, 23]. In transvaginal and transrectal examinations, various guiding devices attached to the transducer and designed to keep the biopsy needle within the scan plane are used. The transducer is placed so that the electronic line of sight (when available) is superimposed onto the structure to be sampled.

Association of a fiberoptic endoscope and ultrasound transducer

Because their information is complementary, fiberoptic and endosonographic examinations are best combined in the evaluation of the upper

6

gastrointestinal tract [24]. Further, optical monitoring facilitates the determination of the scan plane orientation. The major technical problem in developing a sonoendoscope has been the placement of a miniaturized ultrasound transducer at the distal end of a fiberoptic endoscope while preserving instrument flexibility. Fiberoptic sonoendoscopes have been developed using an optical side-viewing fibroscope and either a radial, mechanically activated transducer or a miniaturized linear-array (or convex-array) transducer placed along the axis of the endoscope (Fig. 1.10) [25]. Such configurations allow the overlap of the optical and acoustic fields of view.

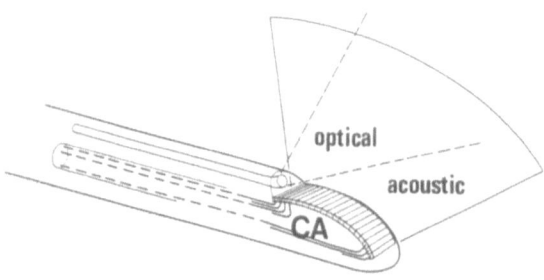

Figure 1.10. Diagram showing the association of a fiberoptic endoscope and side-viewing convex-array ultrasound transducer (CA). The overlapping of both the optical and acoustic fields of view facilitates the localization of the lesion and the orientation of the sonograms.

The fiberoptic—sonoscopic combination has proved particularly valuable in the evaluation of the upper gastrointestinal tract. However, it requires sophisticated, fragile, and therefore expensive transducers. Furthermore, performing the examination requires expertise in both fiberoptic endoscopy and ultrasound, which has limited the use of this technique to dedicated institutions.

Conclusion

Endosonography has recently become popular in such applications as transrectal scanning of the prostate and transvaginal examination of the uterus and adnexa. As shown above, all available ultrasound scanning techniques have been used to solve the specific technical problems encoun-

tered in endosonography. The optimal configuration of the probe (particularly regarding the size and flexibility requirements) depends on the anatomy of the region to be investigated. The combination of fiberoptic and ultrasound endoscopy, the use of Doppler studies (particularly color flow mapping), and multiplanar scanning are each expected in the near future to play a major role in intracavitary sonography.

References

1. Hisanaga K., Hisanaga A., Nagata K., Ichie Y.: Transesophageal cross-sectional echocardiography. Am. Heart J., 1980, 100, 605—609.
2. Di Magno E. P., Regan P. T., Clain J. E., James E. M., Buxton J. L.: Human endoscopic ultrasonography. Gastroenterology, 1982, 83, 824—829.
3. Caletti G. C., Bolondi L., Labo G.: Anatomical aspects in ultrasonic endoscopy of the stomach. Scand. J. Gastroenterol., 1984, 19 (suppl.94), 34—42.
4. Tio T. L., Tytgat G. N.: Endoscopic ultrasonography in the assessment of intra- and transmural infiltration of tumours in the oesophagus, stomach and papilla of Vater and in the detection of extraoesophageal lesions. Endoscopy, 1984, 16, 203—210.
5. Rifkin M. D., Gordon S. J., Goldberg B. B.: Sonographic examination of the mediastinum and upper abdomen by fiberoptic gastroscope. Radiology, 1984, 151, 175—180.
6. Watanabe H., Kato H., Kato T., Morita M., Tanaka M., Terasawa Y.: Diagnostic application of ultrasonotomography to the prostate. Jpn. J. Urol., 1968, 59, 273—279.
7. Resnick M. I., Willard J. W., Boyce W. H.: Recent progress in ultrasonography of bladder and prostate. J. Urol., 1977, 117, 444—446.
8. Gammelgaard J., Holm H. H.: Transurethral and transrectal ultrasonic scanning in urology. J. Urol., 1980, 124, 863—868.
9. Fornage B., Lardennois B.: Ultrasound imaging of the prostate: Recent developments using new equipment. Oral presentation, 67th Annual Meeting of the Radiological Society of North America, Chicago, November 15—20, 1981.
10. Sekine H., Oka K., Takehara Y.: Transrectal longitudinal ultrasonotomography of the prostate by electronic linear scanning. J. Urol., 1982, 127, 62—65.
11. Fornage B. D.: Ultrasound of the prostate. Chichester, John Wiley & Sons, 1989.
12. Rifkin M. D.: Sonourethrography: Technique for evaluation of prostatic urethra. Radiology, 1983, 153, 791—792.
13. Rifkin M. D., Marks G. J.: Transrectal US as an adjunct in the diagnosis of rectal and extrarectal tumors. Radiology, 1985, 157, 499—502.

14. Beynon J., Mortensen N. J. McC., Foy D. M. A., Channer J. L., Virjee J., Goddard P.: Endorectal sonography: Laboratory and clinical experience in Bristol. Int. J. Colorect. Dis., 1986, 1, 212—215.

15. Schwimer S. R., Lebovic J.: Transvaginal pelvic ultrasonography. J. Ultrasound Med., 1984, 3, 381—383.

16. Dellenbach P., Nisand I., Moreau L., *et al.*: Transvaginal, sonographically controlled ovarian follicle puncture for egg retrieval (letter). Lancet, 1984, 1, 1467.

17. Mendelson E. B., Bohm-Velez M., Joseph N., Neiman H. L.: Gynecologic imaging: Comparison of transabdominal and transvaginal sonography. Radiology, 1988, 166, 321—324.

18. Holm H. H., Northeved A.: A transurethral ultrasonic scanner. J. Urol., 1974, 111, 238—241.

19. Nakamura S., Niijima T.: Staging of bladder cancer by ultrasonography: A new technique by transurethral intravesical scanning. J. Urol., 1980, 124, 341—344.

20. Hotzinger H., Becker H.: Intrauterine Ultraschalltomographie (IUT). ROFO, 1984, 140, 66—68.

21. Martin R. W., Bashein G., Zimmer R., Sutherland J.: An endoscopic micromanipulator for multiplanar transesophageal imaging. Ultrasound Med. Biol., 1986, 12, 965—975.

22. Fornage B., Pourcelot L.: Perfectionnement aux sondes d'échographie médicale endocavitaire. European Patent, 1988, No. 0139574.

23. Fornage B. D., Touche D. H., Deglaire M., Faroux M. J., Simatos A.: Real-time ultrasound-guided prostatic biopsy using a new transrectal linear-array probe. Radiology, 1983, 146, 547—548.

24. Farrenkopf E.: [Sonography and endosonoscopy as mutually complementary diagnostic methods]. Ultraschall Med., 1983, 4, 52—56.

25. Pourcelot L., Fleury G., Berson M.: Ultrasonic sweep echography and display endoscopic probe. United States Patent, 1986, No. 4605009.

2. Upper abdominal endoscopic sonography

MATTHEW D. RIFKIN

Conventional ultrasound, developed in the 1960s and the equipment since modified, has proven useful for the evaluation of a variety of disease processes. The first devices produced crude images. The more sophisticated equipment now in use for conventional diagnostic ultrasound yields far better studies but still has limitations. Various inaccessible areas such as the dome of the liver, the spleen, and perigastric and periesophageal regions, may not be clearly identified with conventional sonography. Additionally, the gastric wall, whether normal or pathologically invaded, is not clearly seen. There is suboptimal visualization in obese individuals — where penetration is limited — and in those patients with many air-filled loops of bowel. Thus, adequate diagnostic studies are not always obtained. Various techniques have been developed in an attempt to overcome these limitations. One, which has had significant clinical implications in preliminary research trials and is now a clinically applicable technique in certain areas, is endoscopic ultrasound of the upper gastrointestinal tract.

Instrumentation

Endoscopic ultrasound (endosonography, sono-endoscopy) utilizes various types of ultrasound transducers incorporated into the tips of conventional endoscopes (gastroscopes). Conventional endoscopes have a variety of direct-visualization arrangements and are either end-viewing or side-viewing. Different types of ultrasound scanning systems have been used but size limitations have made mounting the transducer so that the sonographic beam is end-viewing (i.e., the transducer is directly at the tip of the endoscope and 'looks forward') an unusual one.

A radial-type imaging device, which utilizes a transducer that rotates through 360°, has been developed. The imaging is perpendicular to the axis of the endoscopic tip (side-viewing). While 360° images can be obtained, modifications have been made in some instruments so that images between 90° and 180° are presented. Sector scanning, which also 'fires' from the side of the endoscope, also orients the image perpendicular to the endoscopic tip [1—8].

If the scan plane is oriented along the axis of the endoscope, an image of different orientation is obtained. Although a phased-array or convex-array sector transducer can be used, linear-array equipment has most frequently been incorporated in clinical practice (Fig. 2.1) [9—12].

In design, the placement of any type of side-viewing transducer can be varied, from a few to many centimeters, in relation to the tip of the endoscope. But the transducer is fixed in position in any given instrument. If the transducer is placed directly at the tip, the flexibility of the tip is markedly limited. If the transducer is situated slightly away from the tip, the portion of the endoscope where the transducer is placed will be relatively inflexible but the flexibility of the end of the instrument will not be altered.

Most prototype and commercially available sonoendoscopes have incorporated 3.5—12-MHz transducers. In general, the higher the frequency used, the better the resolution obtained. However, higher frequency also correlates with decreased penetration. Thus, results are usually limited when structures deep below the luminal surface are evaluated.

Bruno D. Fornage (ed.), *Endosonography*, pp. 9—23.
© 1989 *Kluwer Academic Publishers*.

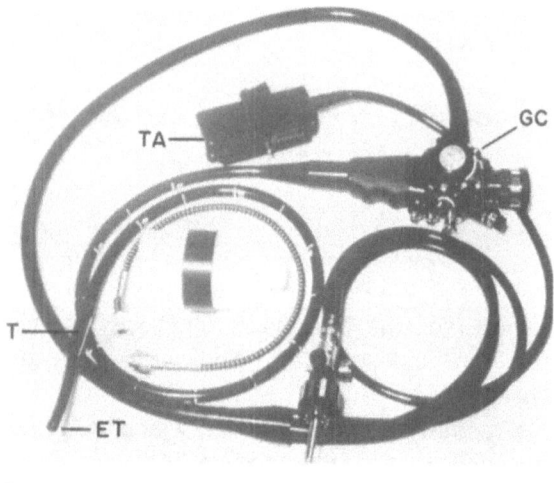

a

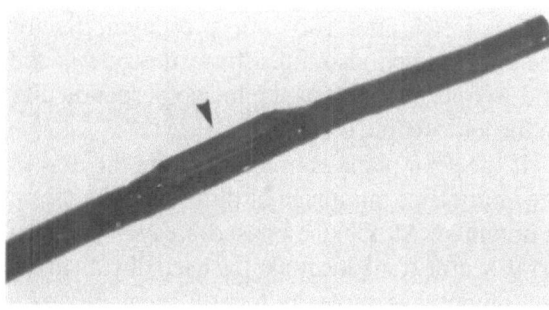

b

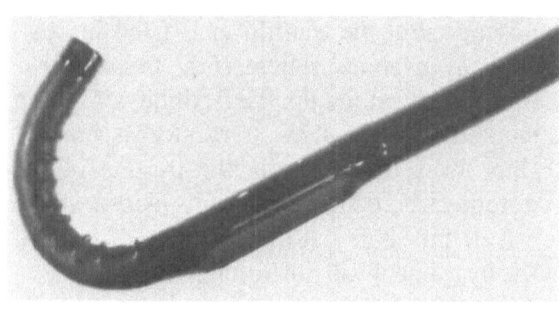

c

Technique of examination

The patient is usually given a mild sedative. While a variety of patient positions are workable, our experience has been that comfort is maximized (taking into account both patient and operator perspectives) with the patient in the left lateral decubitus position [13]. After topical anesthesia is applied to the oropharynx and hypopharynx, the sonoendoscope is positioned in the mouth and then sequentially in the esophagus, fundus and body of the stomach, and, if indicated, the duodenum (Fig. 2.2). Throughout the study, direct visual endoscopic control is retained. It is essential to either place the transducer portion of the sonoendoscope directly on the luminal wall, taking advantage of retained gastric secretions, or to instill fluid into the lumen via the gastroscope suction channel (most sonoendoscopes contain the conventional suction and biopsy channels). With some sonoendoscopes, an exact visual determination of the position of the transducer portion may be possible if the tip of the sonoendoscope can be curved back upon it.

Different structures can be evaluated from

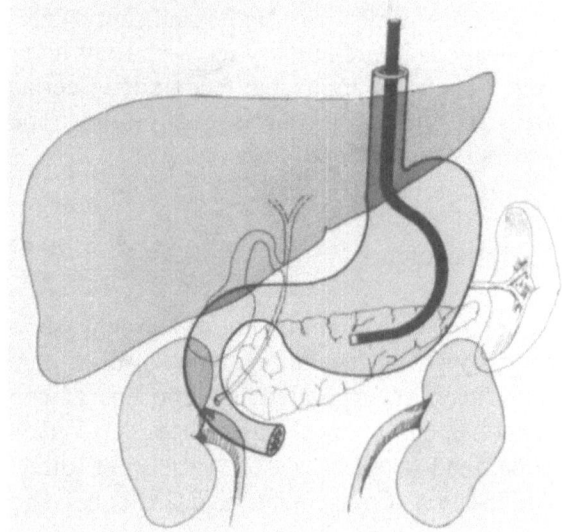

Figure 2.1. Sonoendoscope.
(a) Overall view of the sonoendoscope.
(b) The transducer (arrowhead) in this unit is situated 8 cm from the end of the endoscope.
(c) The tip of the sonoendoscope is still flexible.
ET = Endoscopic tip; GC = gastroscope control; T = transducer; TA = transducer attachment to sonographic unit.

Figure 2.2. Technique of examination. A line diagram shows placement of the sonoendoscope in the stomach. The adjacent organs can be visualized as the transducer is moved sequentially to different areas. (From reference 13, with permission.)

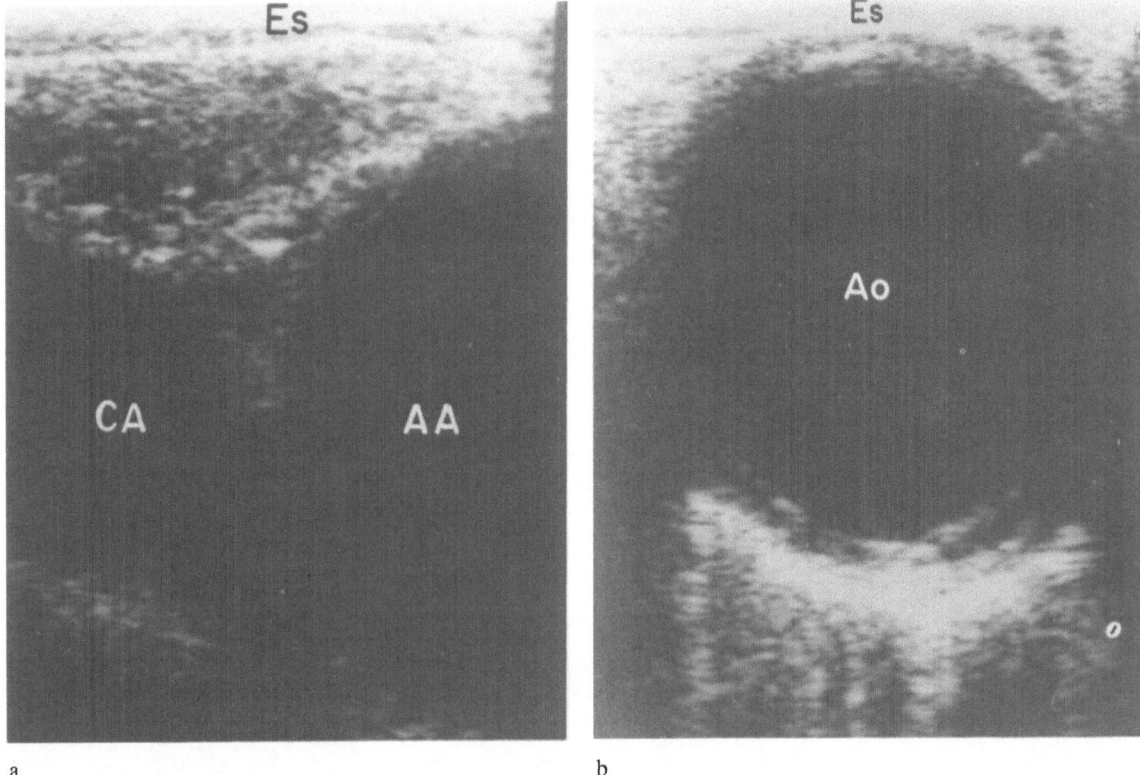

Figure 2.3. The supracardiac vessels.
(a) A longitudinal scan of the aortic arch (AA) shows the origin of the left common carotid artery (CA).
(b) An image oriented transverse to the aorta (Ao) demonstrates the anterior and posterior aortic wall. Es = esophagus.

within the alimentary lumina in accordance with the positioning of the transducer portion of the sonoendoscope. The mediastinal (Fig. 2.3) and cardiac structures are identified by placing the transducer portion within the esophagus. As the sonoendoscope is moved into the stomach, the esophagogastric junction is identified. The spleen is best seen from the superior aspect of the greater gastric curvature toward the fundal and body portions of the stomach. The liver can be identified, usually from the lesser curvature of the stomach or from the duodenum: the left lobe from the body of the stomach, the midportion from the antrum, and the right lobe usually best seen from the duodenum. Depending upon the equipment utilized and its ability to ultrasonically penetrate tissue, both kidneys may be identified, as may portions of the abdominal aorta and other retroperitoneal structures. The pancreas is seen from the posterior aspect of the stomach; according to the positioning of the transducer there, imaging can be in an orientation parallel to the long axis of the pancreas (an axial image) or in a sagittal plane [12].

The normal gastric wall

Extensive work has been done on the sonoendoscopic evaluation of the gastric wall. Better delineation of the normal wall is obtained by having the transducer slightly separated from the mucosal surface. This is easily attained by utilizing retained gastric secretions or by introducing nonaerated water through the suction channel of the sonoendoscope [14]. When the transducer is placed directly onto the mucosal surface, the various layers of the gastric wall may not be as clearly defined as when liquid is interposed (Fig. 2.4 a, c).

There has been some controversy over the

12

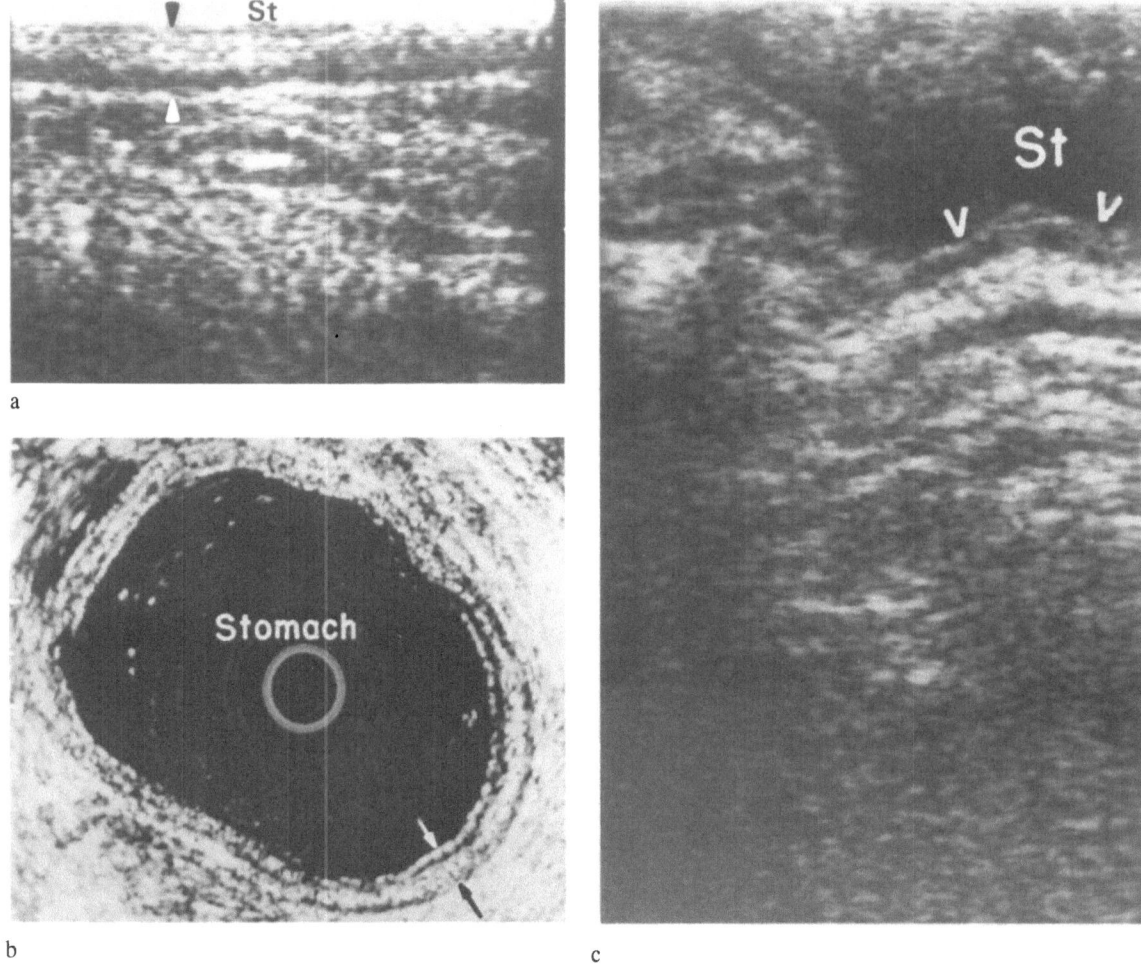

Figure 2.4. Stomach.

(a) A linear-array scan obtained by direct apposition of the transducer and the wall (arrowheads) poorly delineates the different gastric wall layers. St = gastric lumen.

(b) A transversely oriented radial image made in another patient demonstrates the different layers of the wall better (arrows). Courtesy of Dr. G. Tytgat. (From reference 13, with permission.)

(c) A scan made with a linear-array unit and retained secretions in another patient demonstrates fluid in the stomach (St) and the inner (arrowheads) and outer (arrows) layers of the gastric wall. (From reference 13, with permission.)

exact nature and sonographic characteristics of the various layers of the wall [15—20]. In some in vivo studies the correspondence of actual and sonographic layers has been inexact. However, elegant in vitro studies have accurately delineated the various layers [17, 18, 20]. Each specific layer of sonographic reflectivity has been correlated with histologic sections. Five ultrasonic layers have been defined (Fig. 2.4 b):

1. The innermost echogenic layer corresponds to the innermost portion of the gastric mucosa.

2. The next-innermost layer is slightly hypoechoic and corresponds to a combination of the deep mucosa and the muscularis mucosae.

3. The next (the third, or middle) layer is echogenic and corresponds to the submucosa.

4. The fourth layer is hypoechoic and corresponds to the muscularis propria.

5. The outermost layer is brightly echogenic.

This corresponds to a combination of the serosa and perigastric fat.

In vivo studies are not always able to define all of the layers.

Clinical uses

Chest pathology

Cardiac pathology may be identified [10, 21—25], although such findings are most commonly seen when a study of another organ is under-taken. Pericardial effusions (Fig. 2.5 a) can often be seen. Also commonly seen are mitral and aortic valve leaflets (Fig. 2.5 b), and both normal and abnormal excursions of the leaflets have been noted in real-time imaging. Portions of the coronary sinus and coronary arteries may also be noted (Fig. 2.5). However, because visualization is sporadic and incomplete, this technique cannot be utilized as a screening procedure for severe atherosclerotic or other pathologic changes. Endosonoscopic monitoring of cardiac activity during extensive periods of anesthesia has also been utilized by various institutions. This has often been performed by the anesthe-

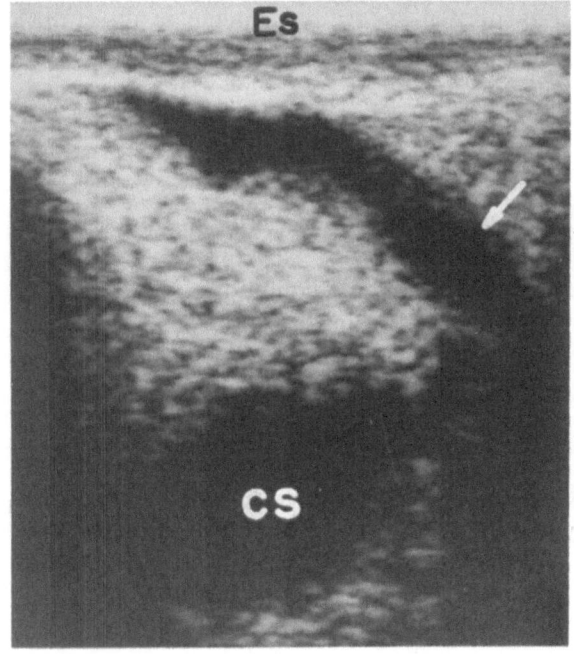

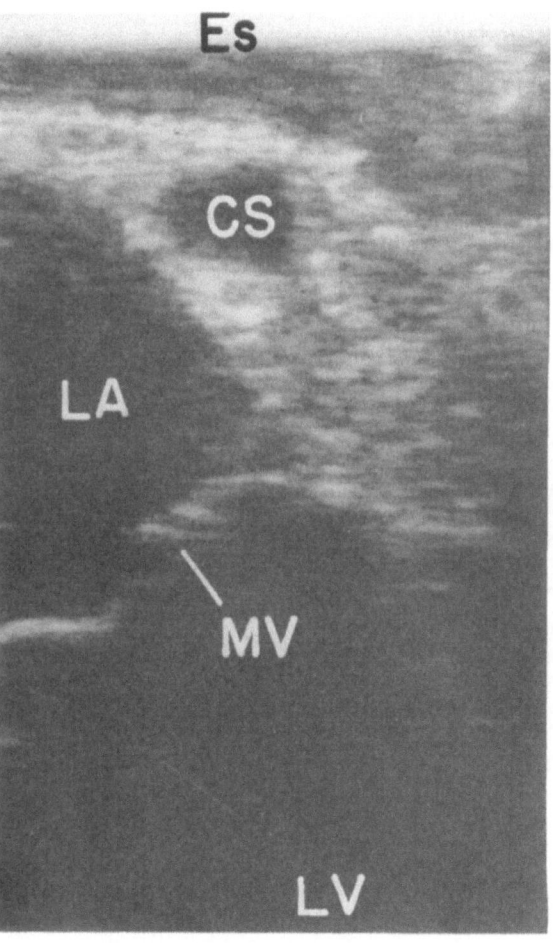

a

b

Figure 2.5. Cardiac studies. (a) A linear-array scan of the heart demonstrates a small pericardial effusion (arrow) between the esophagus (Es) and the coronary sinus (CS). (From reference 13, with permission.) (b) In another patient, the coronary sinus (CS), mitral valve leaflets (MV), left atrium (LA), and left ventricle (LV) are seen. Es = esophagus.

siologist in conjunction with conventional anesthetic monitoring.

The aorta and vena cava may also be identified, as may mediastinal adenopathy (Fig. 2.6) [10, 12]. The endoscan may serve to confirm enlarged lymph nodes suspected either clinically or by previous imaging studies. The sonographic characteristics of adenopathy vary, in accordance with the primary process, but enlarged nodes are typically seen as solid with low- to medium-level acoustic reflectivity.

Esophageal wall lesions can also be evaluated [10–12, 26–28]. Those most commonly seen by endoscopic ultrasound studies have been the

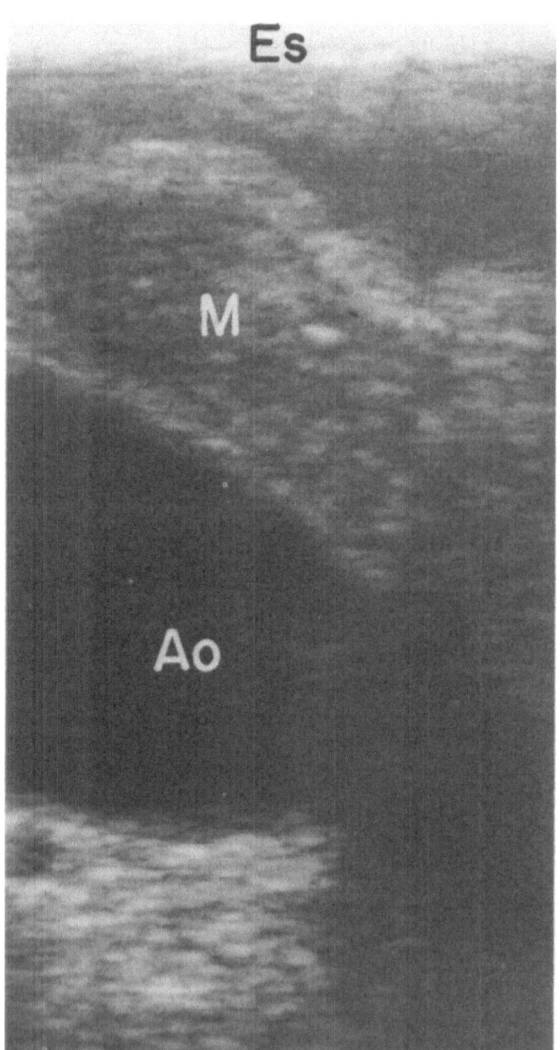

Figure 2.6. Mediastinal adenopathy. A moderately hypoechoic, solid mass (M) is seen between the esophagus (Es) and aorta (Ao).

benign wall lesions — for example, leiomyomata (Fig. 2.7). Leiomyomata have in most cases been seen as well-marginated areas with moderate to low-level acoustic reflectivity, correlating with barium esophagogram findings. Because the insertion of the sonoendoscope can compress much of the lesion, it may appear thinner than on images obtained by other modalities (e.g., esophagography) [12]. This technique is also able to visualize esophageal varices and to identify carcinoma, with staging beyond the wall [26, 27] (see Chapter 3).

Gastric pathology

Gastric wall lesions have been defined and quantitated with sonoendoscopic techniques. Malignant tumors have been seen as masses extending into the gastric lumen. The margins of these relatively hypoechoic but solid lesions are in most cases irregular. While sonoendoscopy alone cannot be used to define these tumors, it can detect extension of cancer into and beyond the gastric wall (Fig. 2.8) more accurately than conventional endoscopy. Malignant ulcerations in gastric carcinomas have also been identified (Fig. 2.9). Endosonography can be used to evaluate the success or failure of treatment administered for gastric carcinoma [29]. Tumors can be identified, measured, and mapped, so that follow-up examinations can delineate shrinkage of tumor (Fig. 2.10), lack of change, or worsening of the patient's condition.

Benign wall lesions as previously described for the esophagus can also be identified in the stomach [30]. Plain endoscopy will only demonstrate extrinsic compression upon the undisrupted mucosa. Conventional radiographic imaging will demonstrate the mass. Exact delineation of the contents of the mass with these approaches is not possible. More importantly, the different types of lesions may be suggested by endosonographic findings. A lesion of low-level echogenicity and with sharply marginated walls is suggestive of a gastric leiomyoma (Fig. 2.11). These findings are similar to those described for esophageal leiomyomata. Duplication cysts may be of more mixed echogenicity because of their mixed cellular elements. Gastric

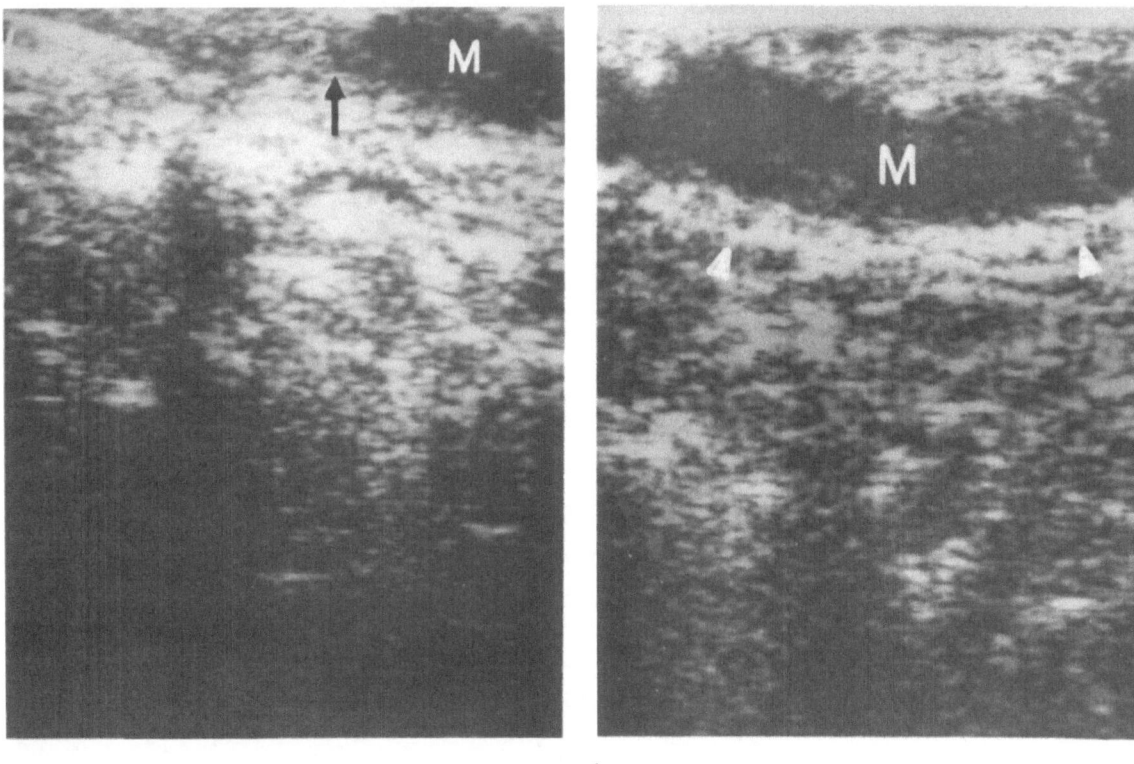

a   b

Figure 2.7. Esophageal leiomyoma.
(a) A hypoechoic wall mass (M) is well delineated from the normal esophageal wall (arrow).
(b) The mass (M) extends caudad. The outer surface (arrowheads) is clearly identified.

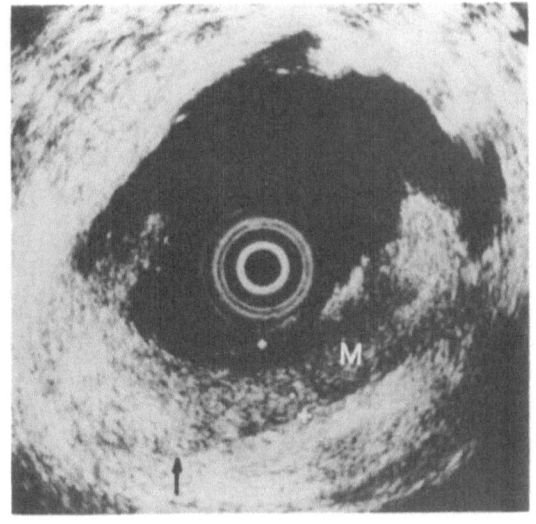

Figure 2.8. Gastric carcinoma. Radial-type scan demonstrates a large, infiltrating mass (M), an adenocarcinoma, with irregularity and invasion beyond the serosa (arrow). Courtesy of Dr. G. Tytgat. (From reference 13, with permission.)

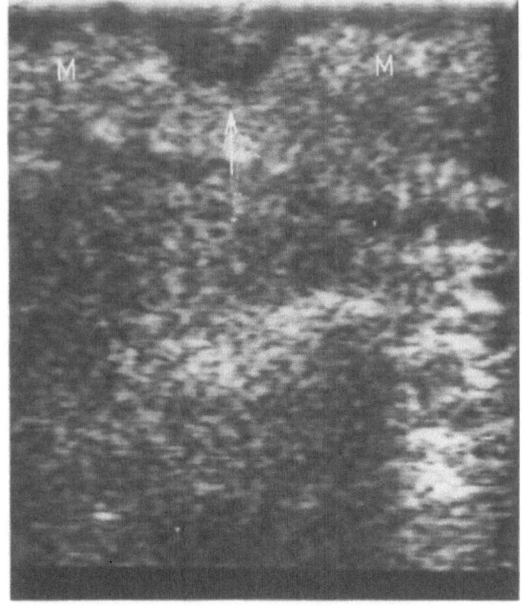

Figure 2.9. Malignant ulceration. A hypoechoic gastric mass (M) with a small ulcer (arrow) is identified.

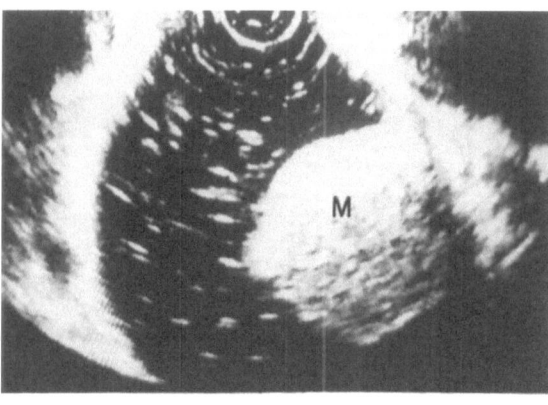

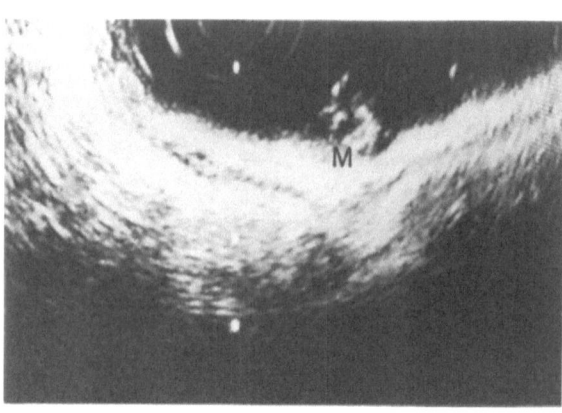

a

b

Figure 2.10. Gastric carcinoma before and after treatment.
(a) Radial scan demonstrates a large mass (M) before treatment.
(b) After radiation therapy, the mass has decreased in size.
Courtesy of Dr. G. Tytgat. (From reference 13, with permission.)

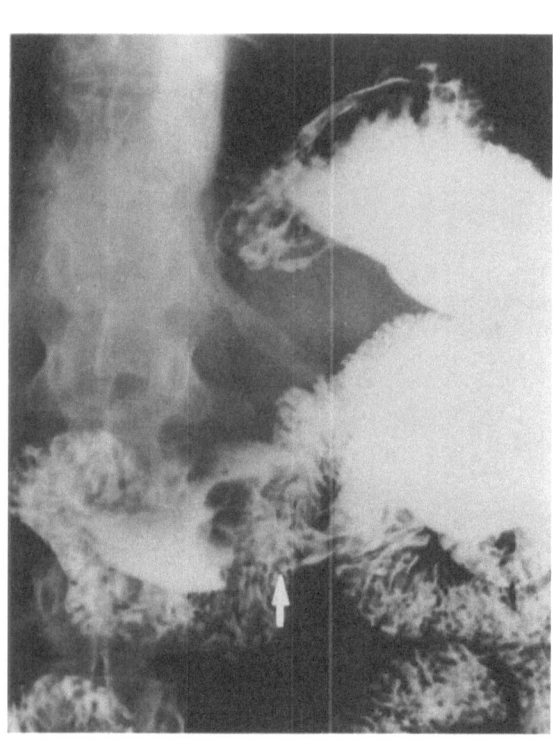

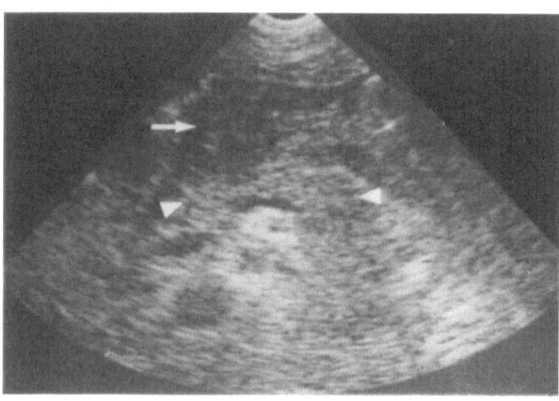

b

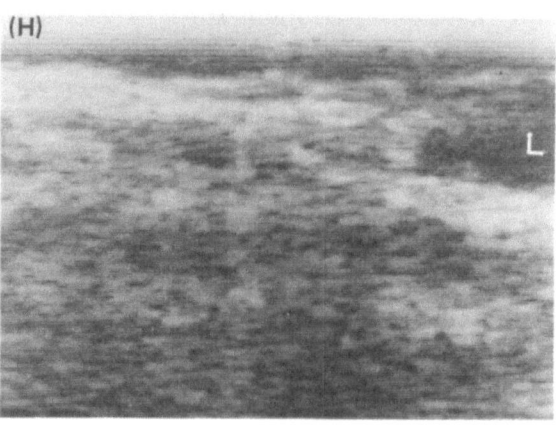

a

c

Figure 2.11. Gastric leiomyoma.
(a) An upper gastrointestinal series demonstrates a wall mass (arrow).
(b) Conventional ultrasound shows an ill-defined mass (arrow) in the region of the antrum of the stomach. The pancreas (arrowheads) appears unremarkable.
(c) An endoscopic sonogram demonstrates a hypoechoic mass (L), a leiomyoma, adjacent to the gastric lumen. H = towards the patient's head. (From reference 13, with permission.)

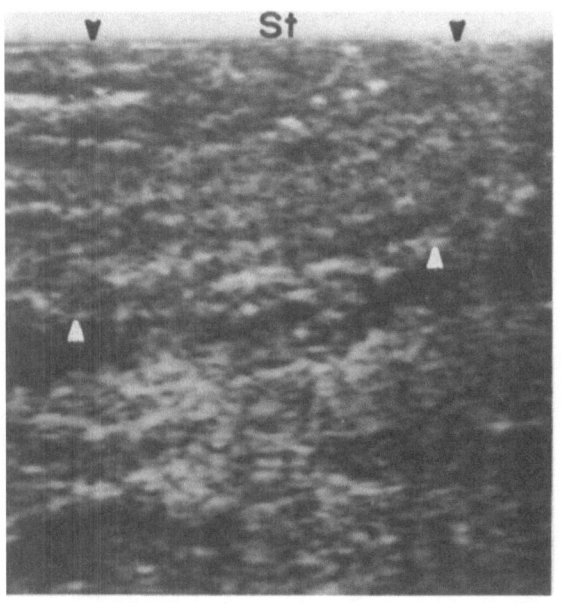

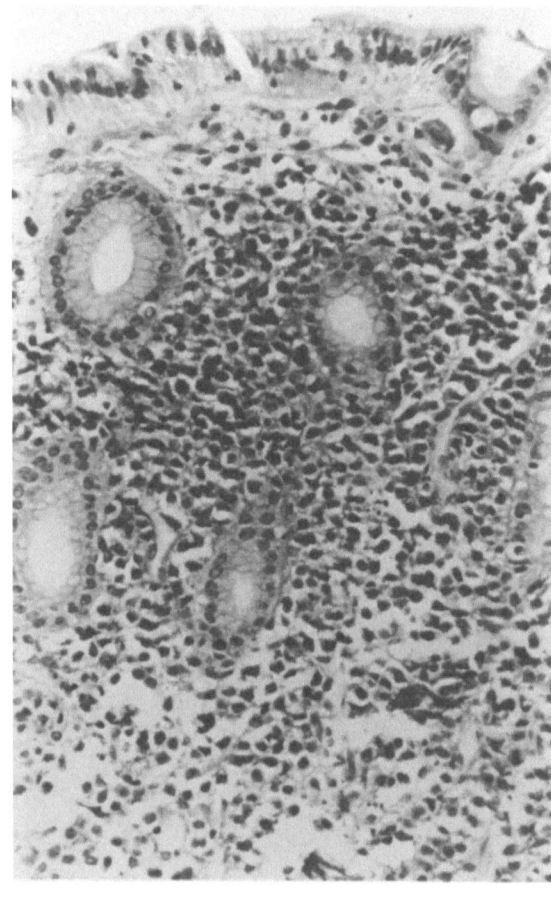

a   b

Figure 2.12. Diffuse gastritis.
(a) The gastric wall (arrowheads) is diffusely thickened as examined from the gastric lumen (St). (From reference 13, with permission.)
(b) Histologic specimen of the thickened wall showing diffuse inflammatory change.

lipomas, because of their fat content, have proven to be slightly more echogenic. While preliminary results are promising about endo-sonography's capability to differentiate the various tumors, more work must be done to prove its ability to do this routinely [10, 30]. Diffuse gastric wall thickening, as seen in gastritis or lymphoma, can also be identified (Fig. 2.12) [31, 32].

Extragastric abdominal pathology

Sonoendoscopic examination of the upper abdomen can visualize perigastric masses [10–12]. The liver is clearly defined, and almost the entire hepatic structure can be delineated from within the gastric and duodenal lumina (Fig. 2.13). The left lobe is best seen from the lesser curvature of the body of the stomach; the right lobe is frequently best seen as the duodenum is cannulated. In cases of massive hepatomegaly, the areas that are farthest from the gastric wall — that is, the subdiaphragmatic and falciform ligament areas — may not be delineated because of the poor deep penetration of the high-frequency transducers. However, given 7.5–10-MHz equipment, careful placement of the transducer, so that it is adjacent to the various portions of the liver, usually allows most small parenchymal abnormalities to be clearly seen.

While large masses (Fig. 2.14) can be delineated, with the same variety of appearances as in conventional ultrasound, endosonography is of particular interest in its ability to image smaller

18

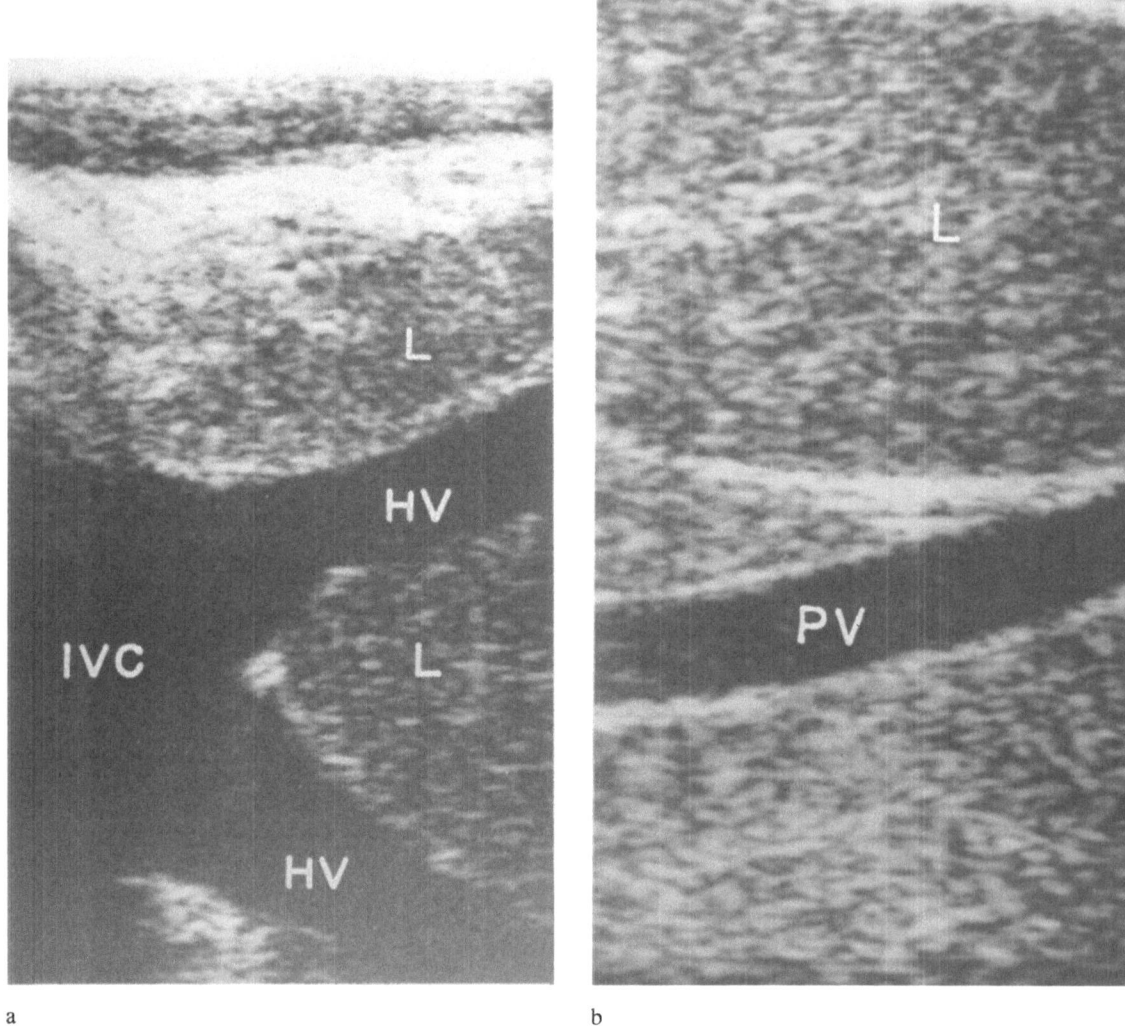

a   b

Figure 2.13. Normal liver.
(a) Normal homogeneous liver texture is identified. The hepatic veins (HV) are seen draining into the inferior vena cava (IVC). The liver (L) texture is normal.
(b) A second scan demonstrates a portal vein (PV), with thick, echogenic walls, traversing the normal hepatic parenchyma (L).

focal lesions (Fig. 2.15). These smaller lesions may have been clinically unsuspected, undiagnosed by conventional imaging studies, or even not palpated during surgery.

The normal gallbladder (Fig. 2.16) and bile ducts and unsuspected pathology, including stones, polyps, and malignant tumors have been identified [11, 33, 34]. The sonographic characteristics are identical to those in conventional ultrasound.

While certain authors have been able to identify the kidneys as the transducer is angled posteriorly and posterolaterally in relation to the gastric lumen [9], other researchers have not been as successful in defining these organs.

The spleen (Fig. 2.17) can also be identified. Abnormalities of texture and focal masses are clearly demonstrated. When using a high-frequency transducer, the deeper areas in the spleen may not be seen if the organ is massively

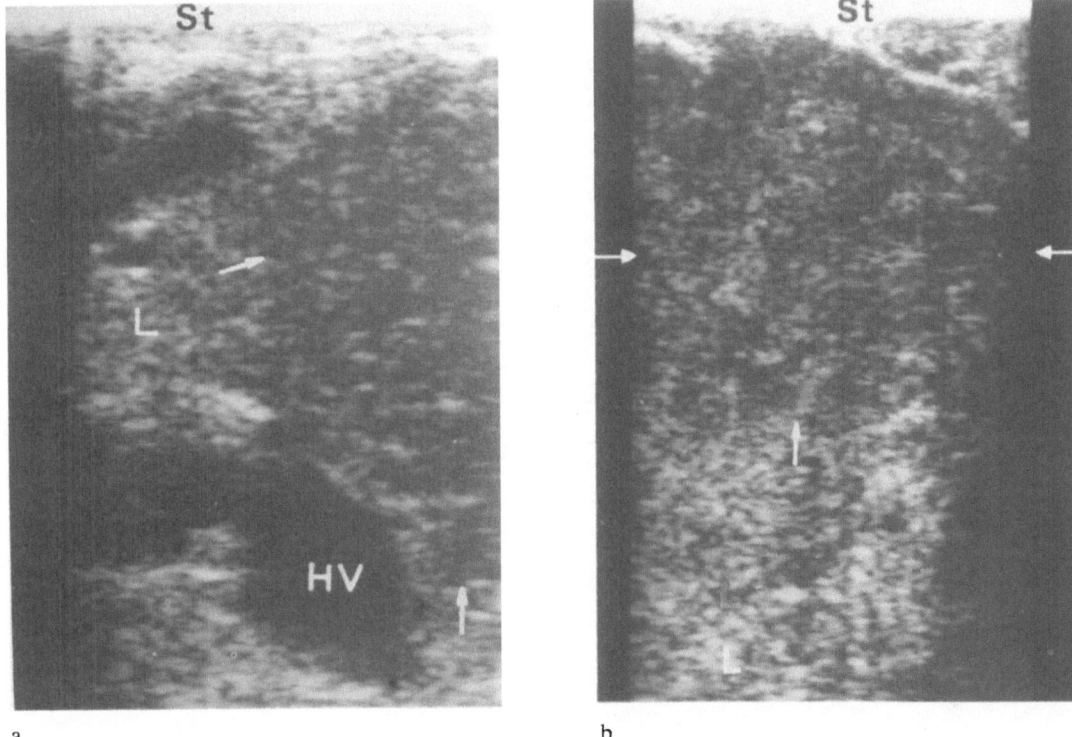

a   b

Figure 2.14. Liver metastases.
(a and b) Scans obtained from the gastric lumen (St) show infiltrating, irregular hypoechoic masses (arrows) representing ill-defined liver metastases. Portions of the normal liver parenchyma (L) are seen, as is a portion of a hepatic vein (HV).

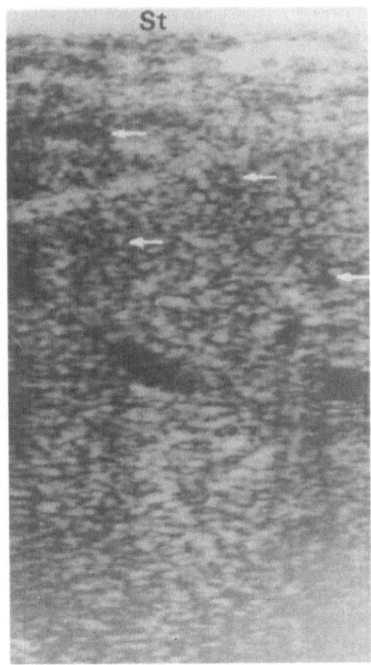

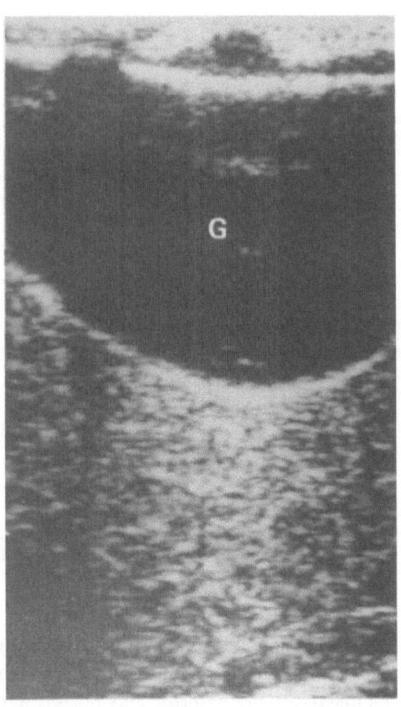

Figure 2.15. Subtle liver metastases. Endoscopic sonogram performed through the gastric lumen (St) shows clinically unsuspected liver metastases (arrows), all measuring less than 5 mm.

Figure 2.16. Normal gallbladder (G) is identified through the duodenum. No echogenic foci, to suggest gallstones or polyps, are identified.

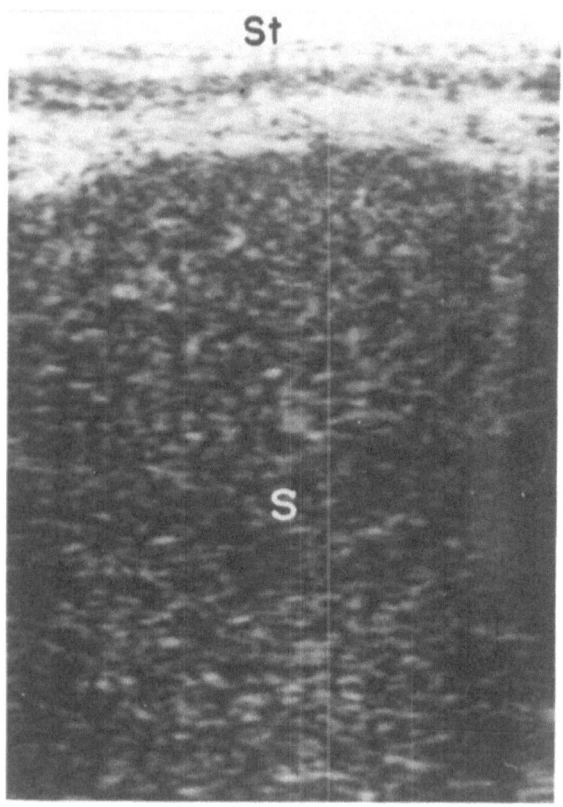

Figure 2.17. Normal spleen. With the sonoendoscope in the fundus of the stomach, normal spleen (S) with homogeneous echotexture is seen. St = stomach.

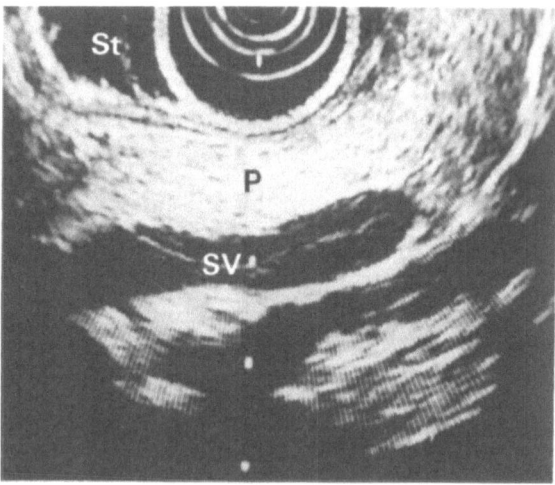

Figure 2.19. Normal pancreas. Radial scan demonstrates a normal pancreas (P) between the gastric lumen St) and the splenic vein (SV). The pancreatic duct is not identified, but pancreatic texture appears grossly normal. Courtesy of Dr. G. Tytgat. (From reference 13, with permission.)

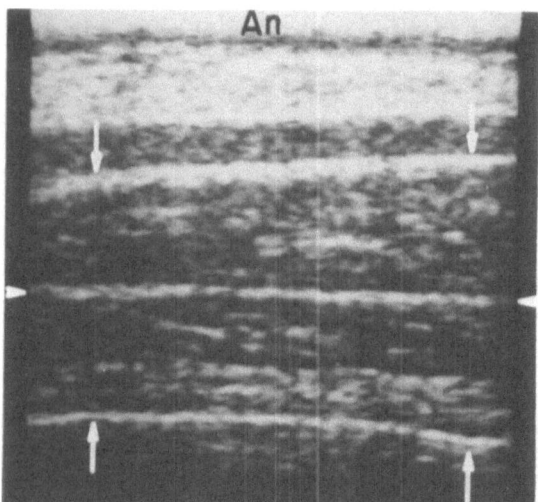

Figure 2.18. Normal pancreas and pancreatic duct. Linear-array scan of the pancreas obtained with transducer in antrum of the stomach (An), parallel to the long axis of the pancreas demonstrates the anterior and posterior margins of the gland (arrows), and a paper-thin, nondilated, normal pancreatic duct (arrowheads). (From reference 13, with permission.)

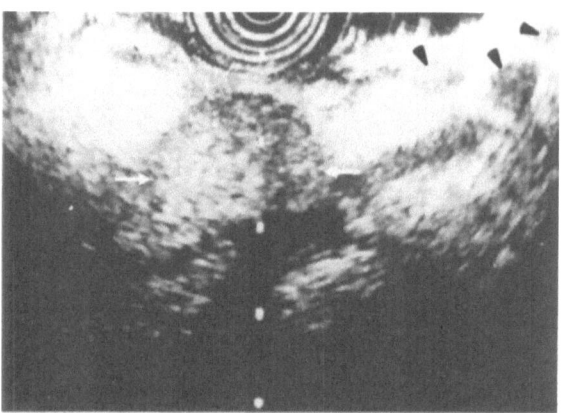

Figure 2.20. Pancreatic carcinoma. Radial scan oriented longitudinal to the pancreas demonstrates an enlarged non-homogeneous pancreatic head (arrows). Note the presence of hypoechoic lymph nodes (arrowheads). Courtesy of Dr. G. Tytgat. (From reference 13, with permission).

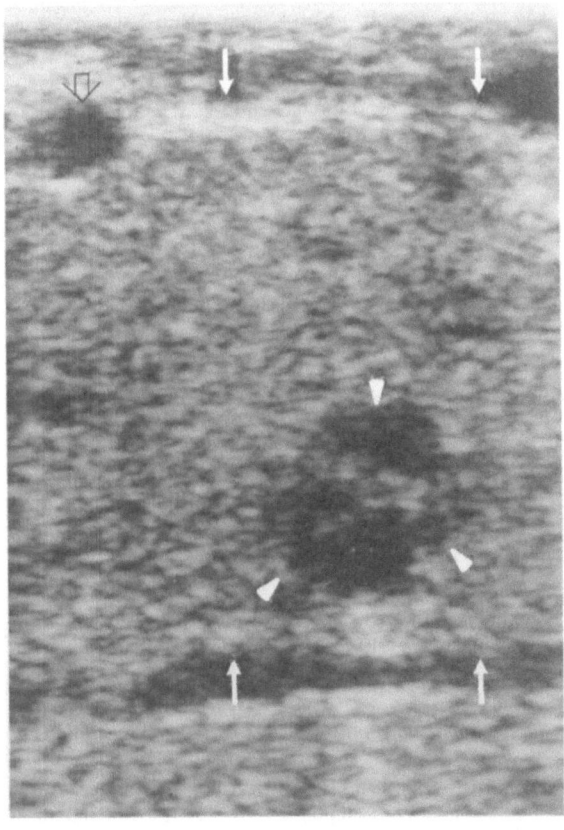

Figure 2.21. Pancreatic carcinoma. A transversely oriented linear-array sonogram demonstrates the pancreas (arrows), a small peripancreatic vessel (open arrow), and an 8-mm hypoechoic, relatively well-defined pancreatic carcinoma (arrowheads). The tumor was confirmed at surgery. (From reference 13, with permission.)

whereas the entire duct can be sequentially imaged with endosonography. The remainder of the pancreas is normally homogeneous on endosonography (Fig. 2.19), the appearance similar to that in conventional sonography.

Abnormal areas that entail subtle echogenicity changes are better defined by endosonography, as are masses. Pancreatic duct dilatation (obvious or subtle), which may be due to malignancy or pancreatitis (or both), is clearly seen. Large pancreatic (Fig. 2.20) or peripancreatic masses (e.g., adenopathy) are also identified at least as clearly as with conventional ultrasound. Unlike other imaging studies, endosonography can follow the abnormal duct, allowing for delineation of subtle intrapancreatic masses that may be overlooked by the other studies. Lesions as small as a few millimeters (Fig. 2.21) have been defined (these proven by surgical exploration). While endosonography has not yet been contemplated as a screening procedure for pancreatic carcinoma, there is potential for such. Further research in this area is indicated.

Preliminary studies using endosonographic Doppler to evaluate abnormalities and therapeutic approaches have been promising as well [44—46]. Further work will elucidate the clinical implications.

Conclusion

The applications of endosonography are becoming clearer as the technique is utilized by more individuals. Luminal and extraluminal anatomy and pathology from the esophagus to the duodenum are being defined with greater clarity than was previously possible with nonoperative techniques. This technique certainly cannot be considered a noninvasive procedure, but the addition of sonographic capability to already scheduled endoscopic examinations greatly increases their value.

References

1. Lux G., Heyder N., Lutz H., Demling L.: Endoscopic ultrasonography. Technique, orientation and diagnostic possibilities. Endoscopy, 1982, 14, 220—225.

enlarged. While the sonographic characteristics of most abnormalities are identical using endosonography and conventional sonography, they are seen more clearly and earlier by the former approach.

The pancreas is another organ that has been defined with great success by sonoendoscopic techniques [10, 11, 35—43]. While the pancreas can be imaged, as with conventional sonography, in a transverse or longitudinal orientation, better results have been achieved when it is imaged parallel to its long axis (i.e., in an axial view). With this approach, the main and secondary pancreatic ducts can be clearly seen. The normal main pancreatic duct is no more than 1 to 2 mm in diameter (Fig. 2.18): with conventional imaging, only a small segment of it will be seen,

2. Lux G., Heyder N., Lutz H.: Ultrasound tomography of the upper gastrointestinal tract. Orientation and diagnostic possibilities. Scand. J. Gastroenterol., 1984, 19 (Suppl. 94), 13—20.

3. Strohm W. D., Classen M.: Anatomical aspects in ultrasonic endoscopy. Scand. J. Gastroenterol., 1984, 19 (Suppl. 94), 21—33.

4. Caletti G., Bolondi L., Labò G.: Anatomical aspects in ultrasonic endoscopy for the stomach. Scand. J. Gastroenterol., 1984, 19 (Suppl. 94), 34—42.

5. Tanaka Y., Yasuda K., Aibe T., Fuji T., Kawai K.: Anatomical and pathological aspects in ultrasonic endoscopy for GI tract. Scand. J. Gastroenterol., 1984, 19 (Suppl. 94), 43—50.

6. Sivak M. V. Jr., George C.: Endoscopic ultrasonography: Preliminary experience. Scand. J. Gastroenterol., 1984, 19 (Suppl. 94), 51—59.

7. Strohm W. D., Kurtz W., Hagenmuller F., Classen M.: Diagnostic efficacy of endoscopic ultrasound tomography in pancreatic cancer and cholestasis. Scand. J. Gastroenterol., 1984, 19 (Suppl. 102), 18—23.

8. Thatcher B. S., Sivak M. V. Jr., George C.: Endoscopic ultrasonography: A preliminary report. Gastrointest. Endoscopy, 1985, 31, 237—242.

9. Di Magno E. P., Regan P. T., Clain J. E., James E. M., Buxton J. L.: Human endoscopic ultrasonography. Gastroenterology, 1982, 83, 824—829.

10. Rifkin M. D., Gordon S. J., Goldberg B. B.: Sonographic examination of the mediastinum and upper abdomen by fiberoptic gastroscope. Radiology, 1984, 151, 175—180.

11. Rifkin M. D., Gordon S. J., Goldberg B. B.: Sonoendoscopy of the mediastinum, upper gastrointestinal tract and upper abdominal contents: Correlation with conventional ultrasound and other imaging modalities. Acta Endoscopica, 1984, 14, 13—22.

12. Gordon S. J., Rifkin M. D., Goldberg B. B.: Endosonographic evaluation of mural abnormalities of the upper gastrointestinal tract. Gastrointest. Endoscopy, 1986, 32, 193—198.

13. Rifkin M. D.: Endoscopic ultrasonography of the gastrointestinal tract. In: Rifkin M. D. (ed.). Intraoperative and endoscopic ultrasonography. New York, Churchill Livingstone, 1987, 167—189.

14. Caletti G. C., Bolondi L., Zani L., Labò G.: Technique of endoscopic ultrasonography investigation: Esophagus, stomach and duodenum. Scand. J. Gastroenterol., 1986, 21 (Suppl. 123), 1—5.

15. Caletti G., Bolondi L., Labò G.: Ultrasonic endoscopy. The gastrointestinal wall. Scand. J. Gastroenterol., 1984, 19 (Suppl. 102), 5—8.

16. Kimmey M. B., Silverstein F. E., Haggitt R. C., et al.: Cross-sectional imaging method: A system to compare ultrasound, computed tomography, and magnetic resonance with histologic findings. Invest., 1987, 22, 227—231.

17. Aibe T., Fuji T., Okita K., Takemoto T.: A fundamental study of normal layer structure of the gastrointestinal wall visualized by endoscopic ultrasonography. Scand. J. Gastroenterol., 1986, 21 (Suppl. 123), 6—15.

18. Bolondi L, Caletti G., Casanova P., Villanacci V., Grigioni W., Labò G.: Problems and variations in the interpretation of the ultrasound feature of the normal upper and lower GI tract wall. Scand. J. Gastroenterol., 1986, 21 (Suppl. 123), 16—26.

19. Tio T. L., Tytgat G. N. J.: Endoscopic ultrasonography of normal and pathologic upper gastrointestinal wall structure. Comparison of studies in vivo and in vitro with histology. Scand. J. Gastroenterol., 1986, 21 (Suppl. 123), 27—33.

20. Silverstein F., Kimmey M., Martin R., et al.: Ultrasound of the intestinal wall: Experimental methods. Scand. J. Gastroenterol., 1986, 21 (Suppl. 123), 34—40.

21. Hanrath P., Schluter M., Langerstein B. A., et al.: Detection of ostium secundum atrial septal defects by transoesophageal cross-sectional echocardiography. Br. Heart J., 1983, 49, 350—358.

22. Reifart N., Strohm W. D., Classen M.: Detection of atrial and ventricular septal defects by transoesophageal two-dimensional echocardiography with a mechanical sector scanner. Scand. J. Gastroenterol., 1982, 19 (Suppl. 102), 101—106.

23. Shrestha N. K., Moreno F. L., Narciso F. V., Torres L., Calleja H. B.: Two-dimensional echocardiographic diagnosis of left atrial thrombus in rheumatic heart disease. A clinicopathologic study. Circulation, 1983, 67, 341—347.

24. Matsumoto M., Hanrath P., Kremer P., et al.: The evaluation of left ventricular function by transoesophageal M-mode exercise echocardiography. In: Hanrath P., Beifeld W., Souquet J. (eds.). Cardiovascular diagnosis by ultrasound. London, Martinus Nijhoff, 1982, 227—236.

25. Matsumoto M., Oka Y., Strom J., et al.: Application of transesophageal echocardiography to continuous intraoperative monitoring of left ventricular performance. Am. J. Cardiol., 1980, 46, 95—105.

26. Caletti G. C., Bolondi L., Zani L., Brocchi E., Guizzardi G., Labò G.: Detection of portal hypertension and esophageal varices by means of endoscopic ultrasonography. Scand. J. Gastroenterol., 1986, 21 (Suppl. 123), 74—77.

27. Tio T. L., Den Hartog Jager F. C. A., Tytgat G. N. J.: The role of endoscopic ultrasonography in assessing local resectability of oesophagogastric malignancies: Accuracy, pitfalls and predictability. Scand. J. Gastroenterol., 1986, 21 (Suppl. 123), 78—86.

28. Strohm W. D., Classen M.: Benign lesions of the upper GI tract by means of endoscopic ultrasonography. Scand. J. Gastroenterol., 1986, 21 (Suppl. 123), 41—46.

29. Heyder N., Lux G.: Malignant lesions of the upper gastrointestinal tract. Scand. J. Gastroenterol., 1986, 21 (Suppl. 123), 47—51.

30. Yasuda K., Nakajima M., Kawai K.: Endoscopic ultrasonography in the diagnosis of submucosal tumor of the upper digestive tract. Scand. J. Gastroenterol., 1986, 21 (Suppl. 123), 59—67.

31. Rifkin M. D., Gordon S. J.: Sonoendoscopic evaluation of extraesophageal and extragastric abnormalities: A review. Scand. J. Gastroenterol., 1986, 21 (Suppl. 123), 68—73.

32. Tio T. L., Den Hartog Jager F. C. A., Tytgat G. N. J.: Endoscopic ultrasonography in detection and staging of gastric non-Hodgkin lymphoma. Comparison with gastroscopy, barium meal, and computerized tomography scan. Scand. J. Gastroenterol., 1986, 21 (Suppl. 123), 52—58.

33. Strohm W. D., Kurtz W., Classen M.: Detection of biliary stones by means of endosonography. Scand. J. Gastroenterol., 1984, 19 (Suppl. 94), 60—64.

34. Yasuda K., Nakajima M., Kawai K.: Technical aspects of endoscopic ultrasonography of the biliary system. Scand. J. Gastroenterol., 1986, 21 (Suppl. 123), 143—150.

35. Fukuda M., Nakano Y., Saito K., Hirata K., Terada S., Urushizaki I.: Endoscopic ultrasonography in the diagnosis of pancreatic carcinoma. The use of a liquid-filled stomach method. Scand. J. Gastroenterol., 1984, 19 (Suppl. 94), 65—76.

36. Classen M., Strohm W. D., Kurtz W.: Pancreatic pseudocysts and tumors in endosonography. Scand. J. Gastroenterol., 1984, 19 (Suppl. 94), 77—84.

37. Okita K., Kodama T., Oda M., Takemoto T.: Laparoscopic ultrasonography. Diagnosis of liver and pancreatic cancer. Scand. J. Gastroenterol., 1984, 19 (Suppl. 94), 91—100.

38. Yasuda K., Tanaka Y., Fujimoto S., Nakajima M., Kawai K.: Use of endoscopic ultrasonography in small pancreatic cancer. Scand. J. Gastroenterol., 1984, 19 (Suppl. 102), 9—17.

39. Lux G., Heyder N.: Endoscopic ultrasonography of the pancreas. Technical aspects. Scand. J. Gastroenterol., 1986, 21 (Suppl. 123), 112—118.

40. Dancygier H., Classen M.: Endosonographic diagnosis of benign pancreatic and biliary lesions. Scand. J. Gastroenterol., 1986, 21 (Suppl. 123), 119—122.

41. Lees W. R.: Endoscopic ultrasonography of chronic pancreatitis and pancreatic pseudocysts. Scand. J. Gastroenterol., 1986, 21 (Suppl. 123), 123—129.

42. Sivak M. V. Jr., Kaufman A.: Endoscopic ultrasonography in the differential diagnosis of pancreatic disease. A preliminary report. Scand. J. Gastroenterol., 1986, 21 (Suppl. 123), 130—134.

43. Tio T. L., Tytgat G. N. J.: Endoscopic ultrasonography in staging local resectability of pancreatic and periampullary malignancy. Scand. J. Gastroenterol., 1986, 21 (Suppl. 123), 135—142.

44. Beckly D. E., Casebow M. P., Pettengell K. E.: The use of a Doppler ultrasound probe for localizing arterial blood flow during upper gastrointestinal endoscopy. Endoscopy, 1982, 14, 146—147.

45. Martin R. W., Gilbert D. A., Silverstein F. E., et al.: An endoscopic Doppler probe for assessing intestinal vasculature. Ultrasound Med. Biol., 1985, 11, 61—69.

46. Silverstein F. E., Deltenre M., Tytgat G., et al.: An endoscopic Doppler probe: Preliminary clinical evaluation. Ultrasound Med. Biol., 1985, 11, 347—353.

3. Endoscopic sonography of the esophagus

LUIGI BOLONDI, GIAN CARLO CALETTI, AND LUIGI BARBARA

The introduction of an ultrasonic transducer into the esophagus allows not only detailed study of the esophageal wall but also visualization of such extraesophageal mediastinal structures as the heart and aorta [1, 2]. Endoesophageal ultrasonography (EU) provides significant additional information in most esophageal wall lesions, and its major applications are in evaluating esophageal carcinoma and esophageal varices.

Instrumentation and technique of examination

Our initial studies were conducted with a 180°-viewing unit, whose technical characteristics have been detailed elsewhere [3]. We now use the Olympus GF-UM 2/EUM 2 endosonoscope with side-viewing optics and a 7.5/10-MHz radial transducer that provides a 360° circular image. The ultrasonic beam generated by the transducer is perpendicular to the axis of the endosonoscope so that radial scanning generates a transaxial cross-sectional image of the esophageal lumen and surrounding structures (Fig. 3.1). Because longitudinal scanning is not afforded by this unit, evaluation of the length of a lesion requires recording the distance of the transducer from the teeth.

A conventional esophagoscopic examination should be performed prior to EU to determine the exact location of the lesion. EU can be performed by direct apposition of the transducer and mucosa, use of a small balloon distended with deaired water, or direct instillation of deaired water into the lumen [4]. The esophagus is usually examined by one of the first two methods; the last method is the routine approach in the evaluation of the stomach. With the direct application of the transducer on the esophageal mucosa, extraluminal structures are adequately displayed but the esophageal wall is not clearly depicted. The balloon technique is superior for visualization of the wall, contingent upon meticulous draining of air from the balloon before starting the examination.

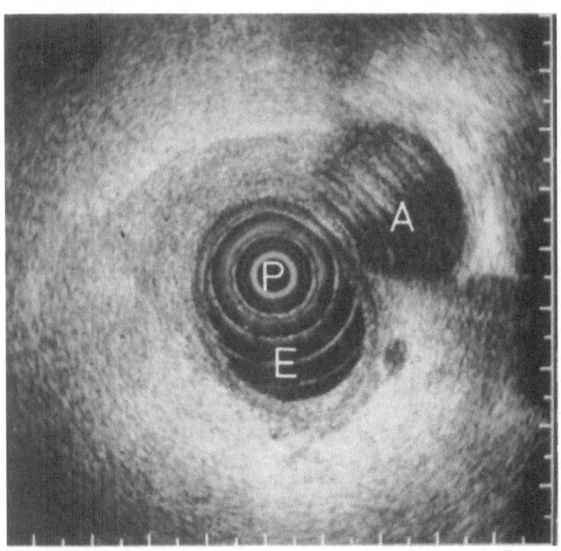

Figure 3.1. Transverse scan made 35 cm from the teeth shows the esophagus and aorta. A = aorta; E = esophagus; P = probe.

Normal ultrasound anatomy

Periesophageal structures routinely demonstrated include the left atrium and the coronary sinus (Fig. 3.2), which are in contact with the

Bruno D. Fornage (ed.), *Endosonography*, pp. 25—34.

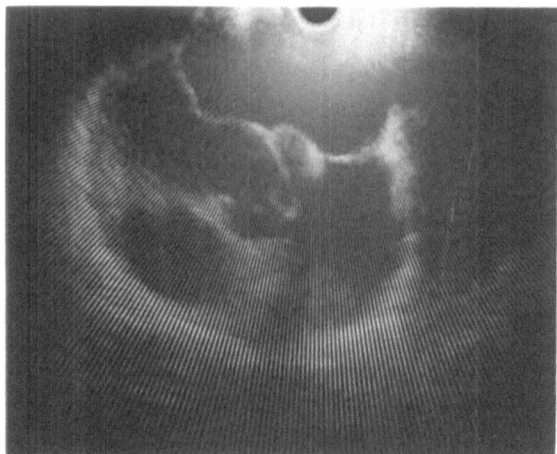

Figure 3.2. Transesophageal four-chamber view of the heart. The esophageal wall is not clearly visualized because the transducer is in direct contact with the mucosa.

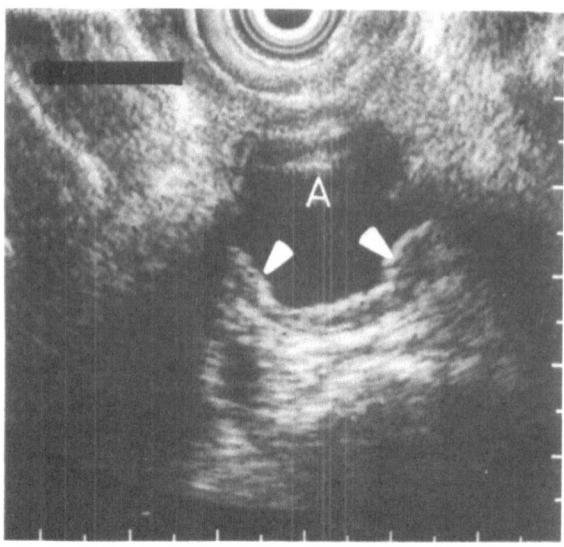

a

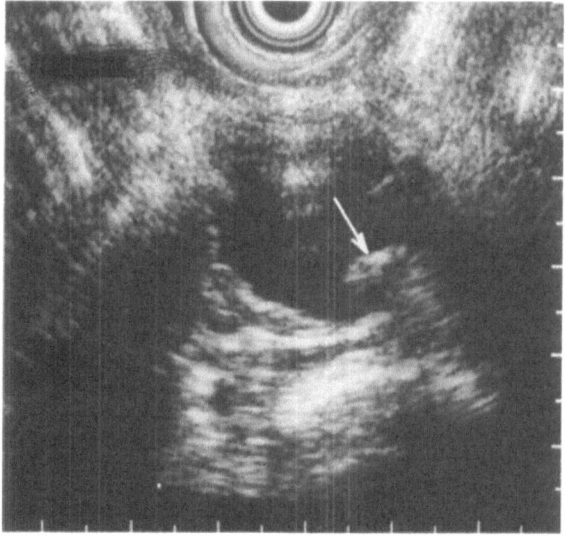

b

Figure 3.3. Transverse sonograms of the aorta. (a) Large, smooth atherosclerotic plaque (arrowheads) is seen in the aorta (A). (b) Sonogram obtained at a lower level demonstrates a calcification (arrow). The layers of the esophageal wall are not visualized because of the direct apposition of the transducer and the wall.

anterior wall, and the aortic arch and descending aorta (Fig. 3.3), adjacent to the posterior wall.

Real-time ultrasound with high-frequency (7.5/10-MHz) transducers delineates layers of varying echogenicity within the wall of the upper and lower alimentary canal [5, 6]. These layers are readily demonstrated in the body of the stomach, but conflicting interpretations have been published regarding their anatomic correspondence [5—8]. The ultrasound appearance of the normal wall has been less extensively investigated in the esophagus. Our preliminary experience has suggested ultrasonic patterns similar to that of the other segments of the upper alimentary tract [5]. Using the direct-contact technique, the multilayer pattern cannot be depicted because the wall is too close to the transducer. The balloon technique allows the visualization of five layers, each of whose thickness may change in relation to the degree of distension of the balloon (Fig. 3.4). Our correlation of the various sonographic layers and anatomic structures is based on the results of in vivo and in vitro investigations [5, 6]. Beginning at the lumen, the first layer (echogenic) corresponds to the interface between the fluid-filled balloon and the esophageal mucosa; the second layer (hypoechoic) corresponds to the deep portion of the mucosa, including the muscularis mucosae; the third layer (echogenic) corresponds to the submucosa and the interface between the submucosa and the muscularis propria; the fourth layer (hypoechoic) correlates with the muscularis propria; the fifth layer (echogenic) corresponds to the interface between the esophageal wall and the peripheral structures and is not clearly visualized in vivo.

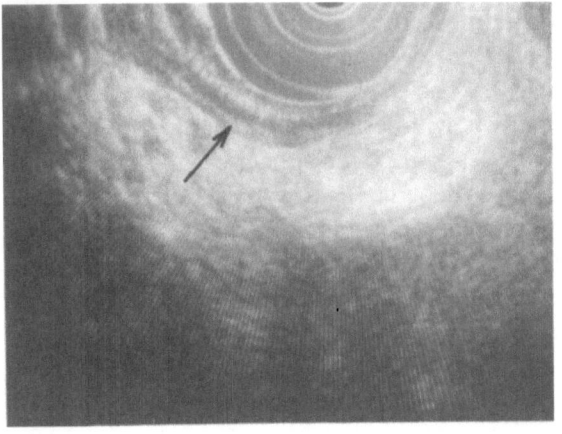

a

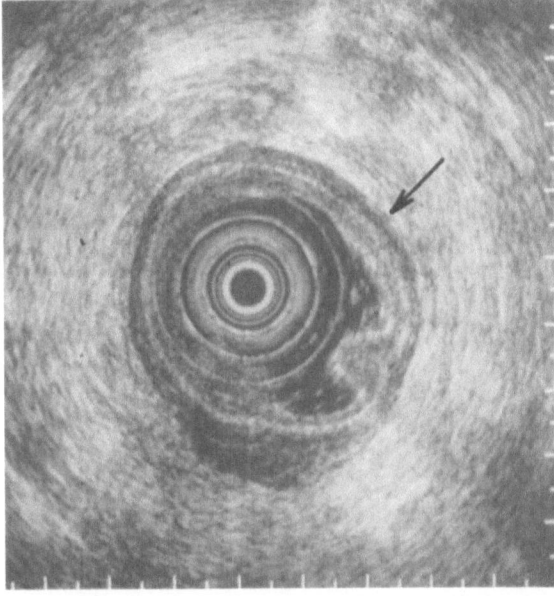

b

Figure 3.4. Transverse scans showing distinct layers in the esophageal wall. (a) The layers are best demonstrated where the wall is least compressed by the balloon surrounding the transducer (arrow). (b) Layers (arrow) are more conspicuous at the gastroesophageal junction.

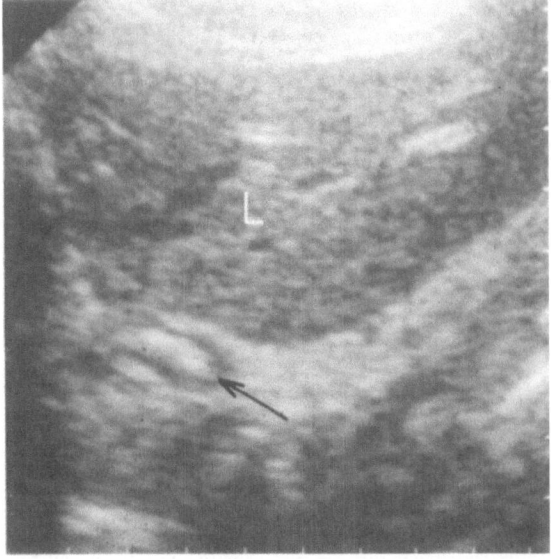

a

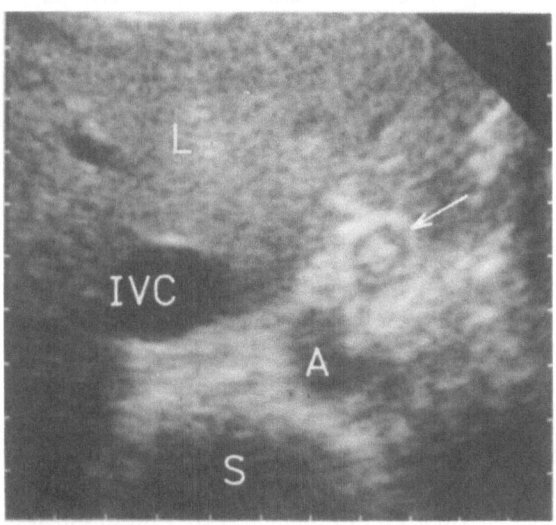

b

Figure 3.5. Conventional transabdominal sonograms of the lower esophagus. (a) Longitudinal scan shows the termination of the esophagus (arrow) posterior to the left lobe of the liver (L). (b) Transverse sonogram shows the cross-section of the esophagus (arrow). A = aorta; IVC = inferior vena cava; L = liver; S = spine.

Esophageal carcinoma

Progressive dysphagia is the usual clinical presentation in both squamous cell carcinoma and adenocarcinoma of the esophagus. Although this symptom can also be associated with benign lesions, cancer should always be suspected until disproven. Only early diagnosis can improve the overall poor prognosis in esophageal carcinoma.

Barium studies are routinely used. Double-contrast imaging is required to detect subtle superficial lesions. *Fiberoptic endoscopy* allows direct visualization of the lesion and the performance of forceps biopsy or brush cytologic study. However, a false-negative rate as high as 6% has been reported for endoscopic biopsy [9]. Cytologic examination increases diagnostic accuracy [10], but its use has been greatly limited

28

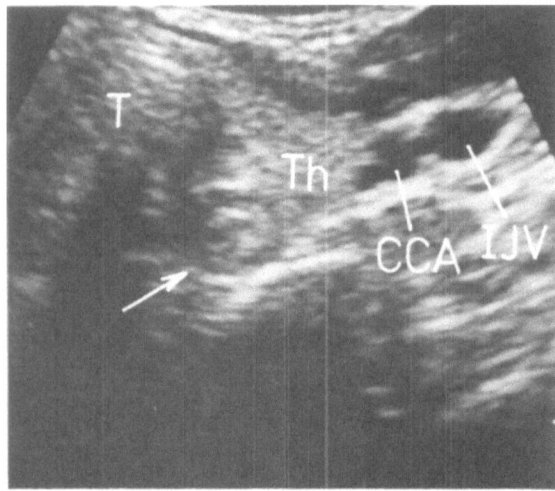

Figure 3.6. Transverse scan of the left cervical region shows normal esophagus (arrow) posterior to the left lobe of the thyroid gland. CCA = common carotid artery; IJV = internal jugular vein; T = trachea; Th = thyroid.

by the requirement of an experienced cytopathologist. *Computed tomography* (CT) has represented a great step forward in both the diagnosis and staging of esophageal carcinoma. Thickening of the esophageal wall due to tumor and extraesophageal tumor infiltration can be evaluated by this noninvasive technique [11]. *Conventional real-time ultrasonography* can visualize the termination of the normal esophagus below the diaphragm (Fig. 3.5) [12] and detect masses at the gastroesophageal junction. A short segment of the normal esophagus is often visualized in the cervical region during examination of the thyroid gland (Fig. 3.6), but the applicability of real-time ultrasound to the detection of esophageal tumors in this region has not yet been evaluated. Encouraging results have also been reported with *radionuclide studies* using [57]Co-labelled bleomycin or ^{67}Ga, each of which is preferentially taken up by squamous cell carcinomas. Invasive techniques such as mediastinoscopy have been abandoned.

In oncology, the therapeutic strategy is primarily based on clinical staging. Many therapeutic regimens involving surgery, chemotherapy, and radiation therapy, alone or in combination, are utilized in esophageal carcinoma. Local factors that significantly influence the results of surgery or radiation therapy include tumor

location (results with surgery being better when cancer develops in the lower third of the esophagus) and longitudinal extent of the tumor (patients with lesions more than 5 cm in length doing less well after either surgery or radiation therapy). The lack of a serosal layer around the esophagus contributes to early local tumor spread, regardless of tumor location. Tracheal or aortic involvement, because of the risk of hemorrhage, contraindicates radical surgery.

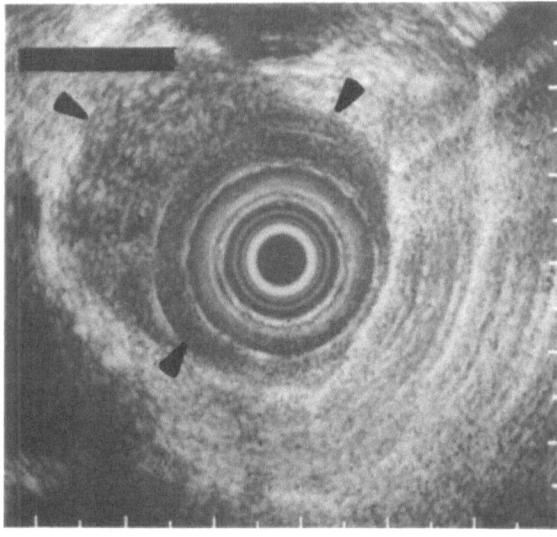

Figure 3.7. Esophageal carcinoma. Tumor appears as a hypoechoic thickening of the esophageal wall (arrowheads).

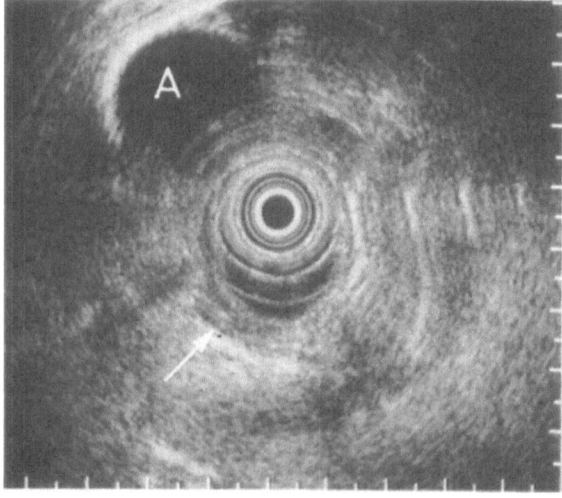

Figure 3.8. Early esophageal carcinoma. Transverse scan shows a localized thickening of the wall (arrow). A = aorta.

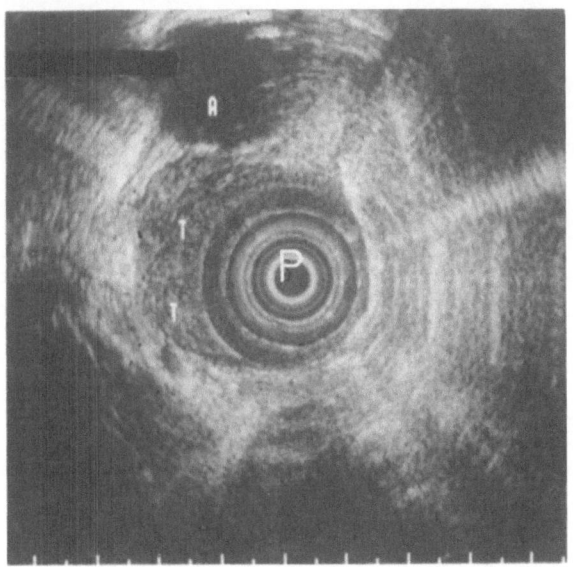

Figure 3.9. Esophageal carcinoma (T) involving half of the circumference of the esophageal wall. A = aorta; P = probe.

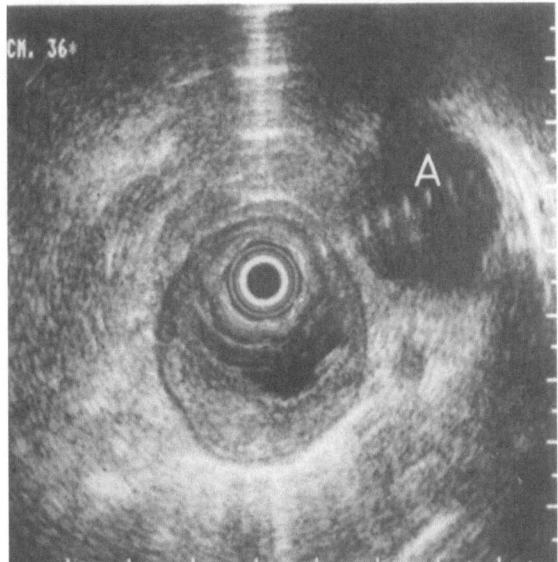

a

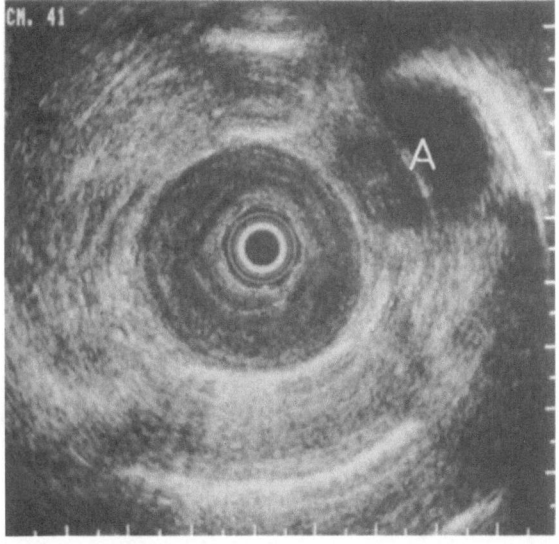

b

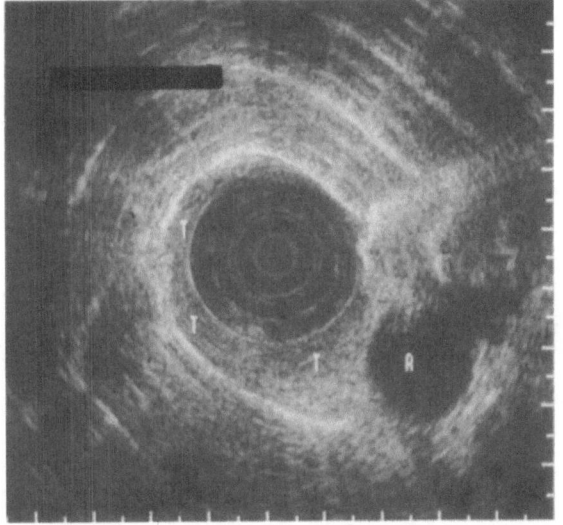

Figure 3.10. Esophageal carcinoma (T) involving more than half of the circumference of the lumen. A = aorta.

Figure 3.11. Esophageal carcinoma. The tumor involves the whole circumference of the lumen and extends more than 5 cm longitudinally. (a) Scan made 36 cm from the teeth. (b) Scan obtained at 41 cm shows the circumferential malignant infiltration around the probe. A = aorta.

Because EU can visualize periesophageal structures in addition to the esophageal wall, interest is growing in the use of EU for the evaluation of esophageal carcinoma.

Endosonographic findings

The typical appearance of an esophageal malignant tumor on EU is a hypoechoic mass with irregular margins that disrupts the multilayered pattern of the normal wall (Fig. 3.7). Some tumors are confined to a limited area of the wall (Fig. 3.8); others involve a variable sector (Figs. 3.9, 3.10) or the whole circumference of the lumen (Fig. 3.11). A prominent centrifugal growth, into the periesophageal tissues, is occa-

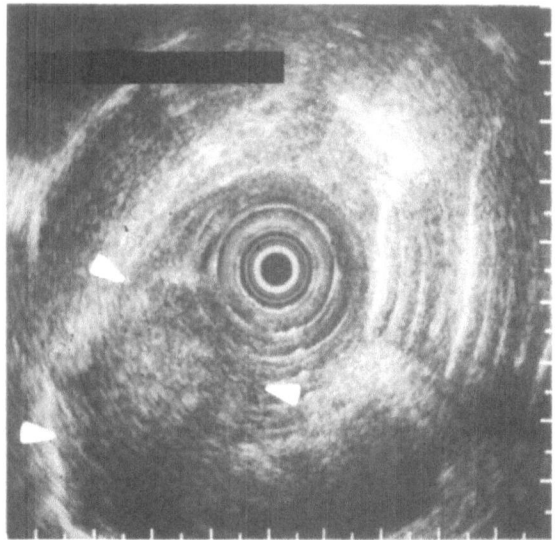

Figure 3.12. Esophageal carcinoma. The tumor is characterized by a prominent centrifugal growth into periesophageal tissues (arrowheads).

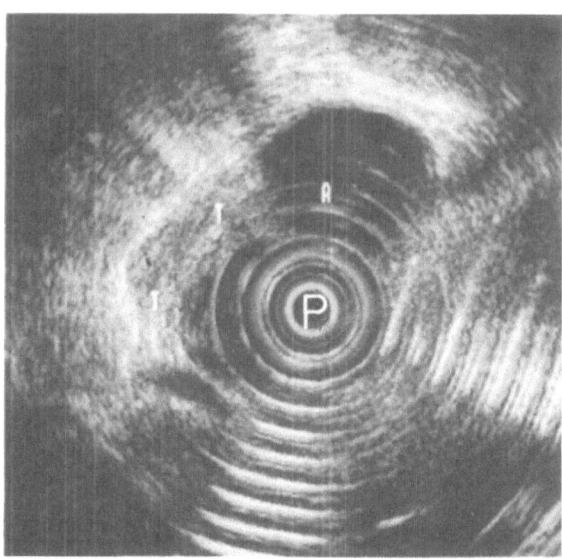

Figure 3.14. Esophageal carcinoma infiltrating the aortic wall. Tumor (T) cannot be differentiated from the wall of the aorta. A = aorta; P = probe.

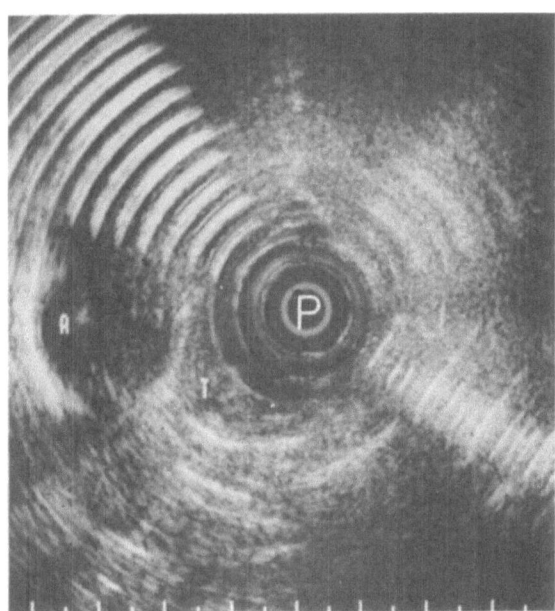

Figure 3.13. Early esophageal carcinoma. The tumor (T) lies in contact with the aorta, which is not infiltrated. A = aorta; P = probe.

sionally seen (Fig. 3.12). Tumor infiltration into the deep layers of the wall may even be demonstrated in areas that appear normal at fiberoptic endoscopy, enabling more accurate staging.

Benign and malignant strictures can be differ-

entiated upon EU examination since benign strictures are not associated with hypoechoic masses within or outside the esophageal wall. Benign esophageal tumors, most of which are leiomyomas, are rare. Differentiation from malignancy on the basis of ultrasound appearance alone is not always possible. Leiomyomas are usually seen as rounded, well-defined, hypoechoic, and homogeneous masses beneath normal mucosa.

Of major concern in the EU evaluation of esophageal carcinoma is the relationship between the tumor and the aortic wall (Figs. 3.13, 3.14). An accurate diagnosis of periaortic invasion is crucial to surgical planning. A second major consideration is metastatic involvement of lymph nodes. Lymph nodes involved by tumor appear as rounded, hypoechoic masses (Fig. 3.15), either solitary or multiple. They are easily differentiated from the enlarged collateral vessels seen with portal hypertension, which often represent a diagnostic problem in CT. EU can detect lymph nodes as small as 3—4 mm.

In a series of 11 patients, Tio and Tytgat showed EU to be superior to barium meal and CT in the visualization of the primary tumor and the detection of lymph node involvement [13]. In many cases, EU provides original, detailed

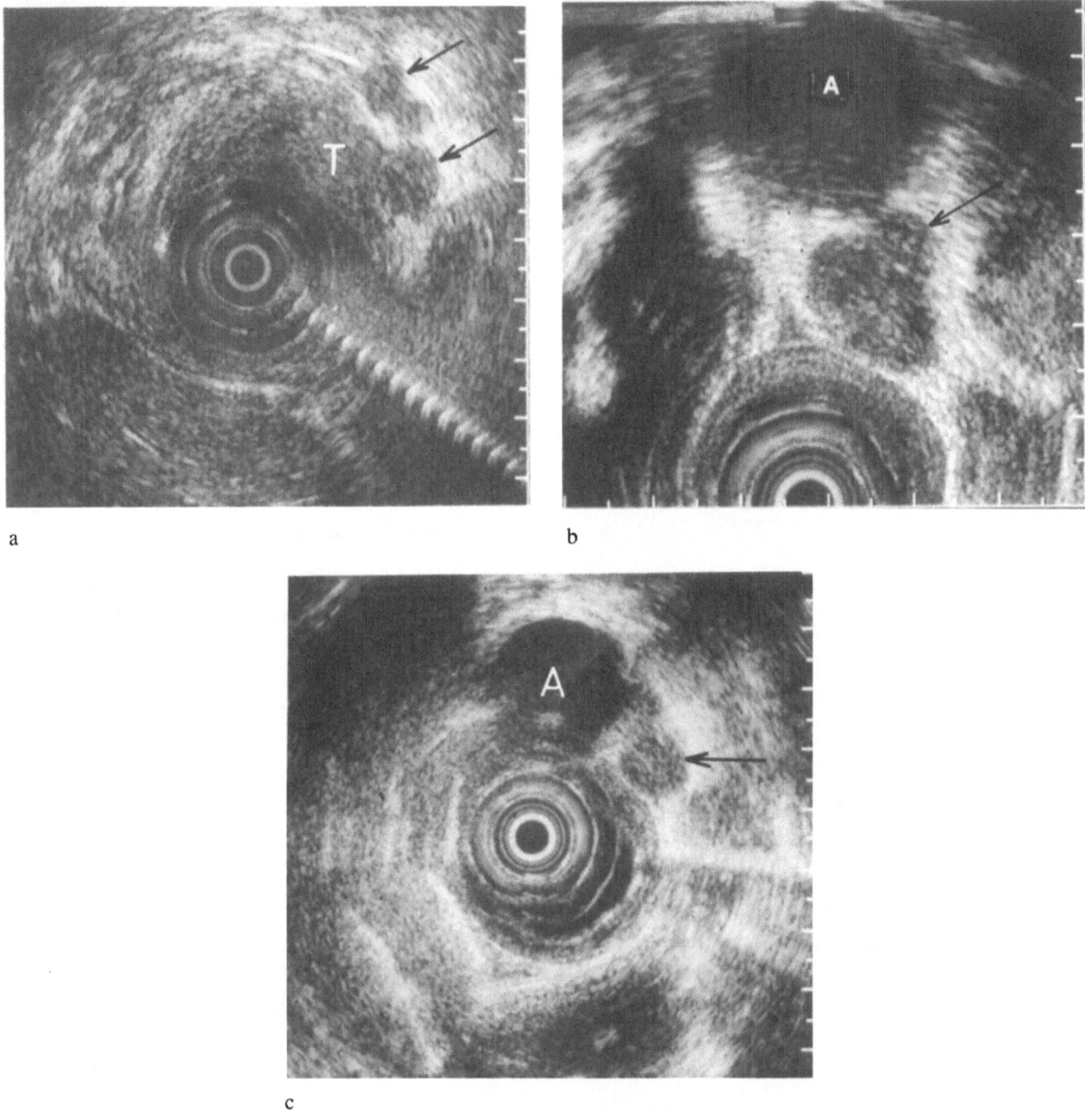

a

b

c

Figure 3.15. Esophageal carcinoma with metastatic lymph nodes in three different patients. (a) Multiple small lymph nodes (arrows) are seen adjacent to the tumor (T). (b) Solitary large metastatic node (arrow) lies between the esophagus and the aorta (A). (c) Metastatic lymph node (arrow) adjacent to the aorta (A).

information aiding in the diagnosis and staging of esophageal carcinoma, including (a) the occasional detection of submucosal masses in patients with negative fiberoptic esophagoscopy and biopsy, (b) the accurate assessment of the longitudinal tumor extent (which parameter has been shown to be of prognostic value), and (c) the detection of periaortic infiltration. The role of EU in the assessment of response to conservative therapy and in follow-up studies for early detection of local recurrence requires further evaluation.

Esophageal varices

Fiberoptic endoscopy is accurate in diagnosing esophageal varices but does not provide information on the portal vein and gastroesophageal collateral veins (on the other hand, it may not

32

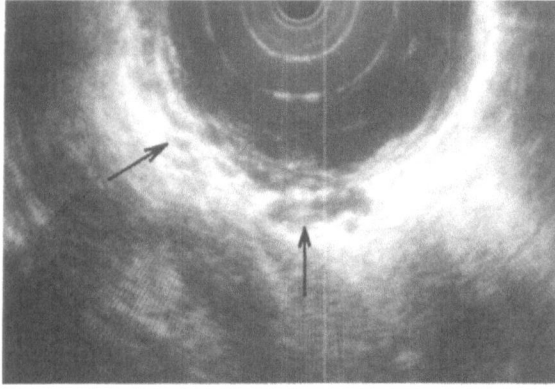

a

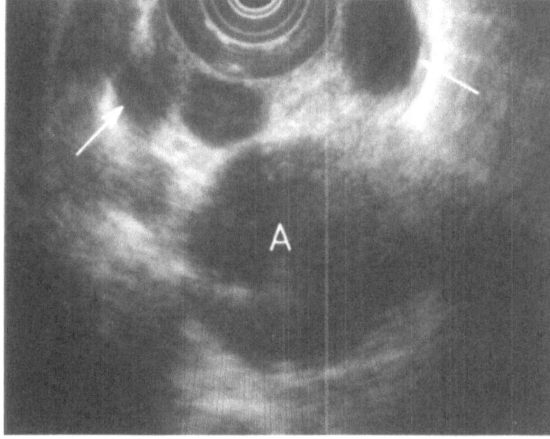

b

Figure 3.16. Esophageal varices. (a) Small submucosal and periesophageal varices (arrows). (b) Large varices (arrows). A = aorta.

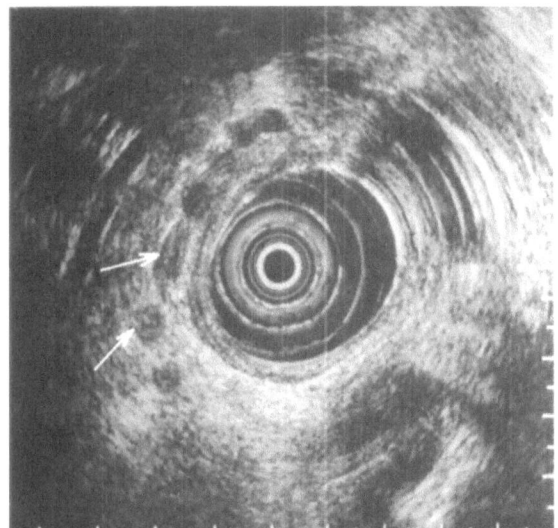

Figure 3.17. Transverse scan shows multiple periesophageal varices whose sections appear as small, hypoechoic, oval to round structures (arrows).

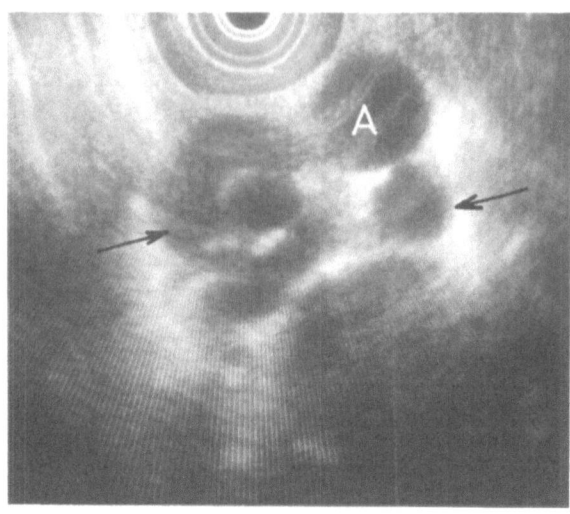

Figure 3.18. Large esophageal varices (arrows) are visualized adjacent to the aorta (A).

easily differentiate between gastric varices and fundic folds) [14]. Transabdominal sonography can visualize the portal system and has been shown to be more sensitive than fiberoptic endoscopy in detecting the early changes of portal hypertension [15, 16], but it usually cannot demonstrate gastroesophageal varices. Angiography also visualizes the whole portal system; unlike transabdominal sonography, it includes small gastroesophageal collateral veins. However, it is a more invasive technique and so cannot be used for follow-up studies. The great advantage of EU in this context is its simultaneous visualization of esophageal varices and deeper collateral vessels. It has not yet been established whether EU could improve on endoscopic assessment of bleeding risk. However, we

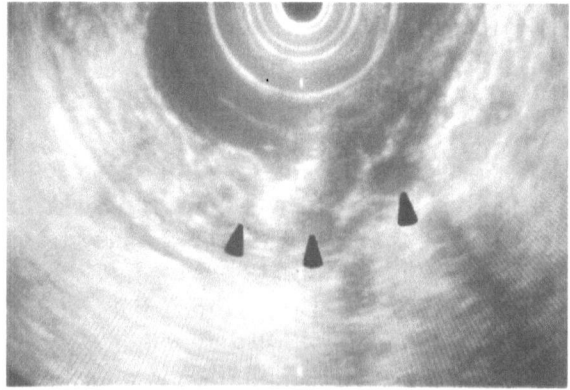

Figure 3.19. Gastric varices. Transverse scan of the fundus shows the dilated veins (arrowheads).

33

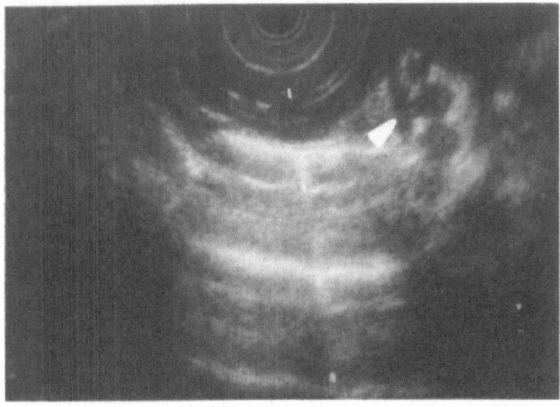

a

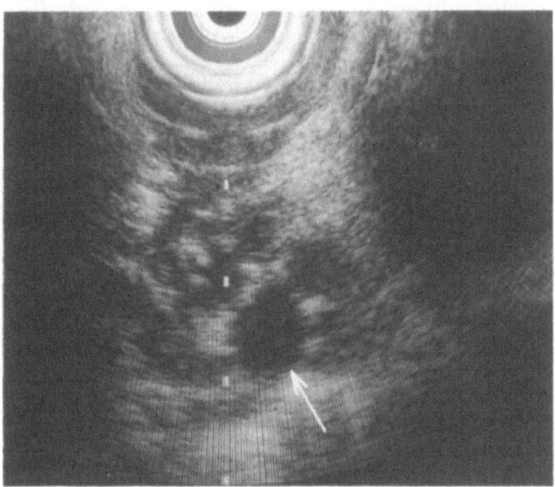

Figure 3.21. Scan shows the azygos vein (arrow) surrounded by multiple collateral veins. Note the centimetric scale.

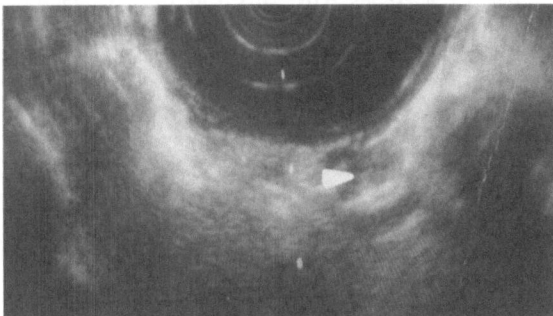

b

Figure 3.20. (a and b) Transverse scans show perforating veins (arrowheads) associated with esophageal varices.

believe that some EU findings in this regard are of clinical significance.

Endosonographic findings

Submucosal esophageal varices are displayed on transverse endoesophageal sonograms as multiple rounded, anechoic structures lying immediately underneath the mucosal layer (Fig. 3.16) [17]. Collateral vessels are demonstrated at variable distances from the esophageal wall (Fig. 3.17) and may be seen adjacent to the aorta (Fig. 3.18). The caliber of enlarged periesophageal veins seen at EU usually correlates well with the size of the esophageal varices as seen at fiberoptic endoscopy; occasionally, however, EU reveals large collateral vessels when fiberoptic endoscopy only shows minimal submucosal varices. Placing the tip of the endosonoscope beyond the cardia allows visualization of the short gastric veins that connect the

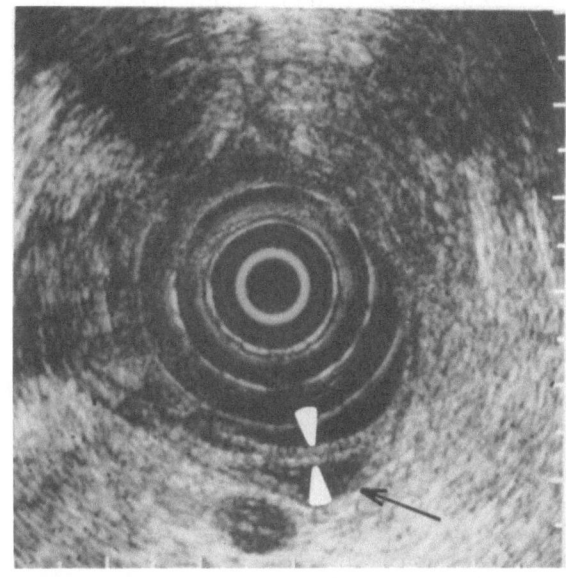

Figure 3.22. Submucosal esophageal varix. Transverse scan shows the varix (arrow) and the overlying superficial layers of the wall, whose thickness can be accurately measured (arrowheads).

esophageal collaterals and the spleen. Examination of the gastric fundus may also demonstrate gastric varices, which are readily differentiated from gastric folds (Fig. 3.19).

Relevant to the risk of hemorrhage, EU is able to (a) exactly determine varix size, (b) visualize perforating vessels (Fig. 3.20), which may play an important role in the mechanism of hemorrhage [18], (c) determine the size of

34

azygos and splenogastroesophageal vessels (Fig. 3.21), and (d) demonstrate the thickness of the esophageal wall over the varix (Fig. 3.22).

After endoscopic sclerosing therapy, fiberoptic endoscopy confirms the regression or disappearance of the varices but cannot evaluate intramural or periesophageal vessels. Transabdominal sonography shows no particular change in the portal system. In our preliminary experience, EU confirmed the disappearance of submucosal veins and demonstrated the maintained patency of collateral vessels.

These preliminary findings indicate a possible role for EU in the management of patients with esophageal varices. Enhanced diagnostic capabilities of EU are expected with the application of pulsed Doppler and color flow imaging [19]. However, further investigation is needed to determine how EU and conventional endoscopy can be combined to provide better assessment of bleeding risk and response to therapy.

References

1. Frazin M. J., Talano J. V., Stephanides L., Loeb M. S., Kopal L., Gunner R. M.: Esophageal echocardiography. Circulation, 1976, 54, 102—107.
2. Bönhof J. A., Frank K., Linhart P.: Transesophageal mediastinal sonography. Ann. Radiol. (Paris), 1985, 28, 15—20.
3. Caletti G. C., Bolondi L., Labò G.: Anatomical aspects in ultrasonic endoscopy for the stomach. Scand. J. Gastroenterol., 1984, 19 (suppl. 94), 34—42.
4. Caletti G. C., Bolondi L., Zani L., Labò G.: Technique of endoscopic ultrasonography investigation: Esophagus, stomach and duodenum. Scand. J. Gastroenterol., 1986, 21 (suppl. 123), 1—5.
5. Bolondi L., Caletti G. C., Casanova P., Villanacci V., Grigioni W., Labò G.: Problems and variations in the interpretation of the ultrasound feature of the normal upper and lower GI tract wall. Scand. J. Gastroenterol., 1986, 21 (suppl. 123), 16—26.
6. Bolondi L., Casanova P., Santi V., Caletti G. C., Barbara L., Labò G.: The sonographic appearance of the normal gastric wall: An in vitro study. Ultrasound Med. Biol., 1986, 12, 991—998.
7. Tanaka Y., Yasuda K., Aibe T., Fuji T., Kawai K.: Anatomical and pathological aspects in ultrasonic endoscopy for GI tract. Scand. J. Gastroenterol., 1984, 19 (suppl. 94), 43—50.
8. Rifkin M. D., Gordon S. J., Goldberg B. B.: Sonographic examination of the mediastinum and upper abdomen by fiberoptic gastroscope. Radiology, 1984, 151, 175—180.
9. Bruni H. C., Nelson R. S.: Carcinoma of the esophagus and cardia. Diagnostic evaluation in 113 cases. J. Thorac. Cardiovasc. Surg., 1975, 70, 367—370.
10. Witzel L., Halter F., Grétillat P. A., Scheurer U., Keller M.: Evaluation of specific value of endoscopic biopsies and brush cytology for malignancies of the esophagus and stomach. Gut, 1976, 17, 375—377.
11. Moss A. A., Schnyder P., Thoeni R. F., Margulis A. R.: Esophageal carcinoma: Pretherapy staging by computed tomography. AJR, 1981, 136, 1051—1055.
12. Bolondi L., Gandolfi L., Labò G.: Diagnostic ultrasound in gastroenterology. Padua, Piccin-Butterworths, 1984, 397.
13. Tio T. L., Tytgat G. N.: Endoscopic ultrasonography in the assessment of intra- and transmural infiltration of tumours in the oesophagus, stomach and papilla of Vater and in the detection of extraoesophageal lesions. Endoscopy, 1984, 16, 203—210.
14. Beppu K., Inokuchi K., Koyanagi N., *et al.*: Prediction of variceal hemorrhage by esophageal endoscopy. Gastroint. Endosc., 1981, 27, 213—218.
15. Bolondi L., Gandolfi L., Arienti V., *et al.*: Ultrasonography in the diagnosis of portal hypertension: Diminished response of portal vessels to respiration. Radiology, 1982, 142, 167—172.
16. Bolondi L., Caletti G. C., Brocchi E., *et al.*: Ultrasonographic findings in portal hypertension: Correlation with the presence and the size of oesophageal varices. In: Lerski R., Morley P. (eds.). Ultrasound '82. New York, Pergamon Press, 1982, 499—503.
17. Caletti G. C., Bolondi L., Zani L., Brocchi E., Guizzardi G., Labò G.: Detection of portal hypertension and esophageal varices by means of endoscopic ultrasonography. Scand. J. Gastroenterol., 1986, 21 (suppl. 123), 74—77.
18. McCormack T. T., Rose J. D., Smith P. M., Johnson A. G.: Perforating veins and blood flow in oesophageal varices. Lancet, 1983, 2, 1442—1444.
19. Sukigara M., Yamazaki T., Takamoto S., Komazaki T., Omoto R.: Color flow mapping of the esophageal varices with transesophageal real-time two-dimensional Doppler echography. In: Proceedings of the Sixth Meeting of the European Federation of Societies of Ultrasound in Medicine and Biology, Helsinki, June 14—18, 1987, 73.

4. Laparoscopic sonography

JÖRG A. BÖNHOF AND PETER LINHART

Laparoscopy allows direct examination of the surfaces of intraperitoneal organs. Biopsies can be performed even with large-bore needles with little risk. It has been said that laparoscopy is "the most reliable technique for closing the diagnostic gap between clinical evaluation and surgical exploration" [1]. That gap is further narrowed when ultrasound is used during laparoscopy. Whereas laparoscopy provides the superficial view of anteriorly located surfaces, structures within and dorsal to intraperitoneal organs are not seen. In most circumstances, the simultaneous visualization of such structures by sonography can be extremely helpful for optimal utilization of laparoscopy. With the ultrasound transducer in direct contact with the intraperitoneal organs, sound wave propagation is optimal and high frequencies can be used, yielding better image quality and more information than in transcutaneous sonography.

The first clinical trials of laparoscopic sonography (or sonolaparoscopy) were performed in Japan in the late 1950s and early 1960s [2—4]. They consisted of the intraperitoneal use of ultrasound probes with an A-mode display. Few additional reports [5] appeared until the early 1980s when Furukawa *et al.* [6] and Fukuda *et al.* [7] presented their preliminary results with the intraperitoneal application of a real-time mechanical sector scanner, while Kodama [8] and Frank [9] and their coworkers reported on laparoscopic sonography utilizing a linear-array transducer. In 1984, we described a technique to perform laparoscopic biopsies under sonographic guidance [10]; subsequently, we reported our experience with linear-array transducers in laparoscopic sonography [11—15]. Several other

investigators have also reported their experience with this technique [16—23].

Instrumentation

Different types of probes have been employed in laparoscopic sonography. The multielement, electronic linear-array transducers represent the most advanced technique available for laparoscopic sonography [9—15, 23]. We have used different prototype linear-array 5.0 and 7.5-MHz probes (Fig. 4.1) connected to commercially available scanners (Siemens). These probes provide a field of view about 3.5 cm in width and 5 to 10 cm in depth depending on the frequency. The angulation of the transducer is controlled by a device at the proximal end of the probe shaft (Fig. 4.1). The outer diameter of the probe is 10 or 11 mm, so that the probe can be inserted into the peritoneal cavity through

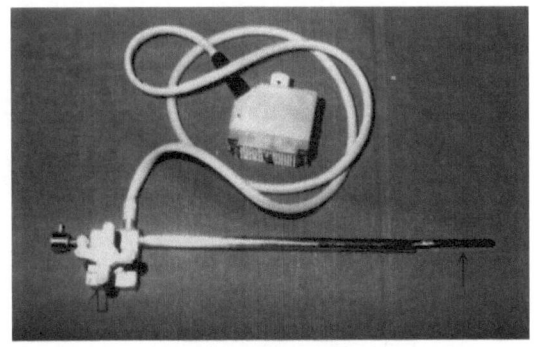

Figure 4.1. Probe for laparoscopic sonography. The linear-array transducer is seen at the tip of the probe (arrow). The open arrow points to the device controlling the angulation of the transducer in relation to the general axis of the probe.

Bruno D. Fornage (ed.), *Endosonography*, pp. 35—41.

36

standard trocar cannulas available from major manufacturers.

Technique of examination

Preparation of the patient for laparoscopic sonography is identical to preparation for conventional laparoscopy, except that additional information must be provided to the patient about the sonographic procedure. First, laparoscopy is performed as usual, according to the recommendations of Beck [24]. Nitrous oxide is insufflated into the peritoneal cavity through a Veres needle after skin anesthetization. A 10-mm trocar cannula for the laparoscope is inserted about 3 cm left and cephalad to the umbilicus. Then, a second incision is made in the right upper quadrant below the ribs to insert a second 10-mm trocar cannula (Fig. 4.2). Optical guidance through the laparoscope inserted through the first incision guarantees that the sonolaparoscopic probe is inserted through the second incision (Fig. 4.3) and placed (Fig. 4.4) without injury to the organs. By this means, optical and sonographic views are obtained during the same procedure. Also, a video camera is attached to the laparoscope, which allows real-time monitoring of the procedure on a separate screen. With the two 10-mm cannulas in place, the sonolaparoscopic probe and laparoscope can be interchanged. This maneuver is often

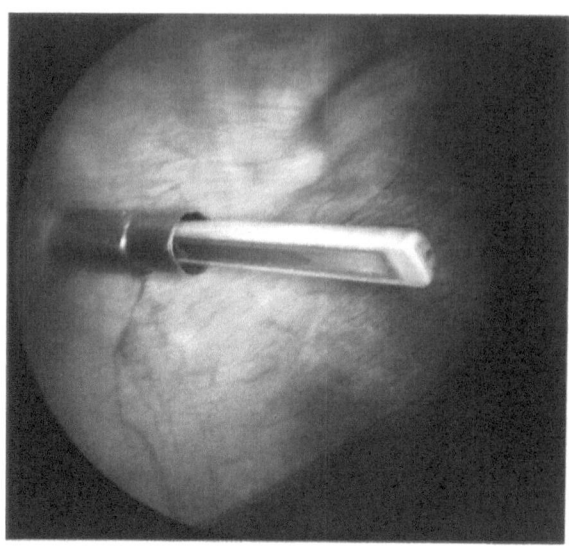

Figure 4.3. Under laparoscopic control, the ultrasound probe is introduced through a 10-mm cannula into the peritoneal cavity.

essential for the evaluation of the upper and lateral portions of the left hepatic lobe.

Attempts have been made to incorporate an optical lens into the shaft of the ultrasound probe to obviate a second incision. Thus far, however, a field of view wide enough to ensure satisfactory control of the movements of the probe has not been attained with this method.

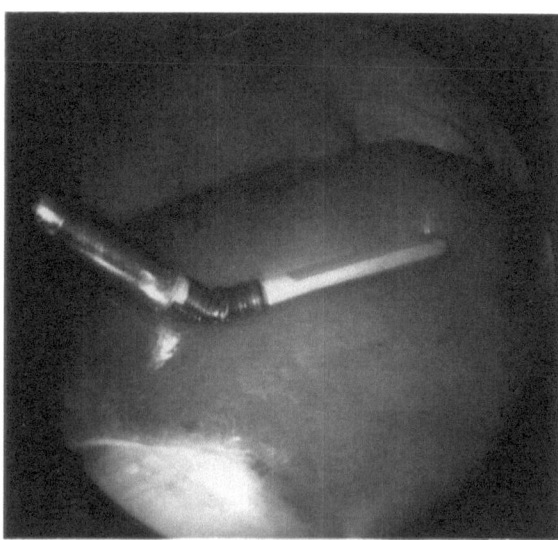

Figure 4.4. Application of the ultrasound probe to the surface of the liver under laparoscopic control. The acoustic coupling is provided by the moisture of the peritoneal surface.

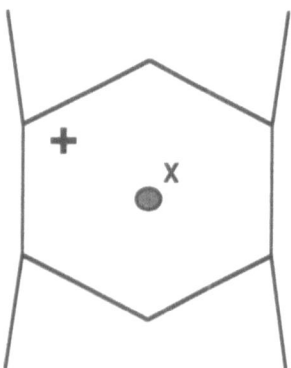

Figure 4.2. Diagram showing the positions of the two incisions (x, first; +, second) used for insertion of the conventional laparoscope and the sonolaparoscopic probe.

Results

As expected from the close proximity of the transducer to the region of interest and the high frequencies used, laparoscopic, like intraoperative sonography, yields images of increased contrast and spatial resolution compared with conventional ultrasound. Consequently, smaller lesions can be detected (Fig. 4.5) and a better characterization of their echotexture can also be achieved (Fig. 4.6).

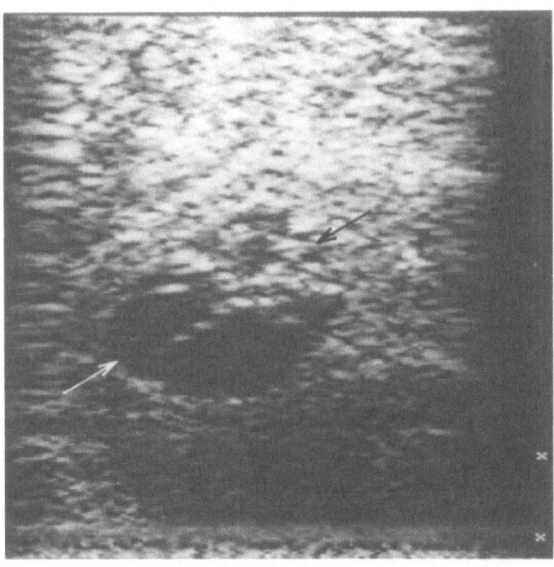

Figure 4.6. Laparoscopic sonogram shows an atypical renal cyst with internal echogenic material (arrows). Conventional sonography and CT showed a focal lesion but failed to characterize it. Calipers in the upper left of the image indicate 5 mm.

Biopsy guidance

The diagnostic workup of abdominal solid masses usually requires a pathologic specimen, often obtained by ultrasound- or computed tomography (CT)-guided biopsy. This can also be obtained by a needle biopsy performed under sonolaparoscopic guidance. Three different techniques are available [10, 13]:

Technique A: The localization of the lesion, the site for biopsy, and the orientation of the needle are determined with laparoscopic sonography. However, the biopsy is performed under optical laparoscopic, not real-time sonographic, control (Fig. 4.7).

Technique B: The lesion is localized with laparoscopic sonography and visualized on the video monitor. Under laparoscopic control, the biopsy needle is placed tangential to the transducer and then inserted toward the lesion (Fig. 4.8). When it has reached the scan plane, the tip of the needle is visualized as a bright echogenic focus. Precise placement of the needle and continuous monitoring of its tip can thus be achieved.

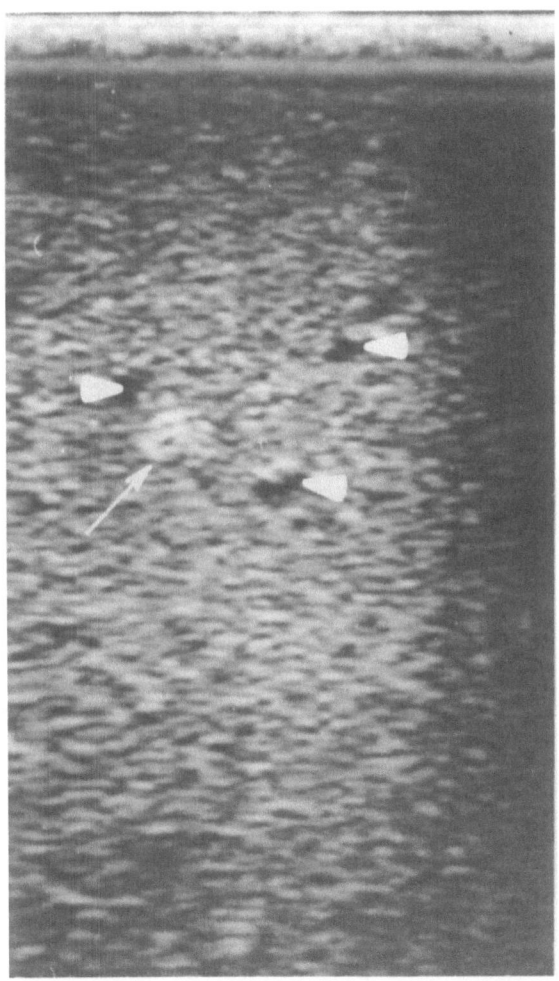

Figure 4.5. Laparoscopic sonogram of the liver using a 7-MHz transducer shows a small, hyperechoic tumor about 3 mm in diameter (arrow), which could not be detected with other imaging modalities. Note the cross sections of vessels (arrowheads).

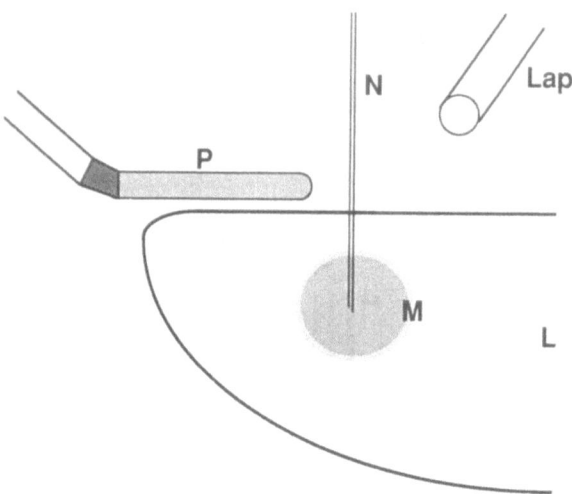

Technique C: A special probe is used, characterized by a longitudinal channel through its shaft for the biopsy needle. Since their linear-array transducer is oblique to the shaft of the probe, the biopsy needle, when coming out of the channel, enters the scan plane oblique to the beam and is seen as an echogenic line (Fig. 4.9).

Technique C is the most accurate; the other techniques are used only when it is precluded by the remote location of the lesion. Since biopsies according to techniques B and C are performed under simultaneous laparoscopic and sonographic monitoring, they are referred to as 'double-guided' biopsies.

Figure 4.7. Diagram of ultrasound-guided needle biopsy according to technique A of text. The lesion has been localized by laparoscopic sonography, but the needle is inserted under visual laparoscopic control only. L = liver; Lap = conventional laparoscope; M = mass; N = biopsy needle; P = sonolaparoscopic probe.

Indications

It would be of interest to have sonolaparoscopic equipment available for every laparoscopy, so that unexpected or suspicious laparoscopic findings could be immediately evaluated by

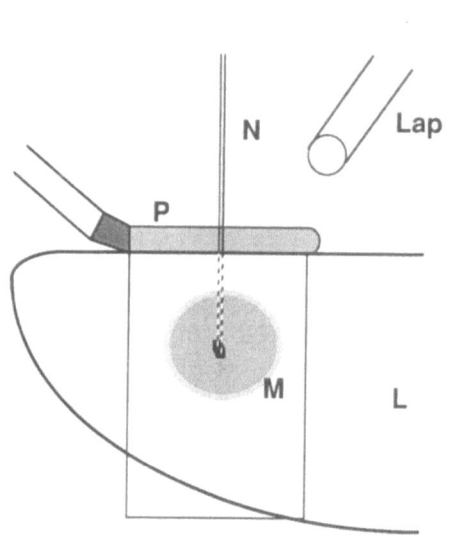

a

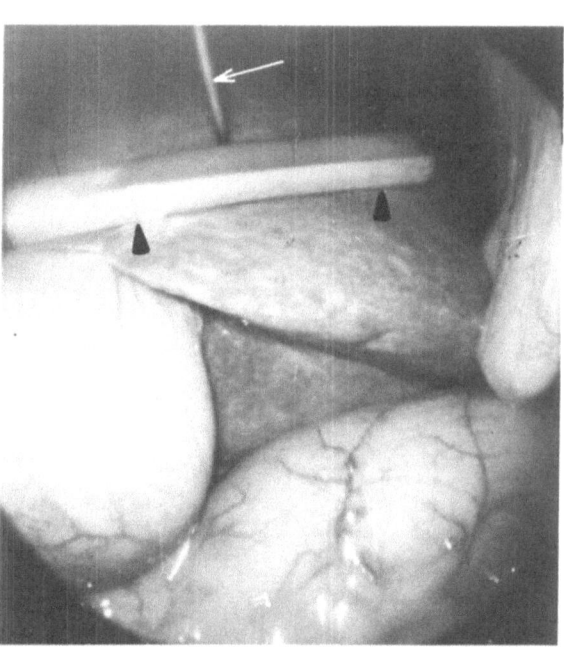

b

Figure 4.8. Ultrasound-guided needle biopsy according to technique B of text. (a) Diagram showing the biopsy needle inserted tangential to the transducer and slightly oblique in relation to the scan plane. When the scanning plane is reached at the level of the lesion, the tip of the needle is clearly visualized as a bright echo. L = liver; Lap = conventional laparoscope; M = mass; N = biopsy needle; P = sonolaparoscopic probe. (b) Biopsy of a liver mass adjacent to the gallbladder. Operative view shows the needle (arrow) tangential to the linear-array transducer (arrowheads) placed on the surface of the liver.

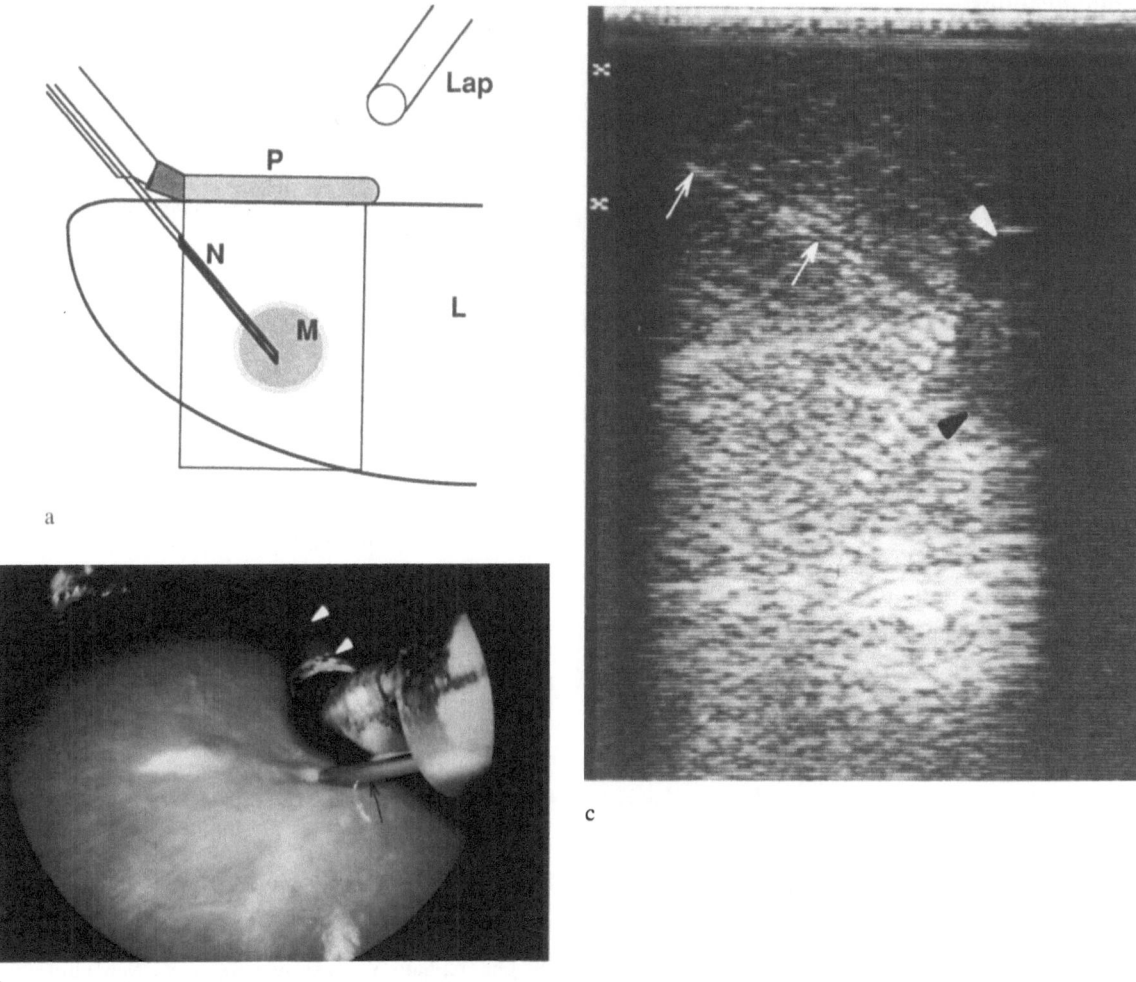

a

b

c

Figure 4.9. Ultrasound-guided needle biopsy according to technique C of text. (a) Diagram showing the biopsy needle entering the ultrasonic scanning plane obliquely. The portion of the needle that is included in the ultrasonic field of view is visualized as an echogenic line. L = liver; Lap = conventional laparoscope; M = mass; N = biopsy needle; P = sonolaparoscopic probe. (b) Ultrasound-guided biopsy of a focal lesion of the liver. Intraoperative view shows the biopsy needle (arrow) coming out of its channel in the shaft of the probe and obliquely penetrating the scan plane of the linear-array transducer (arrowheads). (c) Sonogram shows the oblique echogenic needle (arrows) penetrating a hypo-echoic liver mass (arrowheads).

ultrasound. In general, laparoscopic sonography is helpful whenever laparoscopy cannot confirm the abnormalities seen on previous conventional sonography. However, the major indication for laparoscopic sonography is to guide the large-bore needle biopsy of a focal lesion when (a) repeat percutaneous ultrasound- or CT-guided fine-needle aspirations have failed to yield a specimen permitting diagnosis, (b) a histopathologic specimen is required (e.g., in lymphoma, or in tumors with a large connective tissue component), or (c) the lesion is adjacent to a vital structure that might be damaged during a 'blind' biopsy.

Finally, despite the development of percutaneous ultrasound- and CT-guided needle biopsy, intra-abdominal lesions may still require exploratory laparotomy with open biopsy for diagnosis. Laparoscopic sonography could spare some of these patients surgical exploration.

Complications

The incidence of complications associated with laparoscopy [1, 25] is not significantly higher than that in percutaneous fine-needle biopsies performed under sonographic guidance [26]. There are not yet enough data to estimate risks of laparoscopic sonography, whether or not in the context of biopsy. In our experience, this technique has been as safe as conventional laparoscopy.

Summary

Laparoscopic sonography enhances the capabilities of laparoscopy. Its major application is the sonographic guidance of laparoscopic large-bore needle biopsies of intraperitoneal masses.

References

1. Boyce H. W. Jr.: Laparoscopy. In: Schiff L., Schiff E. R. (eds). Diseases of the liver. Philadelphia, Lippincott, 1982, 333–348.
2. Yamakawa K., Wagai T.: Diagnosis of intraabdominal lesions by laparoscope. 4. Ultrasonography through laparoscope. Jpn. J. Gastroenterol., 1958, 55, 741.
3. Kikuchi Y.: Recent results of research and development in the field of ultrasonics in Japan. In: Cremer L. (ed.) Proceedings of the Third International Congress on Acoustics. Amsterdam, Elsevier, 1959, 2, 1193.
4. Hayashi S., Wagai T., Miyazawa R., et al.: Ultrasonic diagnosis of breast tumor and cholelithiasis. West. J. Surg. Obstet. Gynecol., 1962, 70, 34–40.
5. Look D., Henning H., Yano M.: Direkte Ultraschall-echographie der Gallenblase unter laparoskopischer Sicht. In: Lindner H. (ed.). Fortschritte der gastro-enterologischen Endoskopie. Vol. 6. Baden-Baden, Witzstrock, 1975.
6. Furukawa Y., Kanazawa H., Wakabayashi I., et al.: A new method of B-mode ultrasonography under laparoscopic guidance. In: Classen M., Henning H., Seifert E. (eds.). Abstracts of the 4th European Congress of Gastrointestinal Endoscopy. Stuttgart, Thieme, 1980, 50.
7. Fukuda M., Hirata K., Saito K., et al.: Studies on intraluminal echography in abdominal disease: Echolaparoscopy. In: Kurjak A. (ed.). Proceedings of the 4th European Congress of Ultrasonics in Medicine. Amsterdam, Excerpta Medica, 1981, 109.
8. Kodama T., Okita K., Oda M., Esaki T., Fukumoto Y., Takemoto T.: Development and clinical investigation of ultrasonic laparoscopy. Scand. J. Gastroenterol., 1982, 17 (Suppl. 78), 1.
9. Frank K., Bliesze H., Beck K., Hammes P., Linhart P.: Laparoskopische Sonographie. Eine neue Dimension in der Diagnostik innerer Organe. Dtsch. Med. Wochenschr., 1983, 108, 902–904.
10. Bönhof J. A., Linhart P., Bettendorf U., Holper H.: Liver biopsy guided by laparoscopic sonography. A case report demonstrating a new technique. Endoscopy, 1984, 16, 237–239.
11. Bönhof J. A., Frank K., Loch E. G., Linhart P.: Laparoscopic sonography. Ann. Radiol. (Paris), 1984, 28, 16–18.
12. Bönhof J. A., Linhart P., Beck K., Frank K., Loch E. G.: Laparoscopic sonography (abstract). J. Ultrasound Med., 1984, 3 (Suppl.), 174.
13. Bönhof J. A., Linhart P., Beck K., Loch E. G.: Laparoscopic sonography: A promising approach to optimize an endoscopic technique (abstract). Ultrasound Med. Biol., 1985 (Suppl. 1), 77.
14. Bönhof J. A., Linhart P., Loch E. G.: Laparoskopische Sonographie. In: Popp L. W. (ed.). Gynäkologische Endosonographie. Quickborn, Ingo Klemke Verlag, 1986, 225–231.
15. Frank K., Bliesze H., Bönhof J. A., Beck K., Hammes P., Linhart P.: Laparoscopic sonography: A new approach to intraabdominal disease. J. Clin. Ultrasound, 1985, 13, 60–65.
16. Ohta Y., Yamazaki M., Torii M., et al.: A device of ultrasonic laparoscope. Gastrointest. Endosc., 1981, 23, 1385.
17. Ohta Y., Fujiwara K., Sato Y., Niwa H., Oka H.: New ultrasonic laparoscope for diagnosis of intraabdominal diseases. Gastrointest. Endosc., 1983, 29, 289–294.
18. Ota Y., Sato Y., Takatsuki K., et al.: New ultrasonic laparoscope: Improvement in diagnosis of intraabdominal diseases. Scand. J. Gastroenterol., 1982, 17 (Suppl. 78), 194.
19. Aramaki N., Yoshida K., Yamashiro Y., Namihisa T.: Ultrasonic laparoscopy. Scand. J. Gastroenterol., 1982, 17 (Suppl. 78), 185.
20. Sato W., Komatsu K., Moriai N., Nakanome C., Sasaki M., Hanada M.: Atlas of ultrasonic laparoscope. Honjo, Japan, 1984.
21. Fukuda M.: Intraluminal scanning: Use of the echo-endoscope and echolaparoscope in the diagnosis of intraabdominal cancer. In: Kossoff G., Fukuda M. (eds.). Ultrasonic differential diagnosis of tumors. New York, Igaku-Shoin, 1984, 186–199.
22. Fukuda M., Mima S., Tanabe T., et al.: Endoscopic sonography of the liver: Diagnostic application of the echolaparoscope to localize intrahepatic lesions. Scand. J. Gastroenterol., 1984, 19 (Suppl. 102), 24–38.
23. Vogel H. M., Friedrich K., Henning H.: Laparoskopische Sonographie: Neues Instrumentarium mit erleichterter Untersuchungstechnik. In: Otto R., Schnaars P. (eds.). Ultraschalldiagnostik 85. Stuttgart, Thieme, 1986, 506–507.
24. Beck K.: Farbatlas der Laparoskopie. Pathologische

Anatomie des Abdomens in vivo. Stuttgart, Schattauer, 1980.

25. Henning H., Look D.: Laparoskopie. Atlas und Lehrbuch. Stuttgart, Thieme, 1985.

26. Livraghi T., Damascelli B., Lombardi C., Spagnoli I.: Risk in fine-needle abdominal biopsy. J. Clin. Ultrasound, 1983, 11, 77—81.

5. Endosonography of the rectum

GIULIO DI CANDIO, FRANCO MOSCA, AND BRUNO D. FORNAGE

Wild and Reid in 1956 demonstrated a local recurrence of rectal carcinoma with the use of an experimental intrarectal ultrasound transducer [1]. In 1983, Alzin *et al.* and Dragsted and Gammelgaard reported on their preliminary experiences with endosonography in the preoperative staging of rectal carcinoma [2,3]. However, it is only recently that results of studies focused on rectal endosonography have been published, some correlated with computed tomography (CT) findings [4—14]. It must be emphasized that endosonography of the rectum is still in the developmental phase.

Anatomy

The rectum begins at the level of the third sacral vertebra and terminates at the anus. It comprises pelvic and perineal portions (Fig. 5.1).

Pelvic rectum

The pelvic rectum is 13 to 15 cm long and is oriented obliquely downward and forward with an intra- and an extraperitoneal segment. Only the first few centimeters of the anterior and lateral aspects of the pelvic rectum are covered with peritoneum; the posterior aspect is related to the presacral aponeurosis by loose connective tissue and by the retrorectal fascia. Anteriorly, the peritoneum forms a pouch, the Douglas's pouch or cul-de-sac, between the rectum and the bladder in the male, and between the rectum and the uterus in the female. To this cul-de-sac is attached the rectovesical (Denonvilliers') fascia in the male, and the rectovaginal fascia in the

female. The extraperitoneal pelvic rectum is mainly made up of the rectal ampulla.

The pelvic rectum is characterized by the presence of two or three permanent, semilunar, internal folds about 1 cm in width, known as Houston's valves. These folds correspond to more or less marked grooves at. the external surface of the rectum.

Relationships

Anteriorly *in the male*, below the cul-de-sac, the wall of the pelvic rectum is related to the bladder base, seminal vesicles, ampullae of the vasa deferentia, and posterior aspect of the prostate (Fig. 5.2). The rectum is separated from these organs by the prerectal space and the rectovesical fascia. Anteriorly *in the female*, the pelvic rectum is related to the uterus and vagina by the prerectal space and rectovaginal fascia.

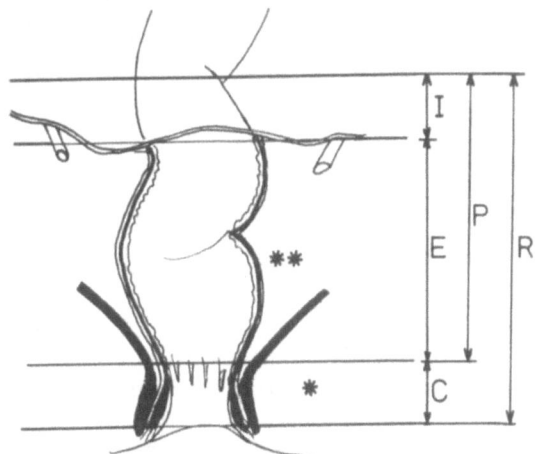

Figure 5.1. Diagrammatic frontal view of the rectum (R). C = perineal rectum (or anal canal); E = extraperitoneal rectum; I = intraperitoneal rectum; P = pelvic rectum; * = ischioanal space; ** = pelvirectal space.

Bruno D. Fornage (ed.), *Endosonography*, pp. 43—69.

44

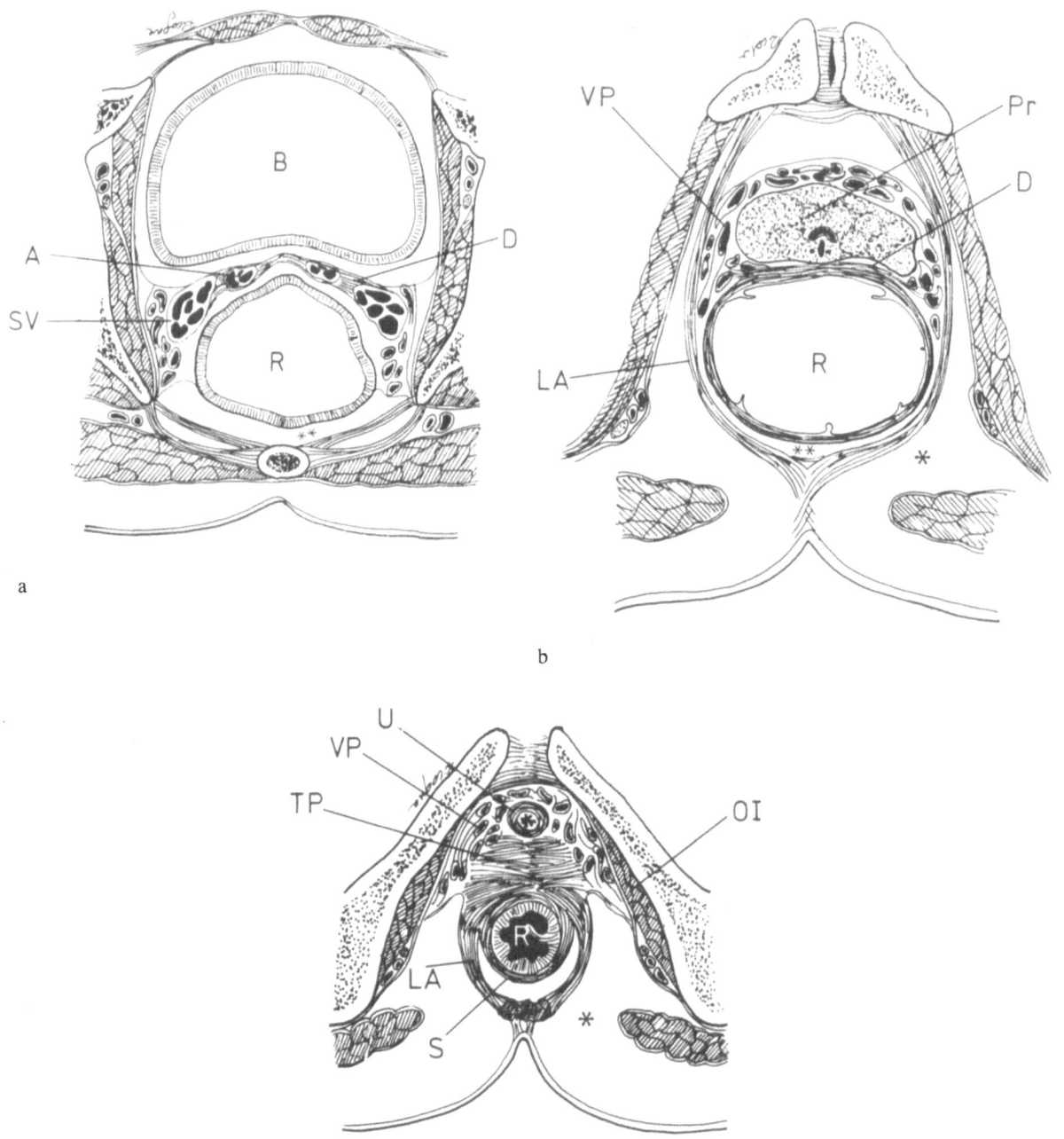

Figure 5.2. Diagrammatic transverse sections of the male pelvis show the relations of the rectum. (a) At the level of the seminal vesicles: A = ampulla of vas deferens; B = bladder; D = Denonvilliers' rectovesical fascia; R = rectum; SV = seminal vesicle; ** = pelvirectal space. (b) At the level of the prostate: D = Denonvilliers' rectovesical fascia; LA = levator ani muscle; Pr = prostate; R = rectum; VP = periprostatic venous plexus; * = ischioanal space; ** = pelvirectal space. (c) At the level of the sphincter: LA = levator ani muscle; OI = obturator internus muscle; R = rectum; S = anal sphincter; TP = transversus perinei profundus muscle; U = urethra; VP = periprostatic venous plexus; * = ischioanal space.

Posteriorly, the pelvic rectum is related to the sacrum and coccyx, which are covered by the presacral aponeurosis and separated from the rectum by the loose connective retrorectal tissue and the pyriformis and coccygeus muscles.

Laterally, the pelvic rectum is related to the

ureters, hypogastric vessels, and levator ani muscles.

Perineal rectum

The perineal rectum, or anal canal, is about 3 cm in length. It is surrounded by the levator ani muscles and is oriented obliquely downward and backward. It is encircled at its termination by the external anal sphincter. An upper mucous and a lower cutaneous portion have been described. The perineal and the pelvic rectum form an angle whose vertex corresponds to the apex of the coccyx. The internal rectal surface is characterized by the presence of 5 to 12 transverse folds, the Morgagni's valves, which are separated from one another by longitudinally oriented crests of mucosa known as Morgagni's rectal columns. The superior limit of Morgagni's columns corresponds to the junction of the perineal rectum and pelvic rectum. The perineal rectum is firmly anchored in the pelvic floor by the transversus perinei profundus muscles (Fig. 5.2c).

Relationships
In the male, the perineal rectum is related anteriorly to the prostatic apex, the membranous urethra, the bulbocavernosus muscles, and Cowper's glands. Below the level of the prostatic apex, the rectum is separated from the urethra by the triangular urethrorectal space, whose size increases toward the anus.

In the female, the posterior wall of the vagina is separated from the anterior wall of the rectum by the rectovaginal fascia, whose thickness increases inferiorly to form the rectovaginal space.

Laterally, the perineal rectum is adjoined by the fat in the ischiorectal fossae.

Structure of the rectal wall

The rectal wall is approximately 2 mm thick and comprises, from the lumen to the periphery, the mucosa (with muscularis mucosae), submucosa, and muscular coat. There is no serosa below the level of the cul-de-sac. The muscular coat consists of an external longitudinal and an internal circular layer of smooth muscle fibers. The circular fibers thicken in the perineal rectum and constitute the internal sphincter. The longitudinal fibers, which are collected into three flat longitudinal bands (or taeniae coli) in the cecum and colon, spread out and form a layer that completely encircles the rectum. These longitudinal muscle fibers can in turn be separated into an outer and an inner layer; the outer layer merges inferiorly with the fibers of the levator ani muscles, whereas the inner layer courses between the internal and external anal sphincters and terminates under the perineal skin.

Normal ultrasound anatomy

Suprapubic examination

The rectum can be visualized on transabdominal sonograms obtained suprapubically through the distended bladder, preferably with sector or convex-array transducers. However, the image quality is often suboptimal because of the distance between the rectum and the probe and the presence of intrarectal gas, which stops the propagation of the ultrasound beam.

The lower rectum is the more readily demonstrated. It is seen posterior to the bladder and the prostate in the male, and to the uterus and vagina in the female (Fig. 5.3). The anterior rectal wall is often visualized as a hypoechoic linear pattern, which actually represents the muscular layer and which delineates the posterior aspects of the bladder and prostate in the male, and of the uterus and vagina in the female. The lumen is occasionally silhouetted by gas. The rectum is best visualized posterior to the vagina or the prostate at the junction between the pelvic rectum and perineal rectum, where the physiologic narrowing of the lumen prevents gas accumulation. In this location, on transverse scans the rectum has a typical target-like pattern, with the outer muscular coat, which is hypoechoic, being particularly well demarcated (Fig. 5.3c).

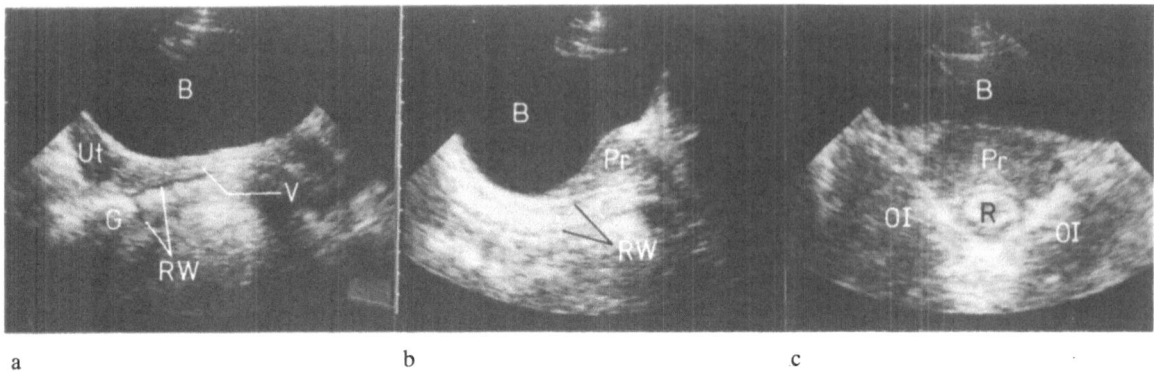

Figure 5.3. Suprapubic sonograms of the rectum obtained with a 3.5-MHz sector transducer in different subjects. (a and b) Longitudinal scans. (c) Transverse scan. B = bladder; G = intrarectal gas; OI = obturator internus muscle; Pr = prostate; R = rectum; RW = rectal wall; Ut = uterus; V = vagina.

Endorectal examination

Although it is not essential, preparation of the rectum can be rapidly achieved with rectal suppositories. A digital rectal examination is first performed to exclude an obstructive mass, stricture, or fissure. Routinely, 5 and 7.5-MHz radial and linear-array transducers are used. Much is expected from the recent commercialization of biplane probes. The intracavitary probe is sheathed with a latex balloon before it is inserted into the rectum. A primary function of the balloon is its prevention of contamination of the transducer. After rectal insertion, the balloon is distended with water so that the rectal wall is moved away from the surface of the transducer and can therefore be visualized. The water distension of the balloon also serves to position the region of interest in the optimal focal zone of the transducer.

Longitudinally and transversely oriented scans obtained, respectively, with linear-array and radial transducers allow similar depictions of the various layers of the rectal wall. However, the interpretation of these images, in particular the correlation between the layers displayed on sonography and their histologic counterparts, has been controversial (Fig. 5.4). Initially, Rifkin recognized two layers: the internal, echogenic, interpreted as the interface of the balloon and the mucosa, and the external, hypoechoic, interpreted as the submucosa and the muscular coat

[4]. Using a 3.5-MHz radial and a 5.0-MHz linear-array transducer, Konishi et al. reported the in vivo demonstration of three layers: hyper-, hypo-, and hyperechoic from the lumen to the periphery, with the hypoechoic, intermediate layer corresponding to the muscular coat [5]. These authors could not distinguish between the mucosa and the submucosa sonographically. All other investigators have described five to seven sonographic layers [6–12, 14]. Given five layers and starting from the lumen, the first, third, and fifth layers are echogenic, and the second and fourth layers are hypoechoic. The fourth layer can in turn be subdivided by a thin echogenic interface into two layers, raising the total number of layers depicted on sonography to seven [10, 11]. According to Boscaini [6] and Hildebrandt [7, 8] and colleagues, the hyperechoic layers represent ultrasound interfaces and only the second and fourth layers correspond to anatomic structures, namely, the mucosa with submucosa and the muscular coat. Beynon *et al.* [10] and Saitoh and associates [11] are in agreement with Boscaini and colleagues and Hildebrandt and coworkers as regards the fourth layer (the muscularis propria). However, they believe that sonography can differentiate the mucosa from the submucosa, the latter corresponding to the third layer (echogenic).

Our interpretation of the endosonographic layers of the normal rectal wall is as follows. The *first layer* (hyperechoic) is a fluid/solid interface,

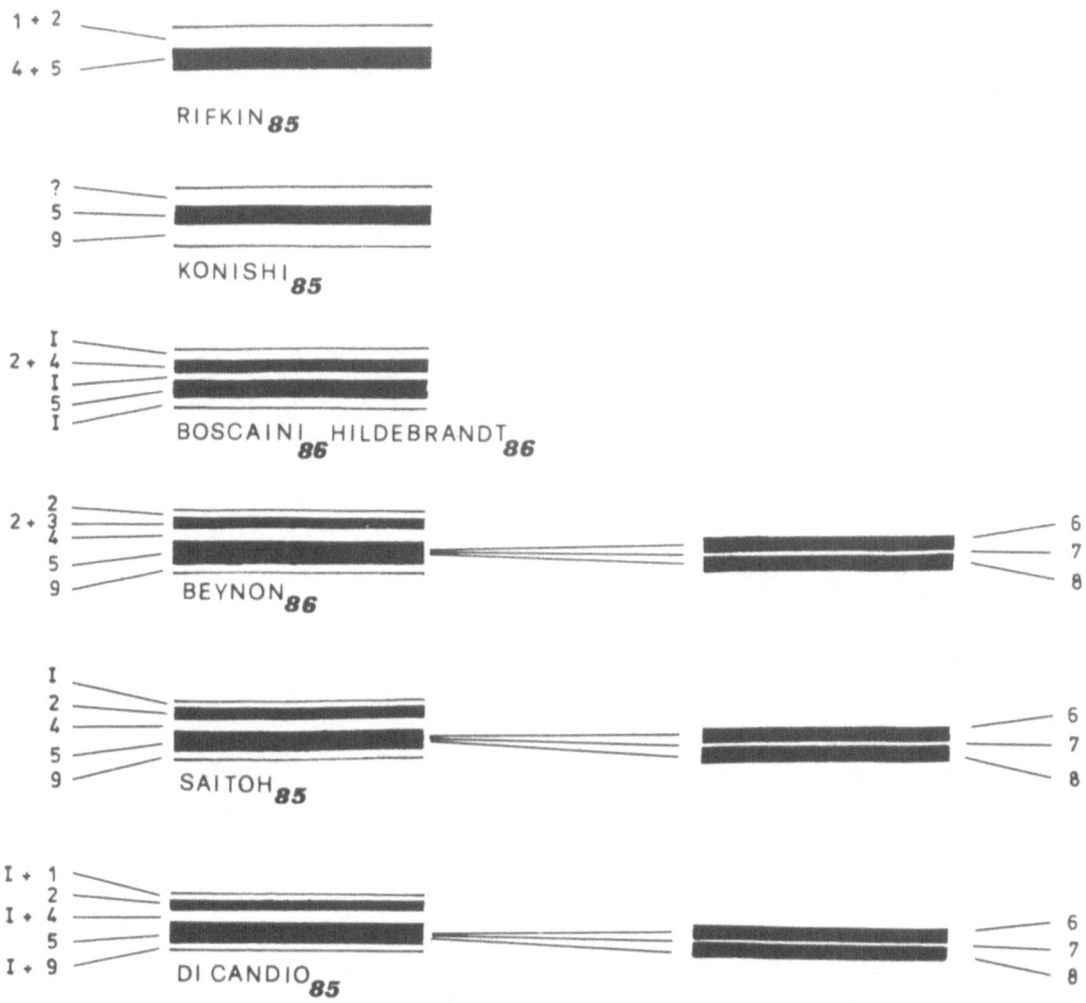

Figure 5.4. Interpretations of the endosonographic appearance of the normal rectal wall according to various investigators. I = ultrasound interface; 1 = latex balloon; 2 = mucosa; 3 = muscularis mucosae; 4 = submucosa; 5 = muscular coat; 6 = internal circular muscular layer; 7 = thin layer of connective tissue; 8 = external longitudinal muscular layer; 9 = loose perirectal tissue.

resulting primarily from the latex balloon. On in vitro studies or when the examination is performed in vivo without a balloon but with a water enema, this first layer is much less conspicuous. Also, it is best seen where the beam is perpendicular to the rectal surface (Fig. 5.5).

The *second layer* (hypoechoic) represents the mucosa, whose classic wavy pattern is well demonstrated on in vitro studies and on in vivo studies performed without the balloon (Fig. 5.6). In our experience, the muscularis mucosae could not be visualized in vivo. On in vitro studies, the second layer is occasionally associated with a

more hypoechoic underlining of its peripheral limit, which might represent the muscularis mucosae.

We believe the *third layer* (hyperechoic) to result from the summation of (a) the interface between the mucosa and the submucosa, (b) the submucosa itself, and (c) the interface between the submucosa and the muscularis propria. When we inserted a 25-gauge needle in the submucosa, it appeared on both longitudinal and transverse scans to be localized in the third sonographic layer (Fig. 5.7), corroborating this belief. Moreover, the third layer is altered in

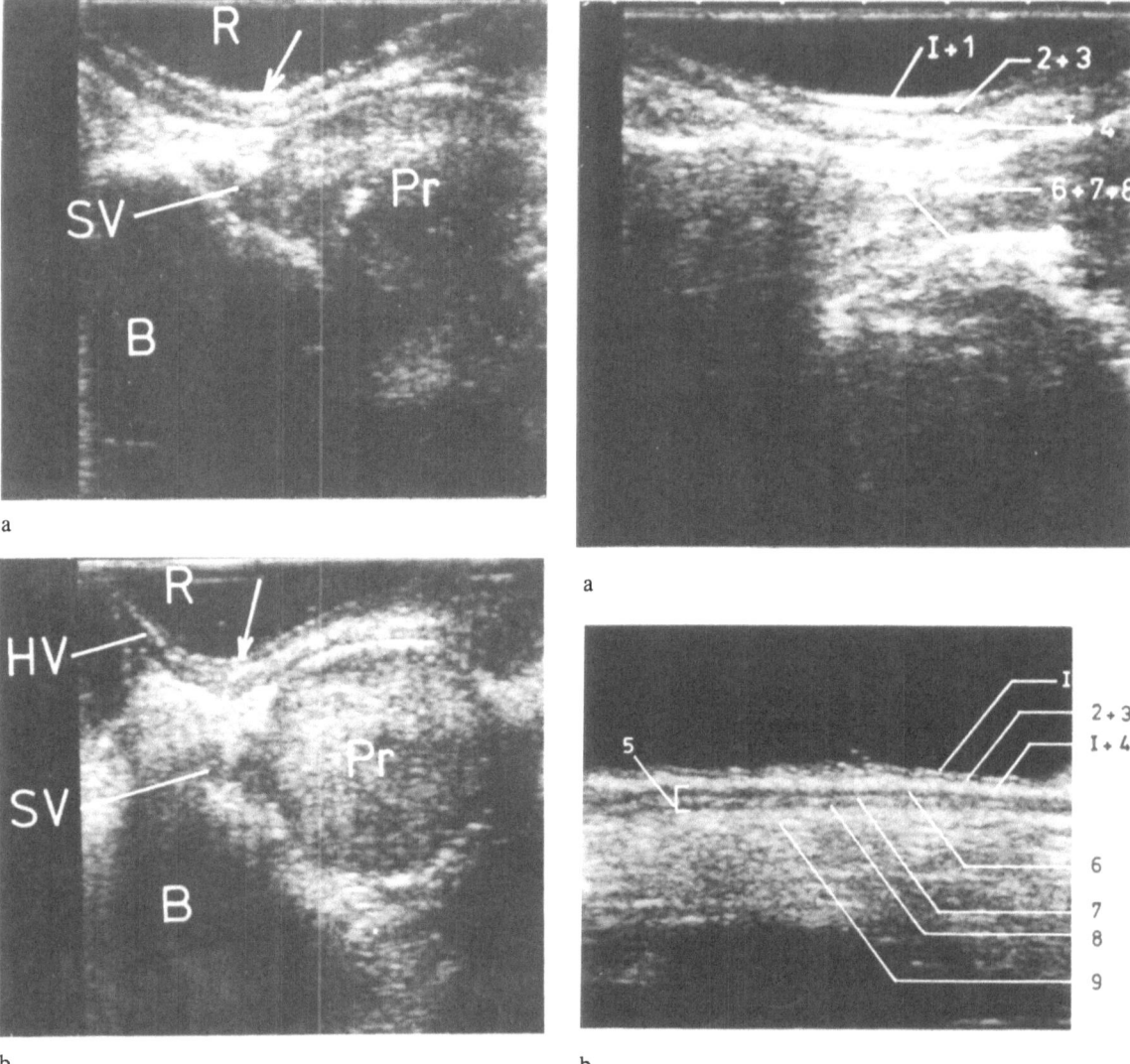

Figure 5.5. Longitudinal endorectal sonograms of the rectum. (a) Sonogram made using a water-distended balloon. (b) Sonogram made with a water enema and without the balloon. The first, echogenic layer (arrow) is much less prominent and a Houston's valve is visualized. B = bladder; HV = Houston's valve; Pr = prostate; R = rectal lumen; SV = seminal vesicle.

Figure 5.6. Longitudinal sonograms of the rectal wall made using a linear-array transducer. (a) In vivo sonogram. (b) In vitro sonogram. Note the subdivision of the muscular coat into two hypoechoic layers separated by a thin echogenic line. Note also the mixed echogenicity of the perirectal soft tissues. I = ultrasound interface; 1 = latex balloon; 2 = mucosa; 3 = muscularis mucosae; 4 = submucosa; 5 = muscular coat; 6 = internal circular muscular layer; 7 = thin layer of connective tissue; 8 = external longitudinal muscular layer; 9 = loose perirectal tissue.

pathologic conditions that specifically involve the rectal submucosa (see below: Inflammatory diseases).

The *fourth layer* (hypoechoic) is the thickest layer. It corresponds to the muscular coat, confirmed in vitro by this layer's absence on sonographic studies of fragments of rectal wall whose muscular coat has been excised (Fig. 5.8).

A subtle echogenic line that subdivides this layer into two layers of roughly equal thickness is occasionally visualized (Figs. 5.6, 5.7a, 5.9, 5.10). According to Saitoh [11], this line represents the connective tissue that separates the planes of the longitudinal and circular muscle

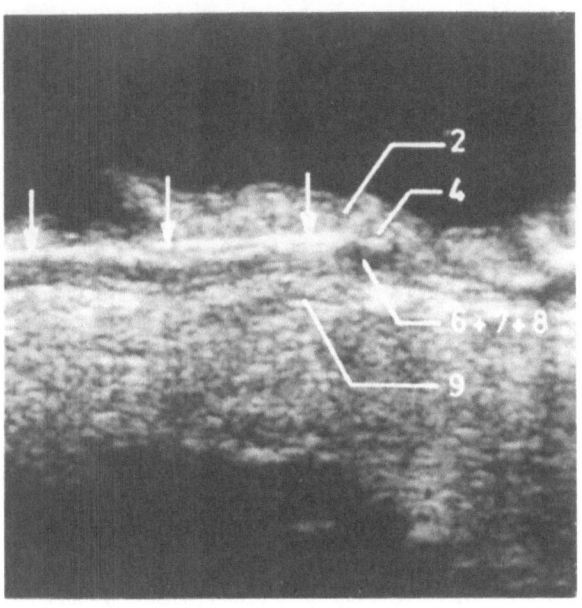 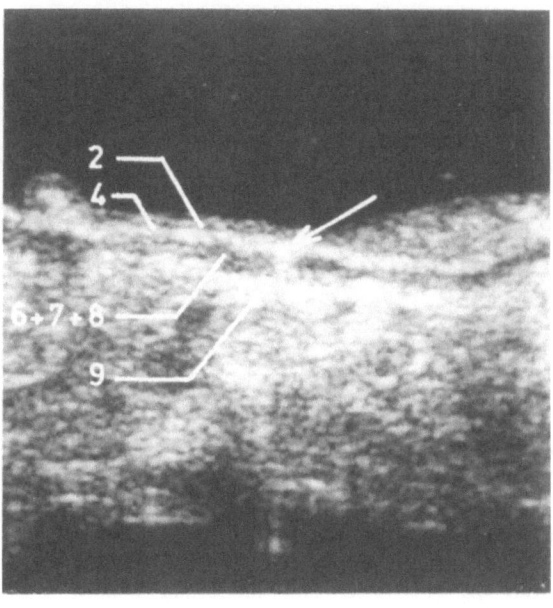

a   b

Figure 5.7. In vitro ultrasound study of the rectal wall after insertion of a 25-gauge needle in the submucosa. Longitudinal (a) and transverse (b) sonograms demonstrate the needle (arrows), which is within the echogenic third layer. 2 = mucosa; 4 = submucosa; 6 = internal circular muscular layer; 7 = thin layer of connective tissue; 8 = external longitudinal muscular layer; 9 = loose perirectal tissue.

fibers. The hypoechoic fourth layer, in particular the sublayer of circular fibers, thickens in the perineal rectum and constitutes the internal sphincter, which is surrounded by the somewhat more echogenic external striated sphincter and which is in close relation with the levator ani and transversus perinei profundus muscles (Fig. 5.11).

The *fifth layer* (hyperechoic) represents the interface between the muscular coat and the perirectal space. In contradistinction to CT [13], sonography cannot distinguish the rectal adipose capsule from the perirectal connective tissue.

Perirectal tissue has a nonhomogeneous echotexture. It contains the pelvic venous plexuses, which appear as anechoic tubular structures. The tissue thickness between the rectum and the prostate does not exceed 1 mm. This area corresponds to the perirectal loose tissue and Denonvilliers' fascia, which cannot be differentiated by sonography (Fig. 5.11).

In vivo endorectal studies made without a water-distended balloon show the typical wavy pattern of the mucosa, and Houston's valves are

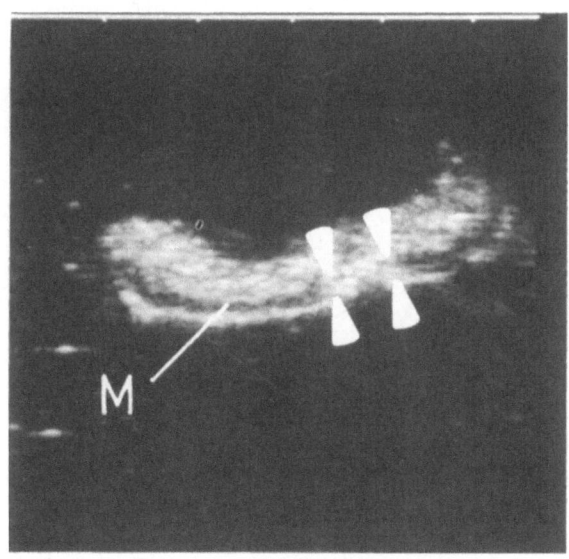

Figure 5.8. In vitro sonographic study of the rectal wall performed after removal of the muscularis propria. Sonogram clearly visualizes the abrupt discontinuity (arrowheads) in the hypoechoic muscular coat (M).

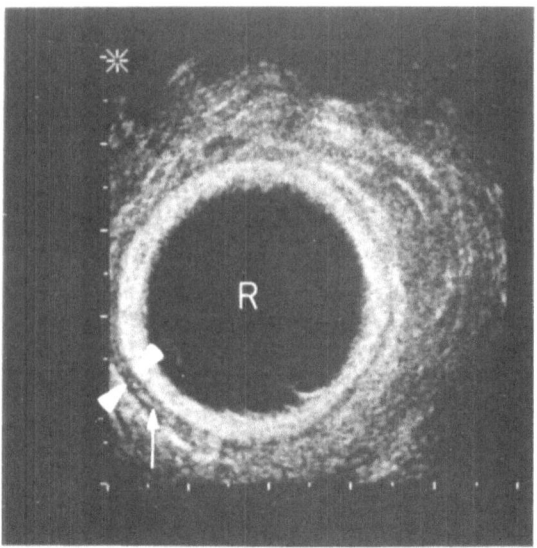

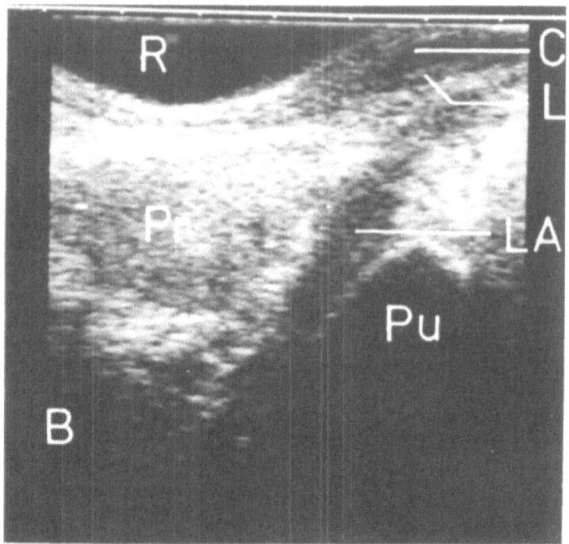

Figure 5.9. Transverse scan of the rectum obtained with a 7.0-MHz radial transducer. Arrowheads point to the hypoechoic muscular coat. Arrow points to the faintly echogenic separation between the circular and longitudinal fibers. R = rectal lumen.

Figure 5.11. Longitudinal parasagittal transrectal sonogram shows the internal anal sphincter. B = bladder; C = circular internal muscular fibers; L = longitudinal external muscular fibers; LA = levator ani muscle; Pr = prostate; Pu = pubic bone; R = rectum.

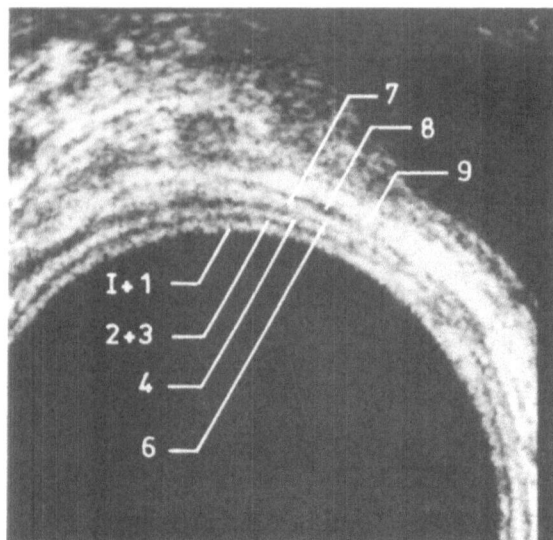

Figure 5.10. Endorectal transverse sonogram of normal rectal wall. Seven sonographic layers can be identified. I = ultrasound interface; 1 = latex balloon; 2 = mucosa; 3 = muscularis mucosae; 4 = submucosa; 6 = internal circular muscular layer; 7 = thin layer of connective tissue; 8 = external longitudinal muscular layer; 9 = loose perirectal tissue.

visualized as folds of the entire wall, including the muscular coat. Real-time examination can demonstrate the motor activity of the rectal wall and the onset of rhythmic peristaltic motion, likely to result from the presence of the transducer or the direct injection of fluid in the rectum (Fig. 5.12).

Rectal cancer

Surgical management of carcinoma of the middle and lower rectum includes local excision, anterior resection, and abdominoperineal resection, each with or without pre- and/or postoperative radiation therapy. The surgical approach is determined by various parameters; some of them are easily evaluated preoperatively, including the general condition of the patient; the presence of other colic tumors; the circumferential extension and length of the tumor, with a special reference to the distance of the tumor from the anal verge; and the histologic grade of the tumor, which is based on the biopsy specimen. However, the degree of deep infiltration into the various layers of the rectal wall or

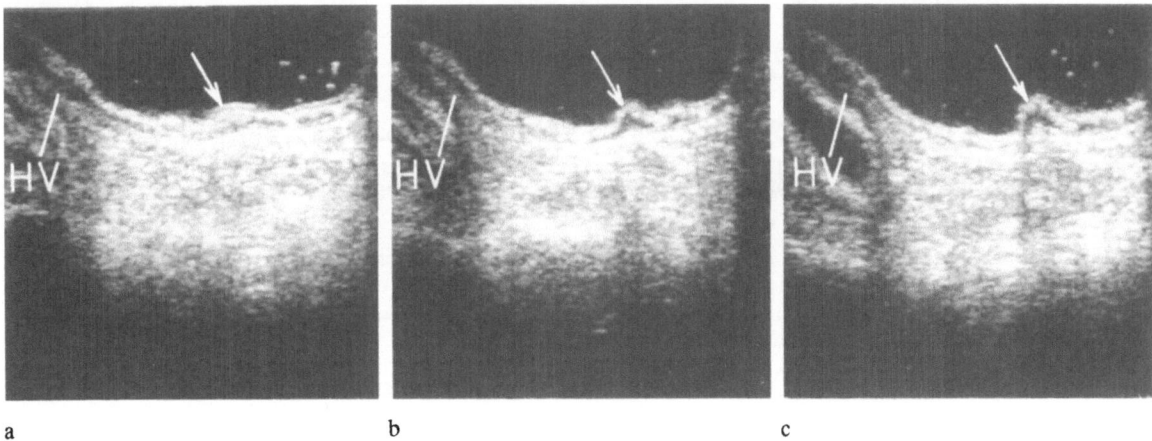

a   b   c

Figure 5.12. (a, b, and c) Longitudinal sonograms made without a balloon but with a water enema show the rectal peristalsis (arrow). Note a Houston's valve (HV).

perirectal lymphatic spread can only be roughly estimated before surgery. The refinement of surgical techniques and the development of end-to-end anastomosis stapling devices have resulted in a wider use of conservative surgery, which, however, keeps to the fundamental principles of radical surgery. A long-standing obstacle to conservative surgery has been the classic requirement that 5 cm of normal rectal wall be excised distal to the lower pole of the tumor, this being thought to provide against occult intramural extension and to minimize the incidence of early local recurrence. However, it has been shown that even if submucosal malignant infiltration is present, it virtually never extends more than 2 cm distally, and that whether the surgical margin is 2 cm, between 2 and 5 cm, or more than 5 cm from the lower pole of the tumor does not significantly influence the incidence of local recurrence.

Prognosis is, however, strongly related to the histologic grade, degree of local infiltration of the tumor, and extent of lymphatic spread [15–21], parameters upon which the staging systems are primarily based.

Staging

The most commonly used classifications are the tumor-node-metastasis (TNM) system, devised by the International Union Against Cancer [22],

and the Dukes classification as modified by Astler and Coller in 1954 (Fig. 5.13) [23]. Five-year survival decreases from 80% to 71% when the tumor has infiltrated the perirectal loose tissue (the stage of the tumor changing from T2 to T3, or from B1 to B2) and drops to 32% when lymph nodes are involved [24].

Examinations used in the presurgical local staging of rectal carcinoma are the digital rectal examination, proctosigmoidoscopy with biopsy, double contrast barium enema, CT, magnetic resonance (MR) imaging [25, 26], and endorectal sonography. The digital rectal examination, to be performed first, allows evaluation of the shape and size of the tumor, its distance from the anal verge, the number of quadrants involved, the degree of rectal stenosis, the mobility of the tumor over the muscular coat, and the mobility of the rectum in relation to the perirectal connective tissue and adjacent organs and pelvic sidewalls. Occasionally, enlarged perirectal lymph nodes can be detected by this examination.

Mason originally defined four stages of rectal carcinoma according to digital rectal examination findings [27]. In stage 1, the tumor is mobile in relation to the muscle wall. In stage 2, the tumor infiltrates into the muscle wall but remains mobile in relation to the perirectal connective tissue. The tumor is confined to the rectum or there is slight extrarectal infiltration.

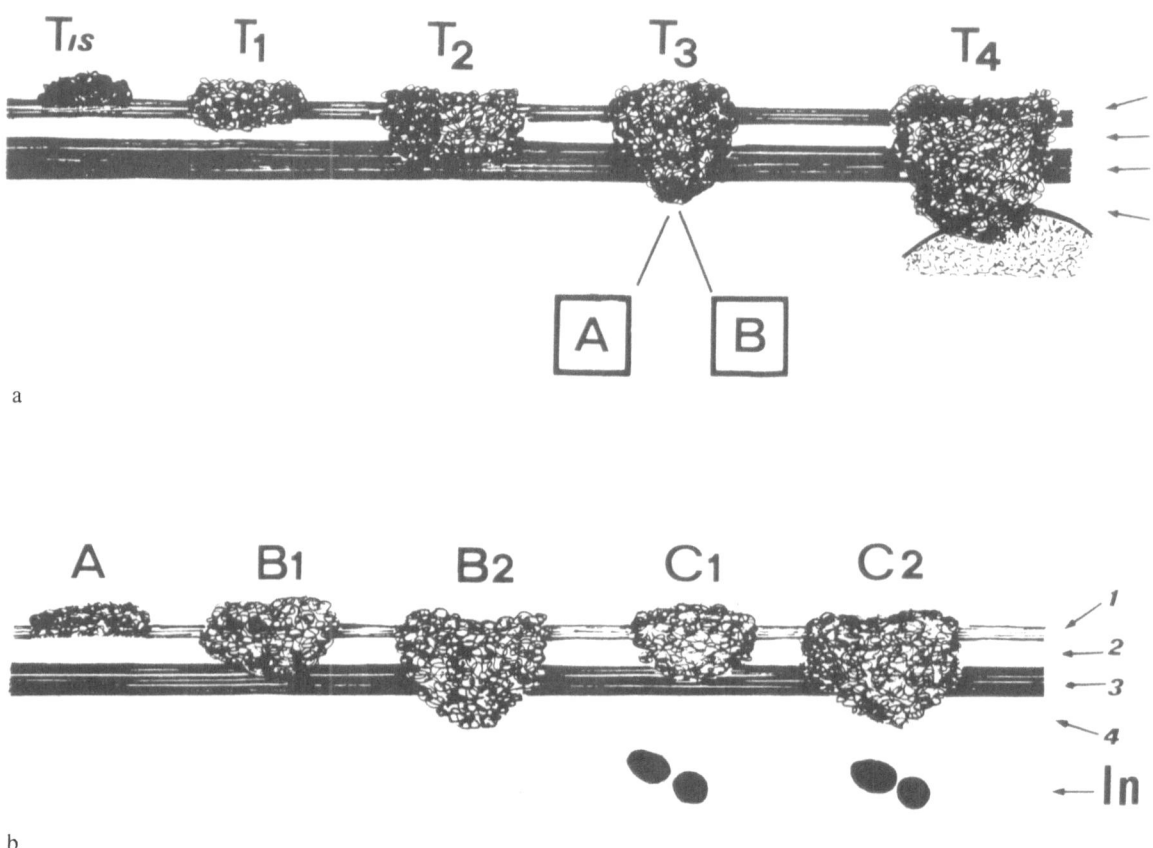

Figure 5.13. Staging systems for rectal carcinoma (see text for details). (a) TNM classification. (b) Astler-Coller modification of Dukes classification. 1 = mucosa; 2 = submucosa; 3 = muscularis propria; 4 = loose perirectal soft tissues; ln = lymph nodes; T3A: absence of fistula; T3B: presence of fistula.

In stage 3, there is limited mobility of the tumor and the rectum, accounted for by a moderate to prominent perirectal infiltration. Finally, in stage 4, adjacent pelvic organs are involved by tumor. Mason additionally proposed two lymphatic stages depending on whether lymph node involvement by tumor was apparent at digital rectal examination.

Recently, Nicholls and Mason and their colleagues also classified rectal carcinomas according to the digital rectal examination into locally confined (Mason's stages 1 and 2) and locally infiltrating (Mason's stages 3 and 4) [28, 29]. In the former group, 5-year survival exceeds 70% and there is a low incidence of local recurrence. In the latter group, 5-year survival is only 30% and local recurrence reaches 20%. Whatever the classification, the circumferential infiltration as determined by the number of lumen quadrants involved is crucial. For instance, any tumor that involves three quarters or more of the rectal circumference should be classified in the second group [28, 29].

Obviously, the results of digital rectal assessment depend on the operator's experience, particularly when the four-stage classification is used. The simplified, two-stage system proposed by Nicholls *et al.* seems to provide more reproducible results. Still, the examination is at best poorly reproducible, a notable problem in the follow-up of tumors treated with preoperative radiation therapy. Further, the approach is of limited value when a tumor is markedly stenotic, and cannot be used when a tumor's lower pole is more than 10 cm from the anal verge.

As regards the imaging techniques utilized, outside of endosonography, satisfactory results have been reported with CT [30—33]. Thoeni *et al.* [30] defined four stages of rectal carcinoma according to CT findings: stage 1, endoluminal mass without thickening of the rectal wall; stage 2, thickening of the rectal wall, to more than 5 mm, without infiltration of the surrounding soft tissues; stage 3, infiltration of the surrounding soft tissues without (stage 3A) or with (stage 3B) involvement of the pelvic sidewalls; stage 4, evidence of distant metastases. The overall accuracy of CT staging in their series was 92%. However, 32 of their 34 patients had a tumor more than 4 cm in diameter, which likely underlies the high accuracy: tumors less than 2 cm in diameter are more difficult to evaluate and may even be overlooked.

CT has the advantage of demonstrating infiltration of the perirectal connective tissue. In this regard, a basic landmark is the perirectal sheath, which separates the capsula adiposa rectalis from the pararectal connective tissue. However, its thickening is still a nonspecific sign, found not only in malignant infiltration but also in proctitis and postirradiation sequelae [34]. A tumor is often unresectable when it has reached this sheath, and never resectable when it has infiltrated through it. On CT, the rectal wall is homogeneous: its various layers — including the muscular coat, which is the barrier to local malignant spread — cannot be differentiated. Tumor and the rectal wall usually display similar densities, which accounts for the limitation of CT in detecting early tumors and in evaluating deep infiltration into the rectal wall. CT is also limited in the diagnosis of metastatic involvement of lymph nodes, usually based on the presence of any lymph node more than 1.5 cm in diameter or the detection of at least three lymph nodes smaller than 1.5 cm. Obviously, the opportunity for false-negative (normal-sized lymph nodes involved by metastasis) and false-positive (benign adenopathy) results exists.

Endosonographic findings

Endosonography is the first imaging technique capable of distinguishing the various layers of the rectal wall [4—14, 35—37]. All investigators now agree upon the visualization of the muscular coat as a hypoechoic layer (the fourth one in our classification). Ultrasound staging of rectal carcinoma is therefore based on the relation of the tumor to this layer.

The patient's position during the examination is determined by the location of the tumor. The tumor should lie under the probe, which position enhances contact between the balloon and the tumor, particularly if the tumor is ulcerated, and prevents interference from residual gas bubbles inside the balloon, these bubbles being collected in the balloon's upper portion.

Rectal carcinoma appears as a generally hypo- or isoechoic mass that abruptly interrupts the regular arrangement of the rectal wall layers and that tends to develop in the direction of the perirectal tissues (Fig. 5.14). We have described a sonographic classification comprising five

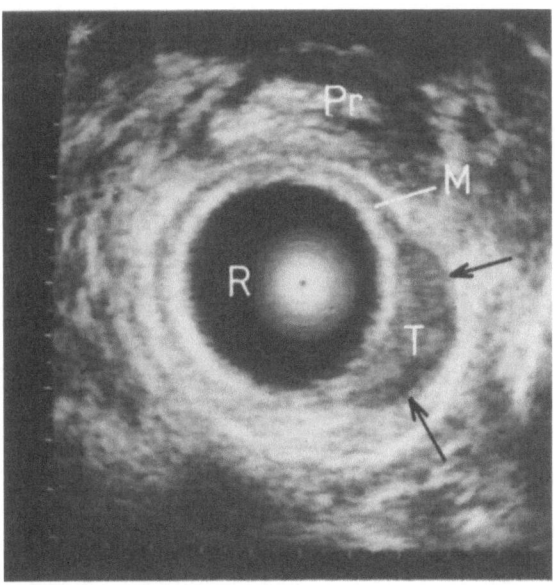

Figure 5.14. Endorectal transverse scan of rectal carcinoma shows a hypoechoic mass (arrows) disrupting the normal multilayer pattern and infiltrating into the perirectal space. M = muscular layer; Pr = prostate; R = rectum; T = tumor. (Courtesy of Dr. V. Arienti.)

stages for the evaluation of the primary tumor (Fig. 5.15) and two stages (N+/N−) for the evaluation of lymph nodes. The primary tumor stages are:

Stage U0. No lesion can be identified by sonography.

Stage U1. The lesion is confined to the mucosa and submucosa and corresponds to the Tis/T1 and A stages of the TNM and Astler-Coller classifications, respectively. These are usually small lesions whose base is still separated from the hypoechoic muscular layer by a thin echogenic line, which represents the preserved submucosa (Figs. 5.16−5.18).

Stage U2. The tumor infiltrates into the fourth layer (the muscular coat), which may be pulled toward the lumen (Fig. 5.19).

Stage U3. The breach into the muscular coat develops progressively (Figs. 5.20, 5.21). In *stage U3A*, tumor is visualized on both sides of the muscular coat, which is irregular and shows displacement toward the lumen (Figs. 5.20c, 5.21c). In *stage U3B*, a discontinuity is seen at the level of maximum infiltration, usually in the center of the malignant ulceration (Figs. 5.20d, 5.21e).

Stage U4. Adjacent spaces/organs are invaded (Figs. 5.22, 5.23).

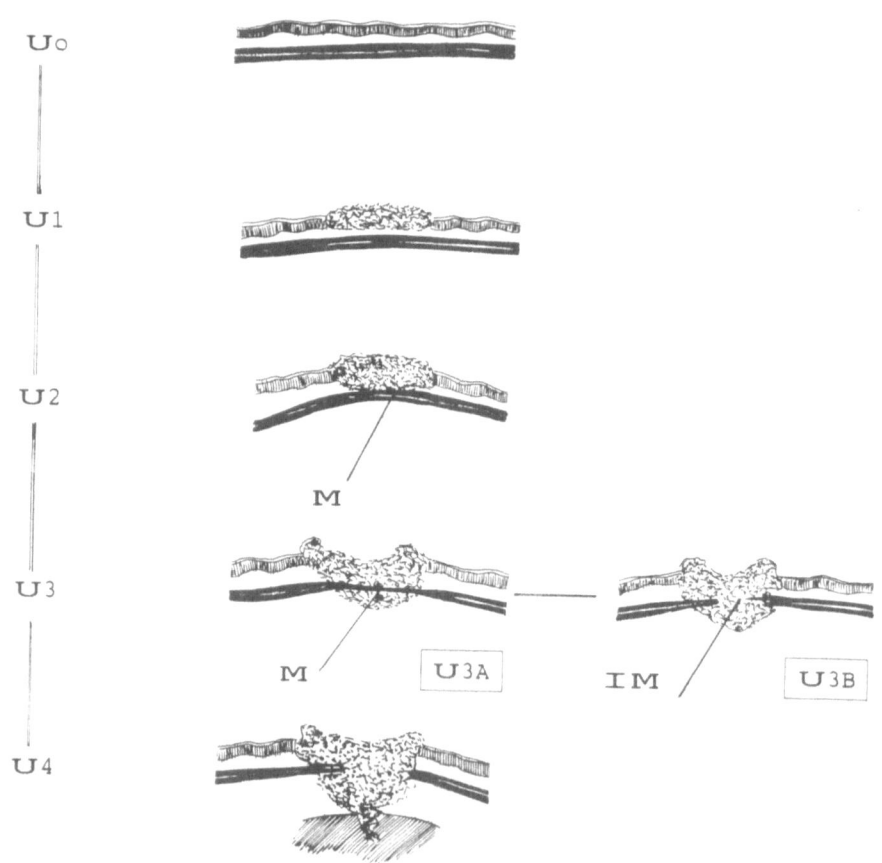

Figure 5.15. Ultrasound staging of rectal carcinoma (see text for details). IM = interruption of the muscular layer; M = muscular layer; U0 to U4 are the endosonographic stages.

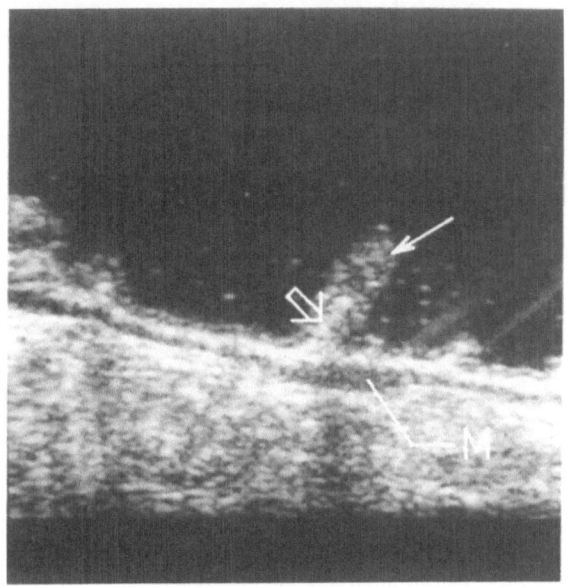

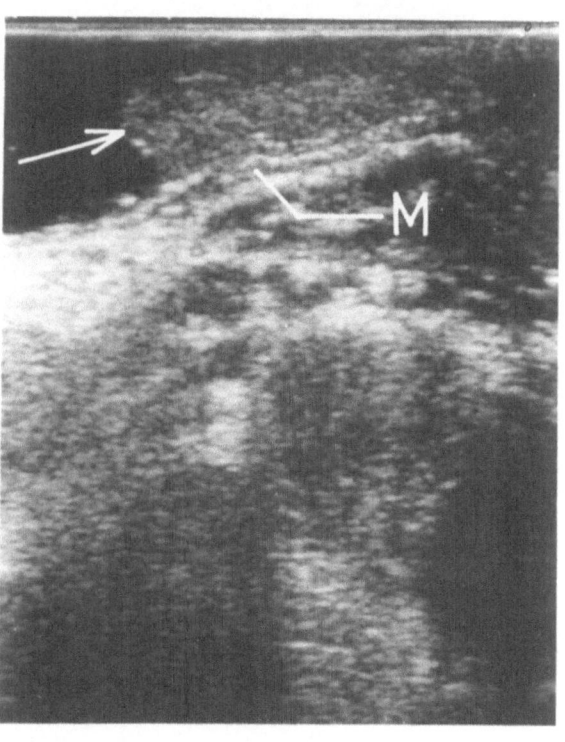

Figure 5.16. Rectal polyp. In vitro longitudinal sonogram of the rectum shows a small, stalked polyp (arrow). The sub-mucosa enters the polyp and forms its connective axis (open arrow). The hypoechoic muscular layer (M) is not involved by the abnormality.

Figure 5.17. Rectal polyp. In vivo longitudinal scan obtained without a balloon shows a sessile polyp (arrow). Note the preserved hypoechoic muscular layer (M).

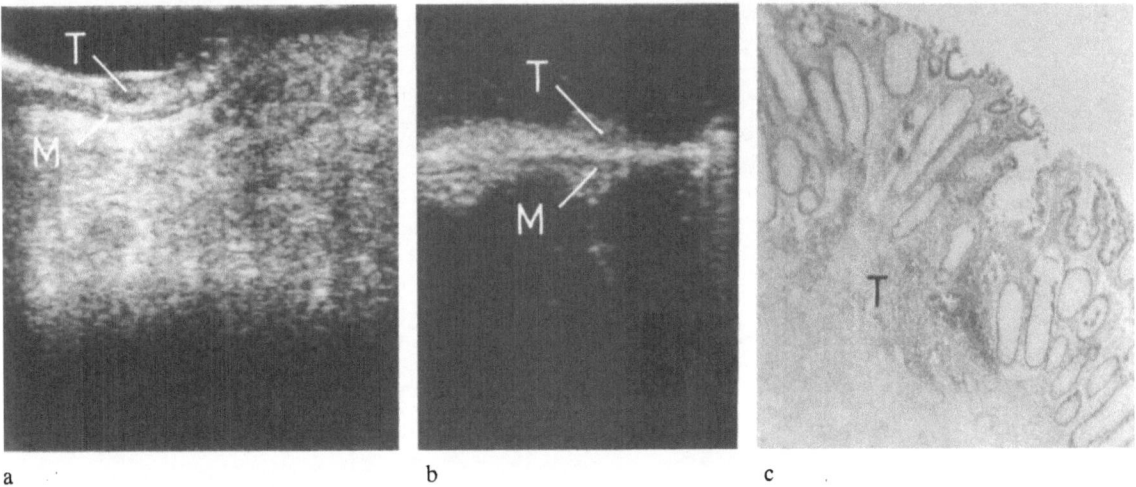

a   b   c

Figure 5.18. In vivo (a) and in vitro (b) longitudinal sonograms of early carcinoma of the lower rectum at stage U1/T1. (c) Histopathologic section. M = muscular layer; T = tumor.

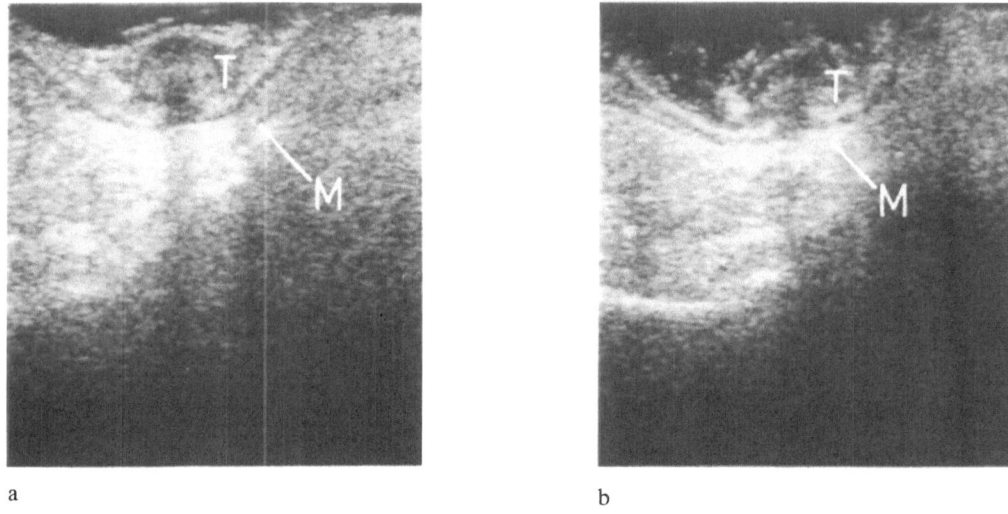

a   b

Figure 5.19. Rectal polypoid carcinoma. Longitudinal sonograms made with (a) and without (b) a balloon. The muscular layer is infiltrated and pulled toward the lumen without evidence of malignant infiltration into the perirectal tissue. Note the disrupted submucosa. M = muscular coat; T = tumor.

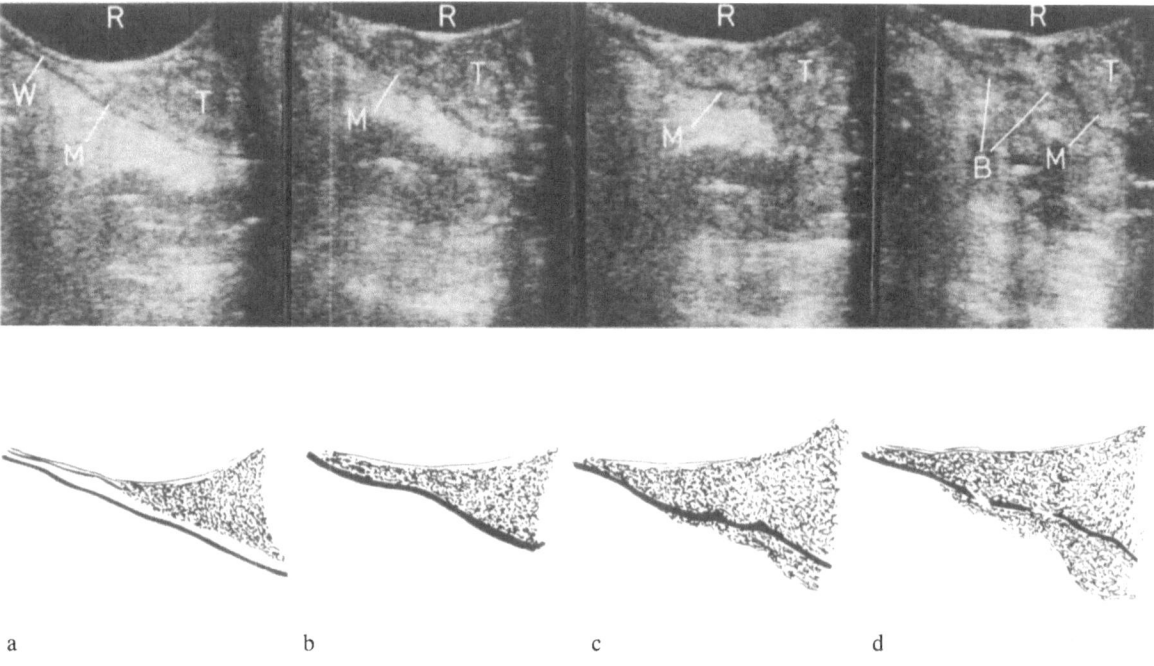

a   b   c   d

Figure 5.20. Rectal carcinoma. (a, b, c, d) Longitudinal sonograms show the malignant infiltration of the muscular layer. B = breach through the muscular layer; M = muscular layer; R = rectal lumen; T = tumor; W = normal wall.

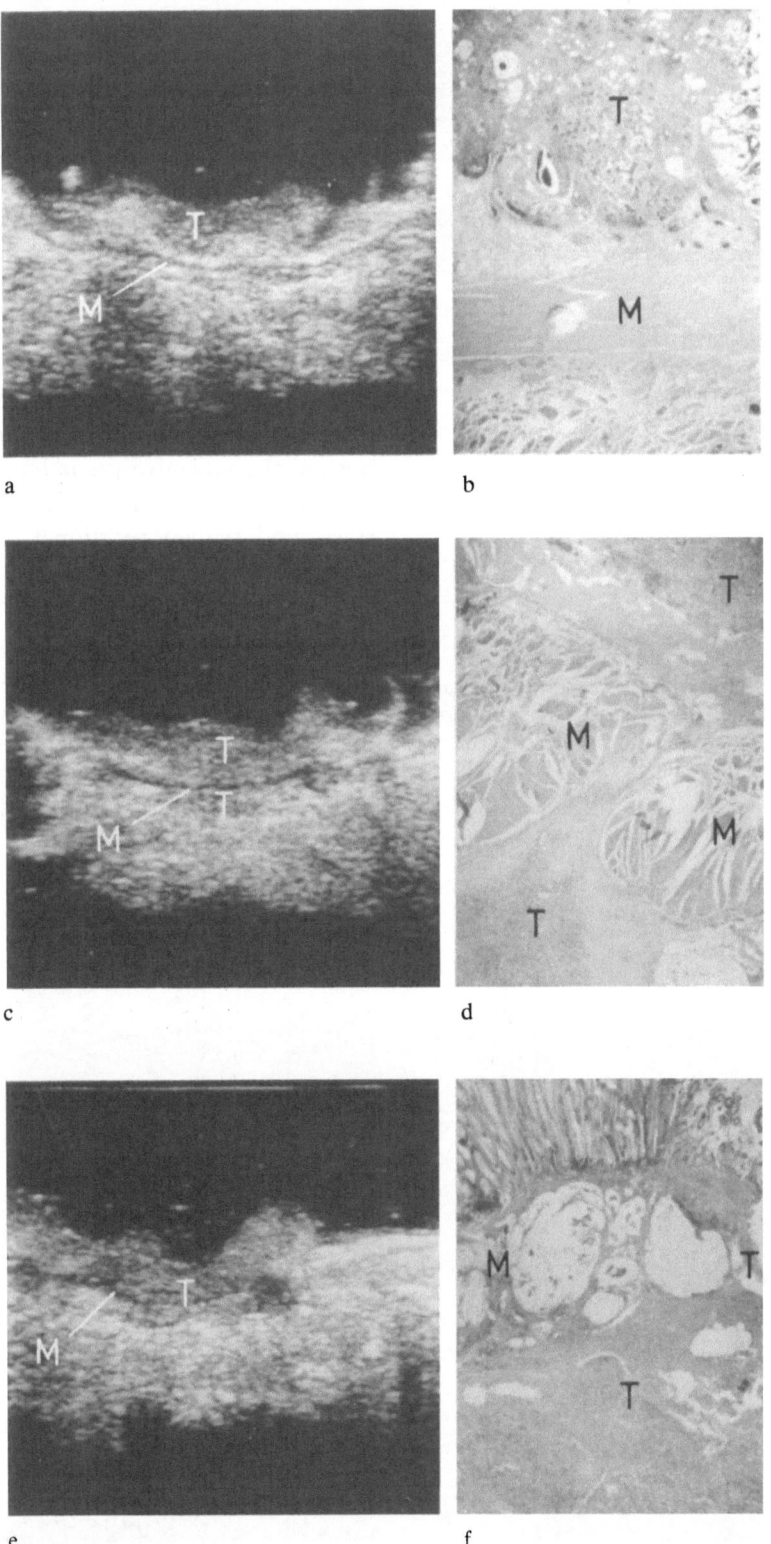

Figure 5.21. In vitro longitudinal sonograms of rectal carcinoma show the pattern of infiltration into the muscular coat. (a) Absence of infiltration. The tumor is confined above the muscular layer. (c) Tumor has infiltrated beyond the muscular layer, which is still visualized (stage U3A). (e) Sonogram shows marked disruption of the muscular coat (stage U3B). (b, d, f) Histopathologic sections corresponding to a, c, e, respectively. M = muscular coat; T = tumor.

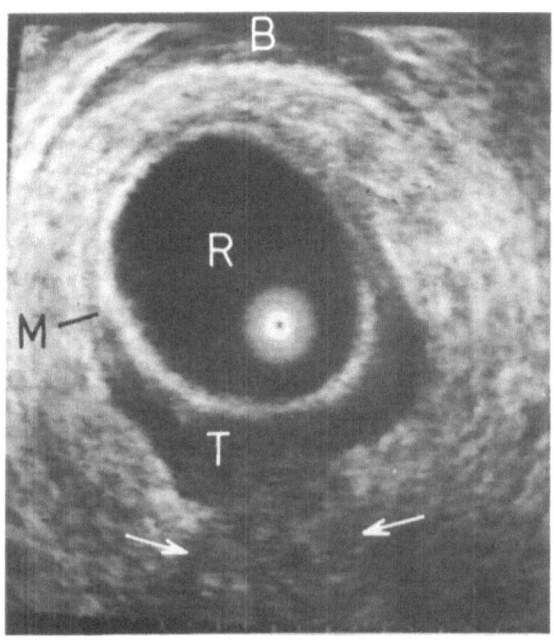

Figure 5.22. Endorectal transverse scan made using a radial probe. The markedly hypoechoic rectal carcinoma infiltrates into the presacral space (arrows). B = bladder; M = muscular coat; R = rectum; T = tumor. (Courtesy of Dr. V. Arienti.)

Particular attention must be paid to the evaluation of the lower edge of the tumor, where longitudinal submucosal extension can be depicted between the mucosa and the muscular coat (Fig. 5.24). Such intramural extension can also be detected at the lateral edges of a tumor which is spreading circumferentially. In this case, endosonography may confirm that the tumor is already circumferential in the deep layers, despite the visualization of areas of normal mucosa at endoscopy (Fig. 5.25).

Endorectal scanning can detect lymph nodes greater than 5 mm in diameter in the loose perirectal connective tissue but cannot differentiate between a lymph node involved by metastasis and benign reactional adenopathy (Fig. 5.26).

Most rectal tumors are hypoechoic. Occasionally, echogenic nodules are visualized. Internal echoes may result from fibrotic changes or calcifications (Fig. 5.27). Following radiation therapy, decreased echogenicity of the tumor may result from necrosis (Fig. 5.28).

Endorectal sonography can detect early

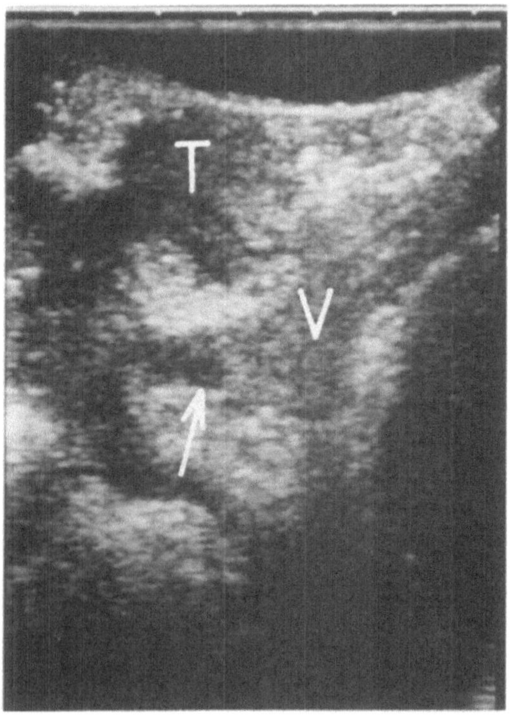

Figure 5.23. Endorectal longitudinal sonogram shows a hypoechoic rectal carcinoma infiltrating into the adjacent structures. The hypoechoic malignant infiltration involves a lateral vaginal fornix (arrow). T = tumor; V = vagina.

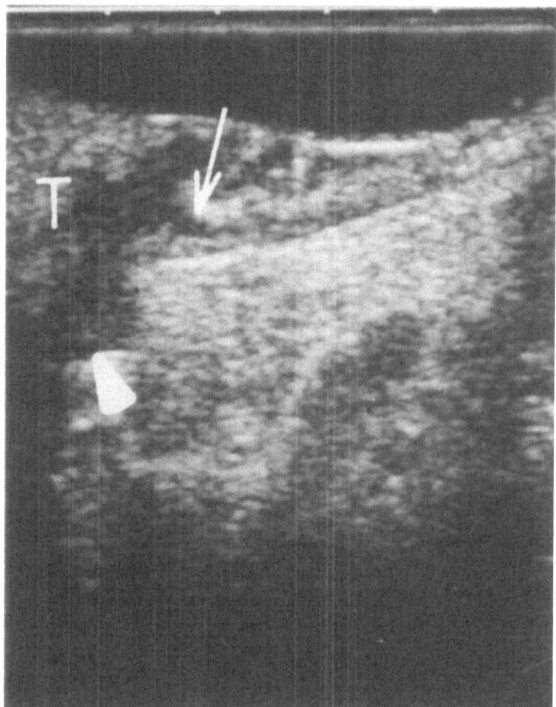

Figure 5.24. Endorectal longitudinal sonogram of a rectal carcinoma (T) that has penetrated the muscular coat (arrowhead). Hypoechoic infiltration into the submucosa can be seen at the lower pole of the tumor (arrow).

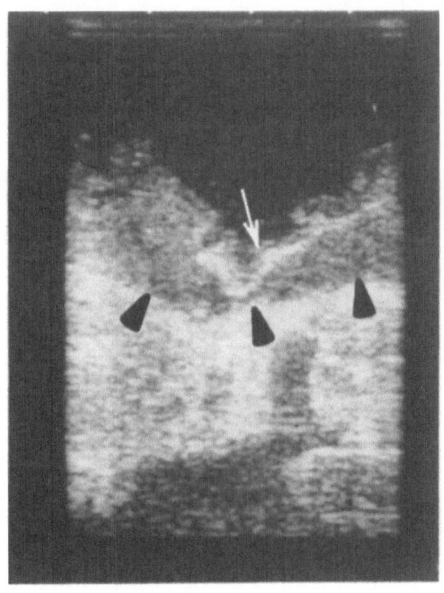 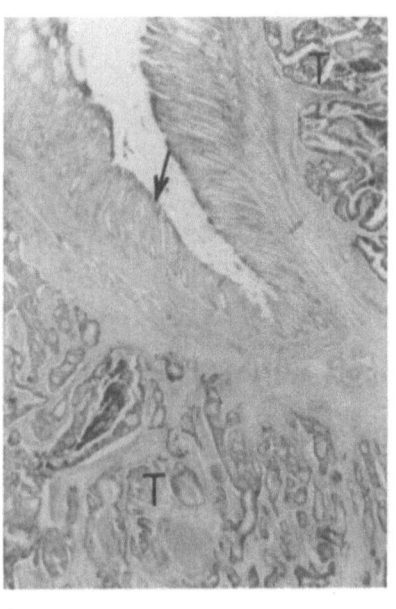

a   b

Figure 5.25. (a) Transverse sonogram made in vitro shows the intramural infiltration of a rectal carcinoma (arrowheads), with overlying normal mucosa (arrow). (b) Histopathologic section confirms normal mucosa (arrow) and underlying tumor (T).

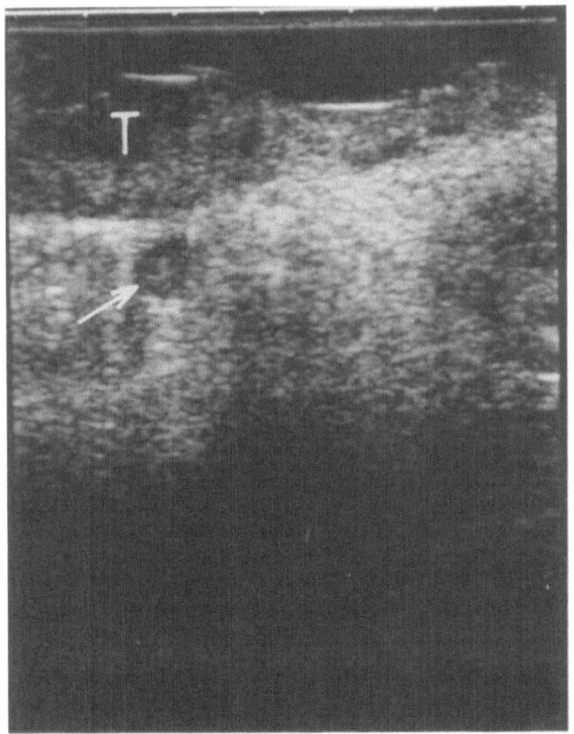

Figure 5.26. Endorectal longitudinal sonogram shows a rectal tumor (T) infiltrating through the wall. A 1-cm lymph node (arrow) is visualized. Pathologic analysis confirmed massive metastatic involvement of the node.

lesions in the rectal wall. Figure 5.18 shows a 4-mm carcinoma confined to the mucosa and submucosa. Bulky tumors, however, are poorly evaluated because rectal stenosis frequently associated with them interferes with the movement of the transducer, while their outer margins usually lie outside of the optimal focal zone and sometimes even out of the field of view of the transducer. Polypoid tumors are best studied without a balloon covering the probe and using the water enema technique; the absence of compression by the balloon allows better evaluation of the relation of the tumor to the various layers of the wall (Figs. 5.16, 5.17, 5.19b). Endosonography can assess the shape, margins, size, and echotexture of the tumors arising in the deep layers of the rectal wall that may go unrecognized at endoscopy. The technique is also used to guide transperineal biopsy (Fig. 5.29).

Diagnostic accuracy

Review of the recent literature confirms the promising results of endorectal sonography in the evaluation of rectal carcinoma. Hildebrandt *et al.* evaluated endorectal sonography in the diagnosis of extrarectal infiltration, that is, in the

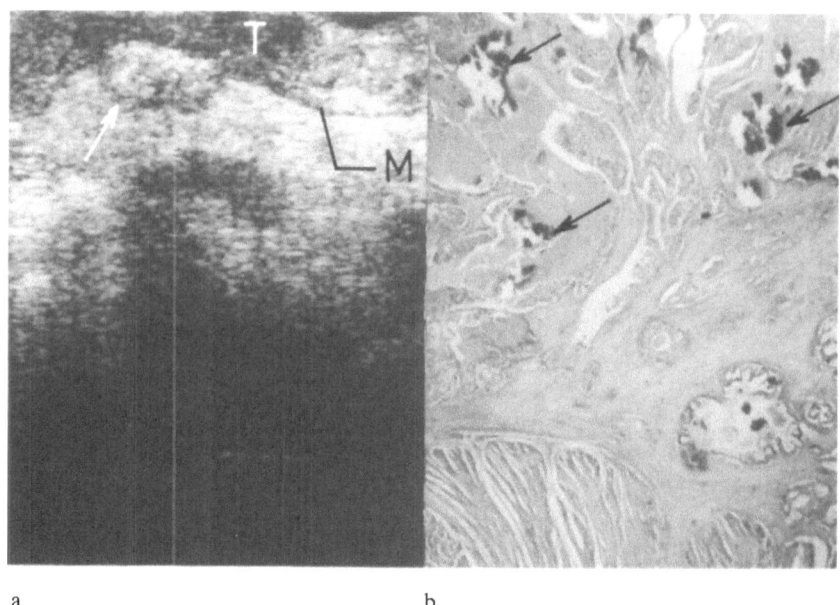

a   b

Figure 5.27. (a) Endorectal longitudinal sonogram shows a hypoechoic rectal carcinoma (T) that has infiltrated beyond the muscular wall (M). At this level, a finely dotted echogenic area is depicted (arrow). (b) Histopathologic analysis confirms the presence of necrosis, fibrosis, and calcification (arrows).

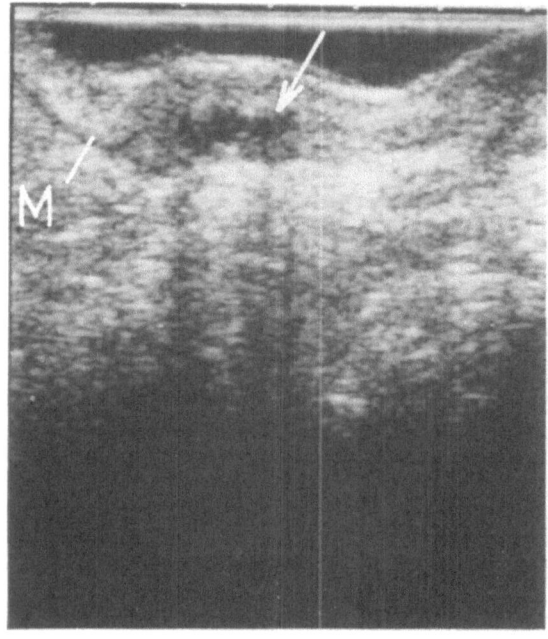

Figure 5.28. Endorectal longitudinal sonogram of a rectal carcinoma infiltrating into the muscular coat after radiation therapy. The lesion is characterized by a hypoechoic central necrotic area (arrow). M = muscular coat.

differentiation of T1/T2 from T3 (or B1/C1 from B2/C2) stages. They found an overall accuracy of 92% (23/25 [7] and 70/76 [8] patients) versus only 60% for the digital rectal examination [7]. Pahlman [9], Rifkin [13], Saitoh [11], and Romano [12] and their colleagues have reported an overall accuracy for endorectal sonography of 55% (6/11 patients), 84% (68/81), 90% (79/88), and 91% (21/23), respectively. Beynon *et al.* have reported an overall accuracy of 91%, with a correlation coefficient of 0.88 ($P < .001$) between the pathologic and endosonographic findings and an accuracy of 95% in the diagnosis of perirectal infiltration [10]. In this study, the sensitivity of digital rectal examination, endorectal sonography, and CT in the detection of infiltration beyond the muscular coat was 65%, 92%, and 84%, respectively, with a specificity of 100%, 100%, and 63%. Other studies have confirmed the superiority of endorectal sonography to CT in staging rectal carcinoma [12—14]. According to Nicholls *et al.*, the accuracy of CT is directly related to the tumor volume and to the extent of perirectal invasion [28]. It drops from 89% for tumors with significant local infiltration to 55% for tumors with limited perirectal infiltration.

Endosonography, like CT, provides limited

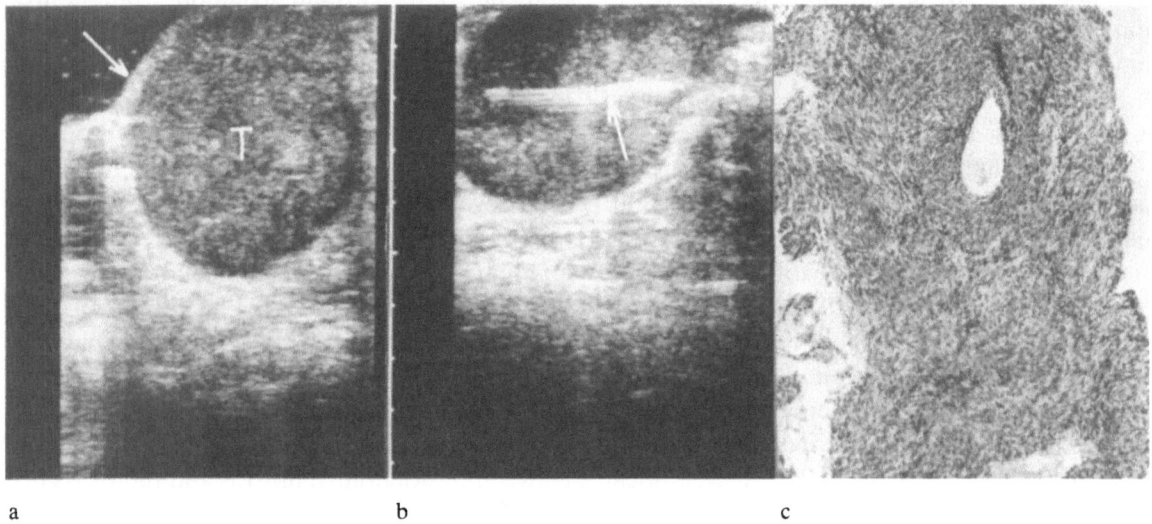

a   b   c

Figure 5.29. Ultrasound-guided large-bore needle biopsy of rectal tumor. (a) Endorectal longitudinal sonogram of a bulky rectal tumor (T). Note the overlying normal mucosa (arrow). (b) Transperineal ultrasound-guided needle biopsy. The 14-gauge Tru-cut biopsy needle is visualized in open position (arrow). (c) Histopathologic specimen is consistent with a leiomyosarcoma.

results in the evaluation of lymphatic spread. However, Saitoh *et al.* have reported a 75% overall accuracy in the sonographic detection of perirectal lymph nodes [11].

We examined 70 patients with carcinoma of the middle or lower rectum with endorectal sonography using a linear-array transducer. Correlation between sonographic and pathologic findings could be obtained in 60 cases. The clinical stage was B1 in 11 of these 60 cases, B2 in 25, C1 in 1, and C2 in 23. In the diagnosis of perirectal infiltration, there were four false-negative and one false-positive results by endosonography, yielding a 91% sensitivity and a 91% specificity. It is to be noted that there were no errors in the last 47 patients. Results are less encouraging as regards the diagnosis of lymphatic spread, with 13 false-negative and 3 false-positive results.

Careful preoperative staging of rectal carcinoma is required to guide the surgical management and to select candidates for anastomosis with anal sphincter preservation. While overstaging results in useless, mutilating surgery, understaging is of greater concern since it leads to insufficient surgery. Small tumors in the lower rectum that are apparently noninfiltrating at physical examination are the best indication for endorectal scanning, to detect an early infiltration of the muscular layer or perirectal structures. In contrast, bulky, stenotic, or fixed tumors or tumors of questionable resectability or for which preoperative radiation therapy is considered should be evaluated with CT or MR, either of which will accurately demonstrate the extension by contiguity into neighboring structures, particularly the pelvic sidewalls.

Local recurrence

Local recurrence is the major concern after surgical treatment of rectal carcinoma. Its incidence varies significantly in the literature. Gunderson and Sosin found that 70% of patients who underwent radical surgery for Dukes stage B or C rectal carcinoma had locally recurrent disease at second-look laparotomy 6 to 12 months later [38]. When treatment was anterior resection, Morson *et al.* found a 7% local recurrence rate [39]; Goligher, 10% [40]; Hurst *et al.*, with an end-to-end anastomosis stapling device used, 32% [41]; and Garlock and Ginzburg, 36% [42]. Pahlman and Glimelius reported that 74 (38%) of 197 patients who had undergone anterior resection ($n = 58$) or abdominoperineal resection ($n = 139$) developed locally recurrent tumor [43].

It seems that neither the surgical technique nor the length of the normal rectum resected distal to the tumor significantly influences the incidence of local recurrence. Morson *et al.* found a 7% local recurrence rate following anterior resection, versus 10% following abdominoperineal resection [39]; Deddish and Stearns [21] and Slanetz *et al.* [44] reported similar results. Williams *et al.* found a 12% local recurrence rate following anterior resection, versus 9% following abdominoperineal resection [15]. The Williams report found a 10% local recurrence rate when the excised segment of normal rectum exceeded 5 cm, versus 15% when this segment was less than 5 cm long. Pollet and Nicholls [19] reported the incidence of local recurrence to be 7.3% with a lower surgical margin of less than 2 cm, 6.2% with a 2—5-cm margin, and 7.8% at more than 5 cm.

In contrast, the incidence of local recurrence strongly correlates with the histologic grade and degree of local infiltration of the tumor, particularly the extent of extramural invasion. Rao *et al.* discovered local recurrence in only 0.1% of patients treated for Astler-Coller stage A tumor [45] and Pahlman and Glimelius showed, in patients with stage B disease, the incidence of local recurrence to be related to the extent of extramural infiltration [43]. In fact, several factors probably influence the development of local recurrence. According to Morson *et al.* [39], the recurrent disease develops in the pelvic connective tissues from a residual cluster of malignant cells; the tumor subsequently invades the rectal wall, with a predilection for the anastomosis. Retrograde lymphatic involvement has also been claimed to play a significant role [46]. Other hypotheses include (a) the graft of malignant cells detached from the primary tumor during surgical manipulation (which would justify operative irrigations with antimitotic agents), (b) an inadequate lower surgical margin in grossly normal-appearing but already microscopically infiltrated wall, and (c) a particular sensitivity of the colorectal anastomosis to chemical carcinogenesis [47], which might be potentiated by chronic irritation from nonresorbing suture material [48].

Most local recurrences are presacral. Symptoms are usually nonspecific and include sacral pain, tenesmus, proctorrhagia, and symptoms of urinary or gastrointestinal tract obstruction. Pain may develop several months prior to the detection of a palpable mass. While not feasible after abdominoperineal resection, digital rectal examination and rectoscopy with biopsy of any suspicious area can still be performed in patients who have undergone anterior resection.

CT readily detects masses more than 2 cm in diameter [31, 49] but often cannot distinguish between postoperative fibrosis and tumor recurrence. Kelvin *et al.* [50] have described CT changes of the pelvic connective tissue following anterior or abdominoperineal resection. Granulation tissue, which is initially isodense, becomes progressively hypodense over a period of several months and turns into a thin, semilunar strip distinct from the sacrum. This pattern is missing in about 10% of cases, in which a persistent isodense pelvic area is noted. Clark *et al.* [51] have stressed the importance of close follow-up of these areas, since only recurrent lesions should increase in size with time. According to Lee *et al.* [52], fibrosis is characterized by minimal streaky densities, whereas local recurrence is associated with more regular shape and margins, and homogeneous density. CT-guided biopsy of suspicious areas can be performed [53, 54]. Once recurrent tumor is pathologically confirmed, CT aids in treatment planning and in monitoring response to treatment.

Endosonographic findings

Endosonography can be used in the follow-up of patients after surgical cure of rectal carcinoma. In the male it is limited to patients who have undergone anterior resection, while in the female endosonographic examination can also be performed after abdominoperineal resection using the vaginal approach.

The normal colorectal anastomosis is slightly scalloped due to the spontaneous contraction of the anastomosis toward the lumen (Fig. 5.30a). Sonographic examination is easily performed

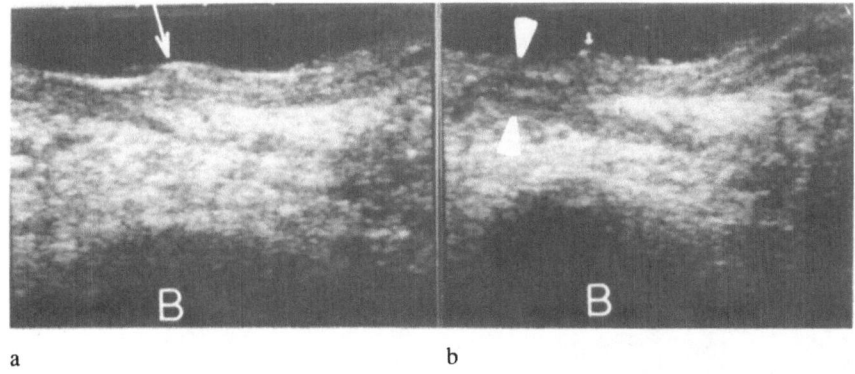

a   b

Figure 5.30. Endorectal longitudinal sonograms made after anterior resection of rectal carcinoma. (a) Normal anastomosis (arrow). (b) Local recurrence (arrowheads) at the anastomosis (small arrows). B = bladder.

when the anastomosis is terminoterminal, but artifacts from gas contained in the blind loop are often encountered in patients with lateroterminal anastomosis.

Sonographically, local recurrence presents as an iso- or hypoechoic, ill-defined, and non-homogeneous area (Fig. 5.30b). The pattern of spread to the rectal wall in early stages may be distinct from that of a primary tumor, since local recurrence usually develops in the perirectal space, whereas primary tumor first develops centripetally. Granulomas associated with sutures can mimic early local recurrence at the level of the anastomosis; ultrasound-guided

transperineal biopsy may clarify the situation (Figs. 5.31, 5.32). In the series of Hildebrandt *et al.*, endorectal sonography was accurate in all 22 patients with proved local recurrence and detected a local recurrence in 6 of them who had no symptoms, a negative endoscopic study, and a normal carcinoembryonic antigen level [8].

Endosonography is expected to be at least as accurate as CT in the early detection of local recurrence, without the disadvantage of irradiation. After abdominoperineal resection, CT or MR imaging is utilized, although in the female endosonography can still be performed transvaginally.

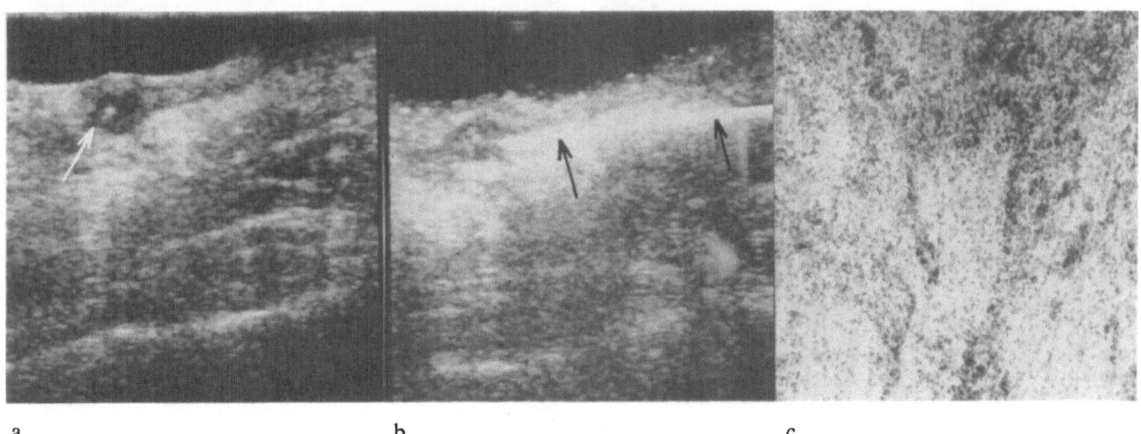

a   b   c

Figure 5.31. Ultrasound-guided fine-needle aspiration of a suture granuloma after anterior resection of rectal carcinoma. (a) Endorectal longitudinal sonogram shows a submucosal nodule (arrow) at the site of anastomosis. Endoscopic examination found a normal overlying mucosa. At palpation, the nodule was suspicious for local recurrence. (b) Transperineal ultrasound-guided aspiration biopsy using a 22-gauge Chiba needle. The needle is clearly visualized (arrows) and its tip has reached the suspicious mass. (c) Cytologic smear shows nonspecific inflammatory changes.

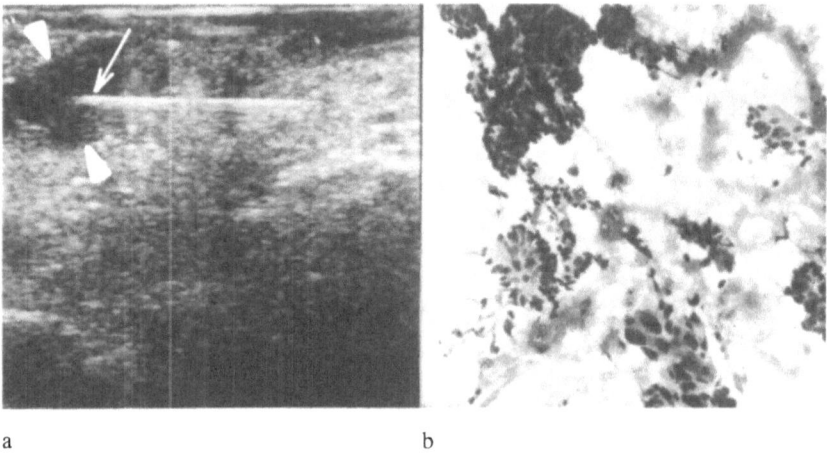

a   b

Figure 5.32. Ultrasound-guided fine-needle aspiration biopsy of local recurrence after anterior resection of rectal carcinoma. (a) Endorectal longitudinal scan obtained during ultrasound-guided transperineal aspiration biopsy shows the tip of the 22-gauge Chiba needle (arrow) in the suspicious hypoechoic mass (arrowheads). (b) Cytologic smear is consistent with local recurrence of rectal adenocarcinoma.

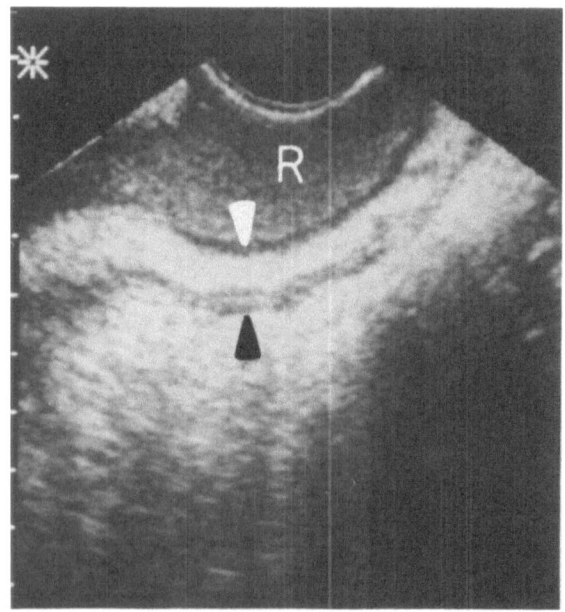

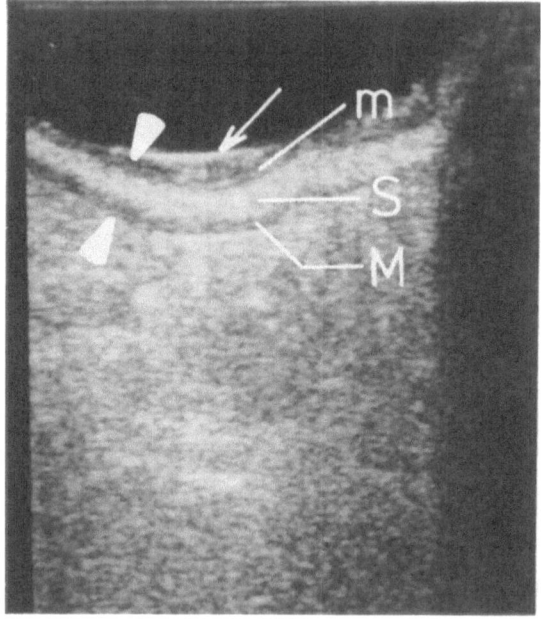

Figure 5.33. Crohn's disease. Endorectal longitudinal sonogram obtained with the use of a sector mechanical probe shows the thickened (13-mm) rectal wall (arrowheads). The multilayer pattern is preserved. Note the markedly thickened echogenic submucosa. R = rectal lumen. (Courtesy of Dr. V. Arienti.)

Figure 5.34. Ulcerative colitis. Endorectal longitudinal sonogram shows an 8-mm-thick rectal wall (arrowheads) with a markedly thickened, echogenic third layer (submucosa). Arrow points to the reflective balloon. m = mucosa; M = muscular coat; S = submucosa.

Inflammatory diseases

Evaluation of inflammatory conditions of the rectum is a recent application of endosonography. A common finding is the thickening of the wall, which may reach 2 cm. This nonspecific finding can be seen in various acute and chronic inflammatory diseases: *Crohn's disease, tuberculosis, postirradiation proctitis, ulcerative colitis,* and other, rare conditions (Figs. 5.33—5.35) [55]. The thickening of the wall involves the various sonographic layers, notably the third one (submucosa), whose echogenicity may decrease because of the edema so that the second and third layers may intermingle (Fig. 5.35). Our early experience indicates that inflammation of the rectum can be sonographically differentiated from malignant tumors. In inflammatory conditions, unlike in carcinoma, the lesion is diffuse and the multilayer pattern preserved. Inflammatory lymph nodes may be visualized in the perirectal tissues.

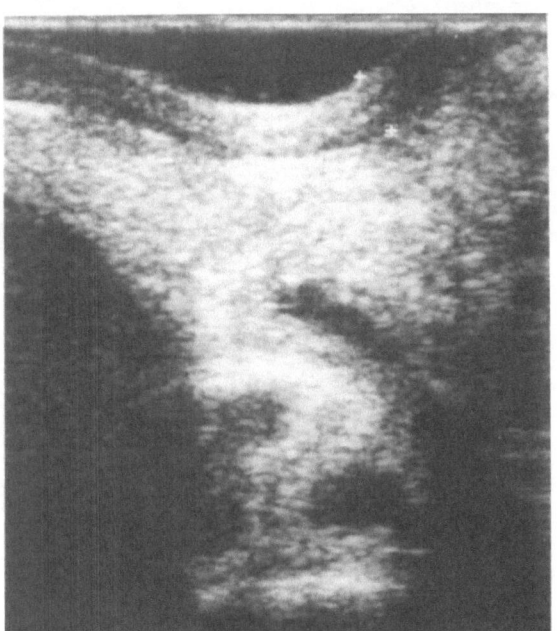

Figure 5.35. Postirradiation proctitis. Endorectal longitudinal scan shows thickening of the rectal wall. The thickness is measured at 9 mm (markers). There is poor delineation between the mucosa and submucosa.

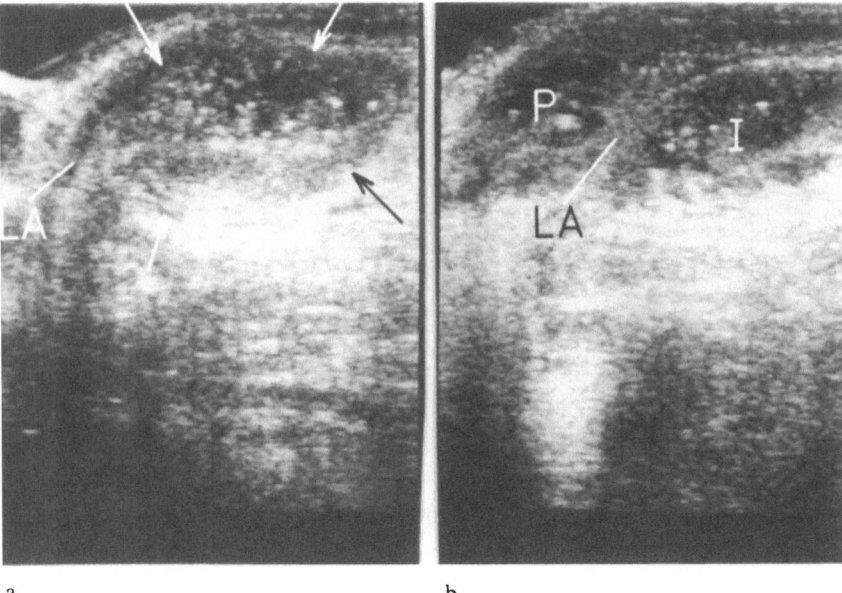

a   b

Figure 5.36. Rectal abscesses. (a) Endorectal longitudinal sonogram shows a primarily hypoechoic complex mass in the ischiorectal fossa (arrows). Note the tiny internal echoes suggesting the presence of microbubbles. (b) Abscess located on either side of levator ani muscle, occupying both the ischiorectal (I) and pelvirectal (P) areas. LA = levator ani muscle.

66

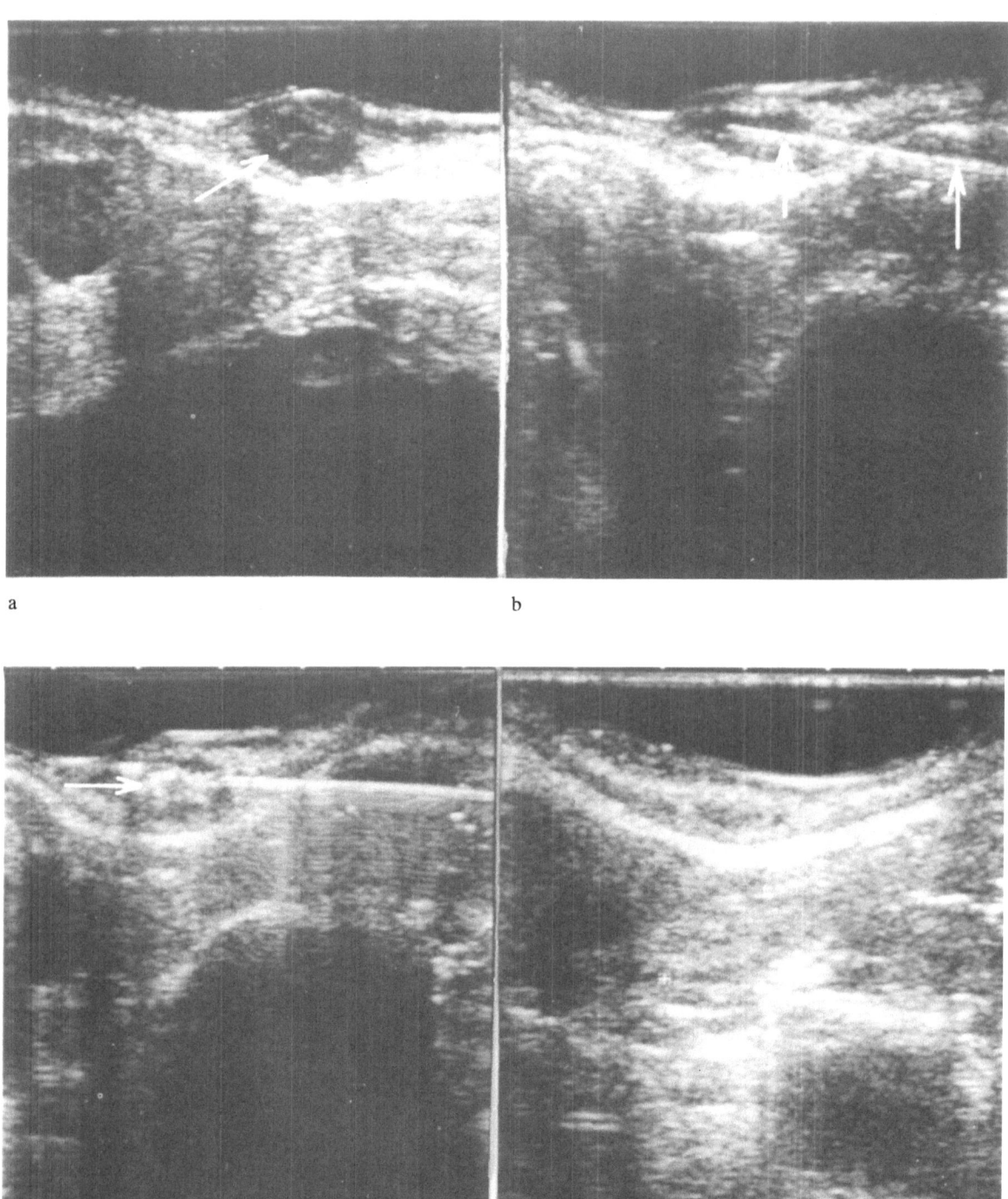

a b

c d

Figure 5.37. Rectal abscess. Ultrasound-guided fine-needle aspiration and antibiotic instillation. Endorectal longitudinal sonograms. (a) Sonogram shows a small, submucosal rectal abscess (arrow). (b) Ultrasound-guided transvaginal fine-needle aspiration. Arrows point to the 22-gauge needle, whose tip has been placed in the center of the abscess. (c) Injection of antibiotic solution creates bright echoes in the abscess cavity (arrow). (d) Follow-up sonogram performed 1 month later confirms the nearly complete regression of the lesion.

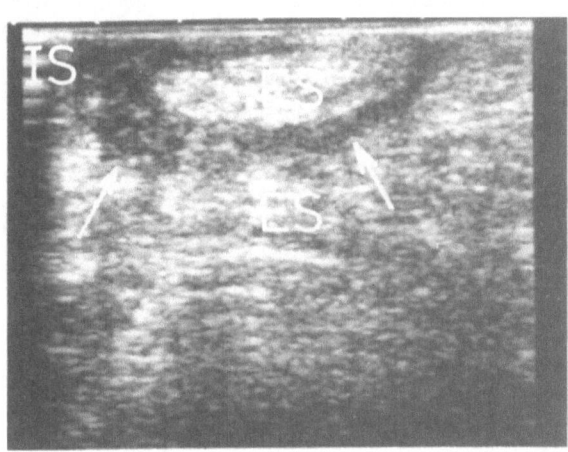

Figure 5.38. Endorectal longitudinal scan shows an anorectal fistula (arrows) originating in the internal sphincter and coursing through the external sphincter. ES = external sphincter; IS = internal sphincter.

Anorectal abscesses develop in superficial (submucous or subcutaneous) or deep (pelvirectal or ischiorectal) locations. Abscesses may also develop between the external longitudinal and internal circular muscular layers. Abscesses may result from infection of a perianal hematoma or hemorrhoid or develop after sclerosing injection of hemorrhoids or as a complication of a deep anal fissure. Usually, neither the patient's history nor physical examination can elicit a particular cause and the point of entry of the infecting agent cannot be demonstrated. The abscess sonographically appears as a primarily sonolucent complex mass with distal acoustic enhancement. It may contain echogenic septa or debris; occasionally, bright internal echoes (Fig. 5.36), which are thought to represent gaseous microbubbles produced by anaerobes, are seen. The size of abscesses is variable. Figure 5.37 shows a small abscess entirely included in the third layer (submucosa). Infrequently, chronic ischio- or pelvirectal abscesses mimic rectal carcinoma. In this situation, ultrasound-guided biopsy is usually diagnostic.

Anorectal fistulas are not easily evaluated by endorectal sonography. A fistulous tract may be visualized as a hypoechoic linear pattern in the ischio- or pelvirectal space. Infrequently, endorectal sonography can demonstrate secondary tracts not visualized at fistulography (Fig. 5.38).

References

1. Wild J. J., Reid J. M.: Diagnostic use of ultrasound. Br. J. Phys. Med., 1956, 19, 248—257.
2. Alzin H. H., Kohlberger E., Schwaiger R., Alloussi S.: Valeur de l'échographie endorectale dans la chirurgie du rectum. Ann. Radiol. (Paris), 1983, 26, 334—336.
3. Dragsted J., Gammelgaard J.: Endoluminal ultrasonic scanning in the evaluation of rectal cancer: A preliminary report of 13 cases. Gastrointest. Radiol., 1983, 8, 367—369.
4. Rifkin M. D., Marks G. J.: Transrectal US as an adjunct in the diagnosis of rectal and extrarectal tumors. Radiology, 1985, 157, 499—502.
5. Konishi F., Muto T., Takahashi H., Itoh K., Kanazawa K., Morioka Y.: Transrectal ultrasonography for the assessment of invasion of rectal carcinoma. Dis. Colon Rectum, 1985, 28, 889—894.
6. Boscaini M., Montori A.: Transrectal ultrasonography: Interpretation of normal intestinal wall structure for the preoperative staging of rectal cancer. Scand. J. Gastroenterol., 1986, 21 (suppl. 123), 87—98.
7. Hildebrandt U., Feifel G.: Preoperative staging of rectal cancer by intrarectal ultrasound. Dis. Colon Rectum, 1985, 28, 42—46.
8. Hildebrandt U., Feifel G., Schwarz H. P., Scherr O.: Endorectal ultrasound: Instrumentation and clinical aspects. Int. J. Colorect. Dis., 1986, 1, 203—207.
9. Pahlman L., Adalsteinsson B., Glimelius B., Lindgren P. G., Scheibenpflug L.: Ultrasound in preoperative staging of rectal tumours. Acta Radiol. [Diagn.] (Stockh.), 1984, 25, 489—494.
10. Beynon J., Mortensen N. J. McC., Foy D. M. A., Channer J. L., Virjee J., Goddard P.: Endorectal sonography: Laboratory and clinical experience in Bristol. Int. J. Colorect. Dis., 1986, 1, 212—215.
11. Saitoh N., Okui K., Sarashina H., Suzuki M., Arai T., Nunomura M.: Evaluation of echographic diagnosis of rectal cancer using intrarectal ultrasonic examination. Dis. Colon Rectum, 1986, 29, 234—242.
12. Romano G., De Rosa P., Vallone G., Rotondo A., Grassi R., Santangelo M. L.: Intrarectal ultrasound and computed tomography in the pre- and postoperative assessment of patients with rectal cancer. Br. J. Surg., 1985, 72 (suppl.), 117—119.
13. Rifkin M. D., Wechsler R. J.: A comparison of computed tomography and endorectal ultrasound in staging rectal cancer. Int. J. Colorect. Dis., 1986, 1, 219—223.
14. Kramann B., Hildebrandt U.: Computed tomography versus endosonography in the staging of rectal carcinoma: A comparative study. Int. J. Colorect. Dis., 1986, 1, 216—28.

15. Williams N. S., Dixon M. F., Johnston D.: Reappraisal of the 5 centimetre rule of distal excision for carcinoma of the rectum: A study of distal intramural spread and of patients' survival. Br. J. Surg., 1983, 70, 150—154.

16. Hughes T. G., Jenevein E. P., Poulos E.: Intramural spread of colon carcinoma. A pathologic study. Am. J. Surg., 1983, 146, 697—699.

17. Black W. A., Waugh J. M.: The intramural extension of carcinoma of the descending colon, sigmoid, and rectosigmoid: A pathologic study. Surg. Gynecol. Obstet., 1948, 87, 457—464.

18. Quer E. A., Dahlin D. C., Mayco C. W.: Retrograde intramural spread of carcinoma of the rectum and rectosigmoid: A microscopic study. Surg. Gynecol. Obstet., 1953, 96, 24—30.

19. Pollet W. J., Nicholls R. J.: Does the extent of distal clearance affect survival after radical anterior resection for carcinoma of the rectum? (abstract). Gut, 1981, 22, 872.

20. Wilson S. M., Beahrs O. H.: The curative treatment of carcinoma of the sigmoid, rectosigmoid, and rectum. Ann. Surg., 1976, 183, 556—565.

21. Deddish M. R., Stearns M. W. Jr.: Anterior resection for carcinoma of the rectum and rectosigmoid area. Ann. Surg., 1961, 154, 961—966.

22. Spiessl B., Scheibe O., Wagner G.: TNM Atlas. Illustrated guide to the classification of malignant tumours. Berlin, Springer-Verlag, 1982.

23. Astler V. B., Coller F. A.: The prognostic significance of direct extension of carcinoma of the colon and rectum. Ann. Surg., 1954, 139, 846—851.

24. Storer E. H., Goldberg S. M., Nivatvongs S.: Colon, rectum and anus. In: Schwartz I. S. (ed.). Principles of surgery, 4th ed. Hightstown, McGraw-Hill, 1984, 1169—1244.

25. Hodgman C. G., MacCarty R. L., Wolff B. G., et al.: Preoperative staging of rectal carcinoma by computed tomography and 0.15 T magnetic resonance imaging. Preliminary report. Dis. Colon Rectum, 1986, 29, 446—450.

26. Butch R. J., Stark D. D., Wittenberg J., et al.: Staging rectal cancer by MR and CT. AJR, 1986, 146, 1155—1160.

27. Mason A. Y.: Rectal cancer: The spectrum of selective surgery. Proc. R. Soc. Med., 1976, 69, 237—244.

28. Nicholls R. J., Mason A. Y., Morson B. C., Dixon A. K., Fry I. K.: The clinical staging of rectal cancer. Br. J. Surg., 1982, 69, 404—409.

29. Nicholls R. J., Galloway D. J., Mason A. Y., Boyle P.: Clinical local staging of rectal cancer. Br. J. Surg., 1985, 72 (suppl.), 51—52.

30. Thoeni R. F., Moss A. A., Schnyder P., Margulis A. R.: Detection and staging of primary rectal and rectosigmoid cancer by computed tomography. Radiology, 1981, 141, 135—138.

31. Zaunbauer W., Haertel M., Fuchs W. A.: Computed tomography in carcinoma of the rectum. Gastrointest. Radiol, 1981, 6, 79—84.

32. Mayes G. B., Zornoza J.: Computed tomography of colon carcinoma. AJR, 1980, 135, 43—46.

33. Van Waes P. F. G. M., Koehler P. R., Feldberg M. A. M.: Management of rectal carcinoma: Impact of computed tomography. AJR, 1983, 140, 1137—1142.

34. Grabbe E., Lierse W., Winkler R.: The perirectal fascia: Morphology and use in staging of rectal carcinoma. Radiology, 1983, 149, 241—246.

35. Di Candio G., Mosca F., Cei A., Campatelli A., D'Elia F.: Stadiazione ecografica del carcinoma del retto. Presented at the 88th Meeting of the Societa Italiana di Chirurgia. Rome, October 12—16, 1986.

36. Di Candio G., Mosca F., Campatelli A., Cei A., Ferrari M., Basolo F.: Endosonographic staging of rectal carcinoma. Gastrointest. Radiol., 1987, 12, 289—295.

37. Di Candio G., Mosca F.: Anatomia ecografica del retto. In: Rizzatto G. (ed.). Anatomia Ecografica. Milan, Masson (in press).

38. Gunderson L. L., Sosin H.: Areas of failure found at reoperation (second or symptomatic look) following 'curative surgery' for adenocarcinoma of the rectum. Clinicopathologic correlation and implications for adjuvant therapy. Cancer, 1974, 34, 1278—1292.

39. Morson B.C., Vaughan E. G., Bussey H. J. R.: Pelvic recurrence after excision of rectum for carcinoma. Br. Med. J., 1963, 2, 13—18.

40. Goligher J. C.: Resection with restoration of continuity in the treatment of carcinoma of the rectum and rectosigmoid. Postgrad. Med. J., 1951, 27, 568—575.

41. Hurst P. A., Prout W. G., Kelly J. M., Bannister J. J., Walker R. T.: Local recurrence after low anterior resection using the staple gun. Br. J. Surg., 1982, 69, 275—276.

42. Garlock J. H., Ginzburg L.: An appraisal of the operation of anterior resection for carcinoma of the rectum and rectosigmoid. Surg. Gynecol. Obstet., 1950, 90, 525—534.

43. Pahlman L., Glimelius B.: Local recurrences after surgical treatment for rectal carcinoma. Acta Chir. Scand., 1984, 150, 331—335.

44. Slanetz C. A., Herter F. P., Grinnel R. S.: Anterior resection versus abdominoperineal resection for cancer of the rectum and rectosigmoid. Am. J. Surg., 1972, 123, 110—117.

45. Rao A. R., Kagan A. R., Chan P. M., Gilbert H. A., Nussbaum H., Hintz B. L.: Patterns of recurrence following curative resection alone for adenocarcinoma of the rectum and sigmoid colon. Cancer, 1981, 48, 1492—1495.

46. Grinnel R. S.: The lymphatic and venous spread of carcinoma of the rectum. Ann. Surg., 1942, 116, 200—216.

47. Filipe M. I., Scurr J. H., Ellis H.: Effects of fecal stream on experimental colorectal carcinogenesis. Morphologic and histochemical changes. Cancer, 1982, 50, 2859—2865.

48. Stanek J. J., Scurr J. H., Ellis H.: Local recurrence and rectal cancer (letter). Lancet, 1983, 2, 1371.

49. Husband J. E., Hodson N. J., Parsons C. A.: The use of computed tomography in recurrent rectal tumors. Radiology, 1980, 134, 677—682.

50. Kelvin F. M., Korobkin M., Heaston D. K., Grant J. P.,

Akwari O.: The pelvis after surgery for rectal carcinoma: Serial CT observations with emphasis on nonneoplastic features. AJR, 1983, 141, 959—964.

51. Clark J., Bankoff M., Carter B., Smith T. J.: The use of computerized tomography scan in the staging and follow-up study of carcinoma of the rectum. Surg. Gynecol. Obstet., 1984, 159, 335—342.

52. Lee J. K. T., Stanley R. J., Sagel S. S., Levitt R. G., McClennan B. L.: CT appearance of the pelvis after abdominoperineal resection for rectal carcinoma. Radiology, 1981, 141, 737—741.

53. Zelas P., Haaga J. R., Fazio V. W.: The diagnosis by percutaneous biopsy with computed tomography of a recurrence of carcinoma of the rectum in the pelvis. Surg. Gynecol. Obstet., 1980, 151, 525—527.

54. Butch R. J., Wittenberg J., Mueller P. R., Simeone J. F., Meyer J. E., Ferrucci J. T. Jr.: Presacral masses after abdominoperineal resection for colorectal carcinoma: The need for needle biopsy. AJR, 1985, 144, 309—312.

55. Di Candio G., Mosca F., Campatelli A., Bianchini M., D'Elia F., Dellagiovampaola C.: Sonographic detection of postsurgical recurrence of Crohn disease. AJR, 1986, 146, 523—526.

6. Transrectal sonography of the prostate

BRUNO D. FORNAGE

Transrectal sonography of the prostate is increasing in popularity as technical improvements, including the development of high-frequency biplane probes, enhance its diagnostic capabilities. The other endosonographic route to the prostate is through the urethra. This approach, however, is subsidiary to imaging of the urinary bladder: as the 24-F transurethral radial probe is withdrawn from the bladder, its rotating tip is placed in the prostatic urethra for transverse scans of the prostate [1—3]. Traumatic and septic risks preclude the use of transurethral sonography for prostatic imaging alone; the technique is discussed in Chapter 7.

Anatomy

McNeal's concepts of the internal structure of the prostate have replaced classic lobar anatomy (Fig. 6.1) [4, 5].

A *fibromuscular stroma* lies anterior to the urethra. It makes up as much as one third of the mass of the prostate and consists mainly of smooth muscle.

The *preprostatic region* comprises the *prostatic sphincter*, a cylindrical smooth muscle that encircles the urethra from the bladder neck to the base of verumontanum and the *periurethral glands*.

The true acinar (functioning) prostate is divided by McNeal into a transition, a central, and a peripheral zone. The *transition zone* represents about 5% of the acinar prostate. It is located on both sides of the urethra, above the verumontanum. The *central zone* is a wedge with its apex at the verumontanum and its base

behind the bladder neck. It surrounds the ejaculatory ducts and is embedded in the *peripheral zone*, which is funnel shaped. The peripheral zone extends inferiorly below the verumontanum.

The anatomic zoning of the prostate is of clinical relevance: it has been shown that carcinoma and prostatitis usually (but not always) arise in the peripheral zone, while benign prostatic hypertrophy (BPH) originates in the transitional zone.

The seminal vesicles lie cephalad to the prostate between the bladder and the rectum. At the point where the ampullae terminate, the vesicles join the vasa deferentia to form the ejaculatory ducts. The size and shape of the seminal vesicles exhibit a great individual variability.

Instrumentation

Transrectal ultrasound was first attempted, using the A-mode technique, in the early 1960s [6—8]. Then Watanabe *et al.* in Japan began to use dedicated endorectal equipment, making B-mode, bistable, radial scans [9, 10]. In 1979, Harada *et al.* reported gray-scale transrectal sonograms of the prostate [11]. In the early 1980s, linear-array endorectal probes that produced longitudinal scans of the prostate became commercially available [12]. The first investigators were urologists [2, 8—17]; radiologists became involved later [18—23].

Different types of endorectal probes are used to obtain differently oriented images. *Transverse scans* are obtained using radial or sector probes.

Bruno D. Fornage (ed.), *Endosonography*, pp. 71—104.
© 1989 *Kluwer Academic Publishers*.

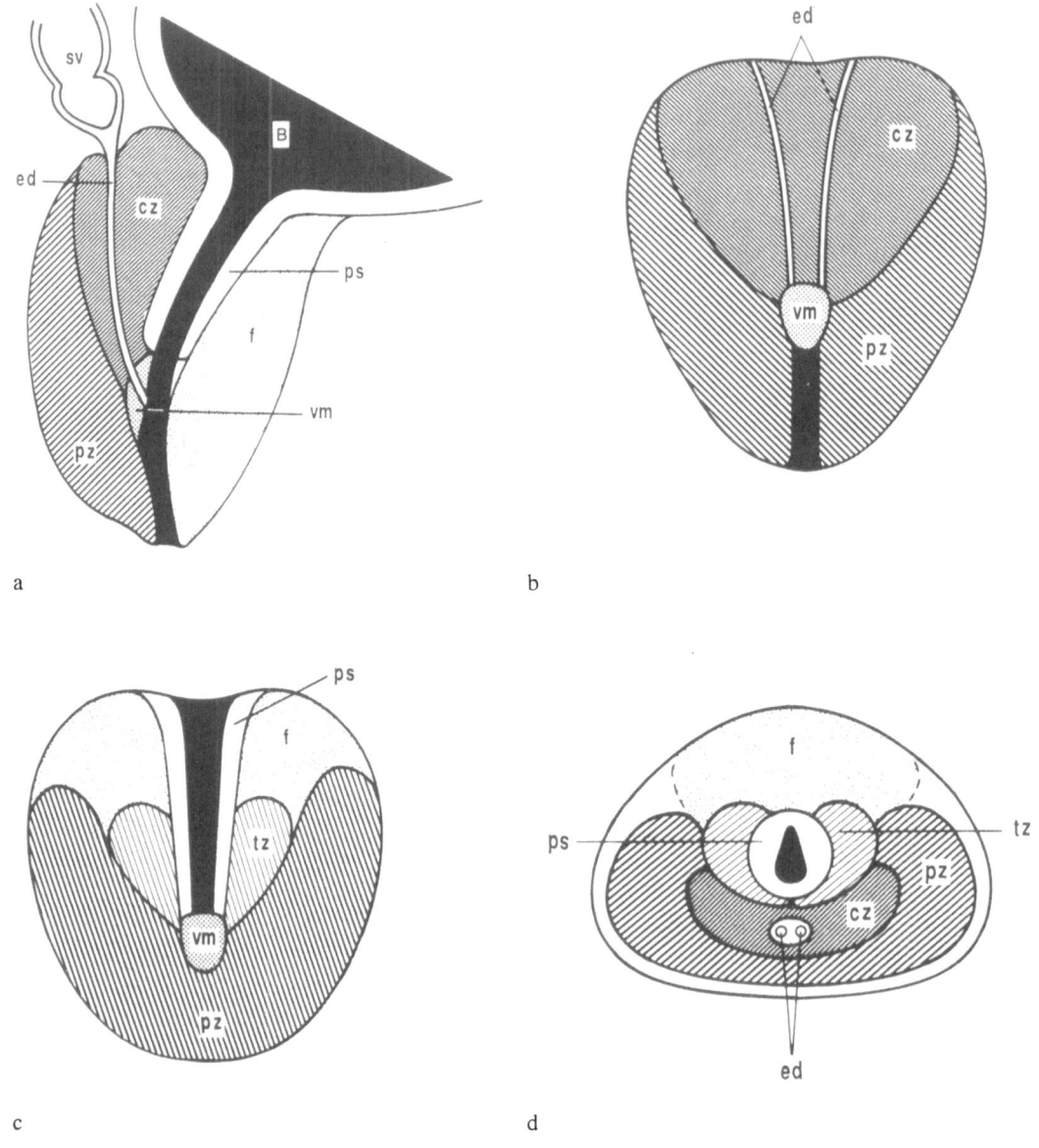

Figure 6.1. Morphology of the prostate. (a) Midsagittal section. (b) Coronal section following distal urethral segment. (c) Oblique coronal section following proximal urethral segment. (d) Transverse section above the verumontanum. B = bladder; cz = central zone; ed = ejaculatory duct; f = anterior fibromuscular stroma; ps = prostatic sphincter; pz = peripheral zone; sv = seminal vesicle; tz = transition zone; vm = verumontanum.

A single rotating transducer is usually employed (Fig. 6.2). Electronic phased-array transducers are also available in this use, but their field of view is limited to 90°. *Longitudinal scans* are typically obtained with linear-array transducers, which provide a rectangular format (Fig. 6.3). However, sector scanning with a mechanical, curved-array, or phased-array transducer can also provide longitudinal sonograms.

Each of these probes scans in a single plane, transverse or longitudinal, so that we soon recommended the consecutive use of both probes in any given patient [20, 24] and presented the concept of transrectal *biplane scanning* [25]. Several designs of biplane probes are currently available.

Biplane probes incorporate either two separate transducers, whose scan planes are fixed

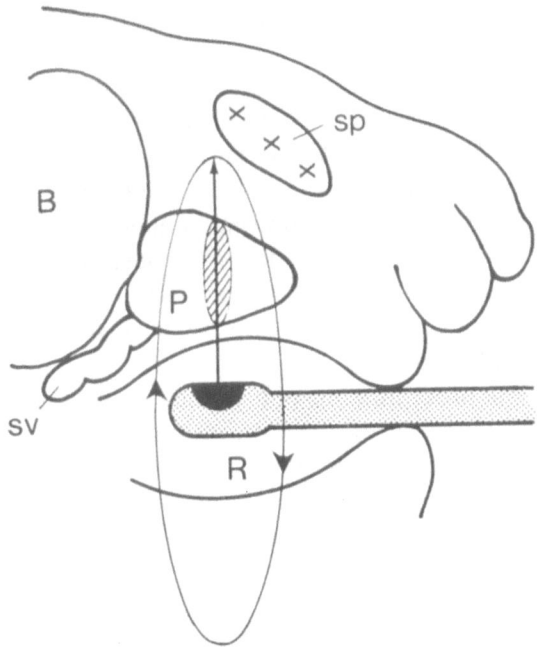

a

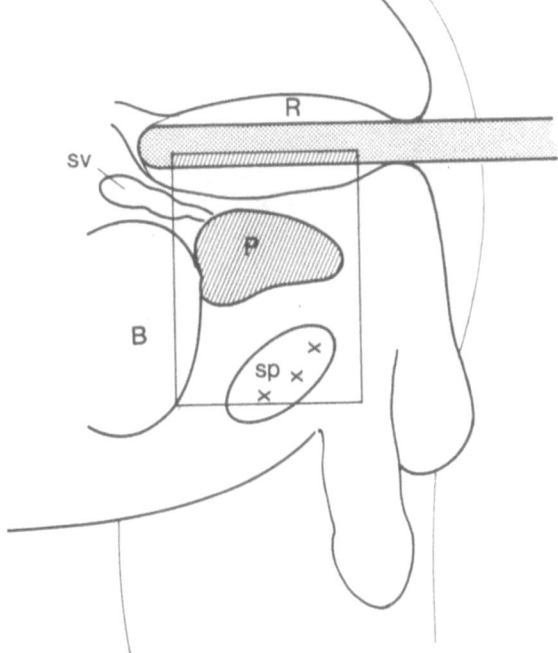

a

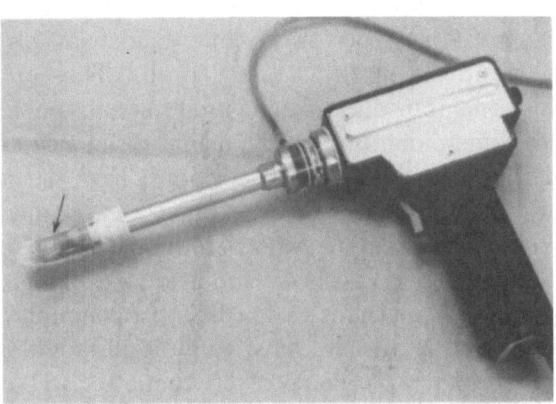

b

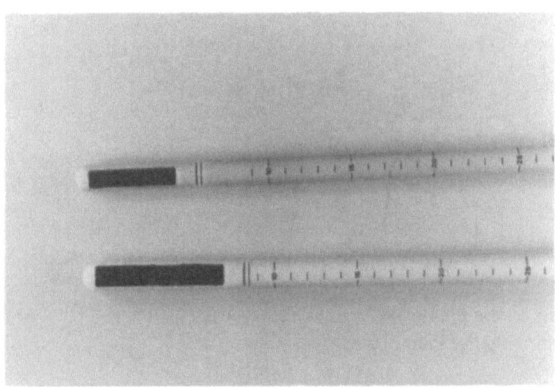

b

Figure 6.2. Transrectal examination of the prostate using a radial probe. (a) Diagram showing the radial probe placed in the rectum. The axial rotation of the transducer generates transverse sections of the prostate. B = bladder; P = prostate; R = rectum; sp = symphysis pubis; sv = seminal vesicle. (b) The transducer is seen at the tip of the probe (arrow), which has been covered by a disposable latex balloon.

Figure 6.3. Transrectal examination of the prostate using a linear-array probe. (a) Diagram showing the linear-array transducer placed in the rectum. B = bladder; P = prostate; R = rectum; sp = symphysis pubis; sv = seminal vesicle. (b) Endorectal linear-array probes. Top: 7.5-MHz probe. Bottom: 5-MHz probe providing a wider field of view.

and in most designs perpendicular to each other (Figs. 6.4, 6.5), or a single, steerable transducer, whose orientation is remote controlled mechanically or electronically. The steerable, single-element transducer allows not only transverse and sagittal sector images but also oblique scans, so that in fact the probe is multiplane (Fig. 6.6).

When two separate transducers are used, the best transducer for longitudinal scanning is a linear-array one (Fig. 6.4), which provides an optimal ultrasonic near-field.

The first commercially available endorectal probes had a frequency of 3.5 MHz. Most of the recent probes are equipped with 7.5 MHz transducers.

74

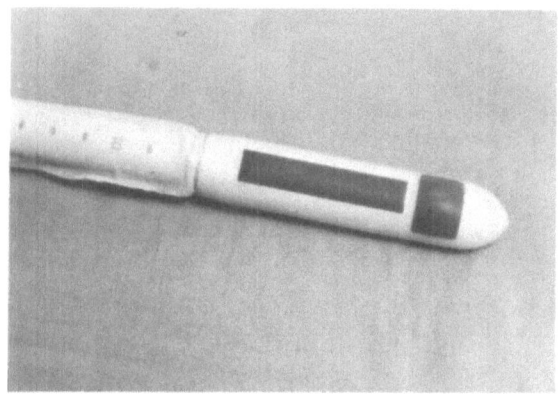

a

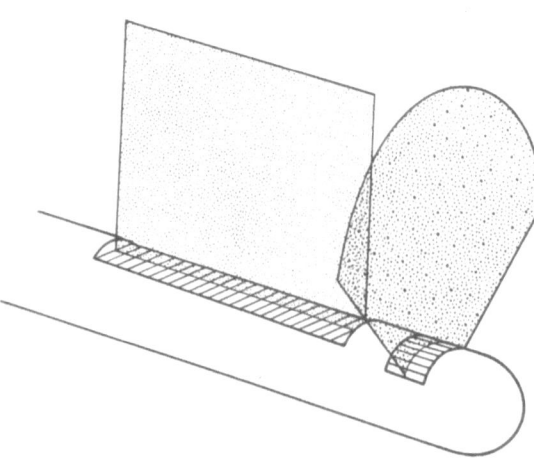

b

Figure 6.4. (a) Biplane endorectal probe associating a transversely oriented curved-array transducer placed at the tip of the probe and a linear-array transducer. (b) Diagram showing the scan planes.

Technique of examination

The tip of the endorectal probe is capped with a thin, disposable latex balloon (usually a condom), which is filled with 20 to 60 mL of deaerated water after its insertion in the rectum. The balloon serves to prevent contamination of the probe, to ensure satisfactory acoustic contact with the rectal wall and displace intrarectal feces and gas, and to place the prostate in the focal zone of the probe.

The procedure must be explained in detail to the patient. A hypertonic sodium phosphate enema or a bisacodyl (Dulcolax) rectal suppository will rapidly prepare the rectum, although satisfactory images are usually obtained without any preparation.

With the patient supine, a rapid ultrasound survey of the abdomen is first performed to rule out any distension of the kidneys. The prostate is examined suprapubically. Next, a digital rectal examination is performed to exclude any obstacle to the insertion of the probe. The conventional transducer can be used for suprapubic real-time monitoring of the digital rectal examination. Various patient positions have been advocated for transrectal prostatic sonography, including the sitting (with dedicated chair-type equipment), knee-elbow, and lateral decubitus positions. The last is by far the most commonly employed and is the most comfortable for the patient (Fig. 6.7). The probe is connected to the

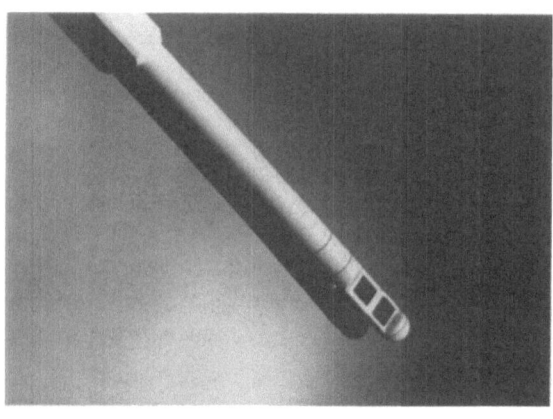

a

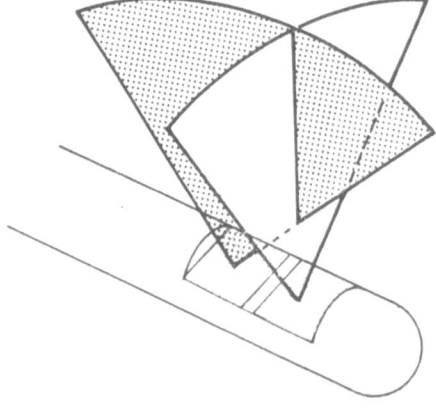

b

Figure 6.5. (a) Biplane probe associating two 7.0-MHz phased-array transducers. (Courtesy of General Electric Medical Systems.) (b) Diagram showing the two transducers with their sector scan planes perpendicular to each other.

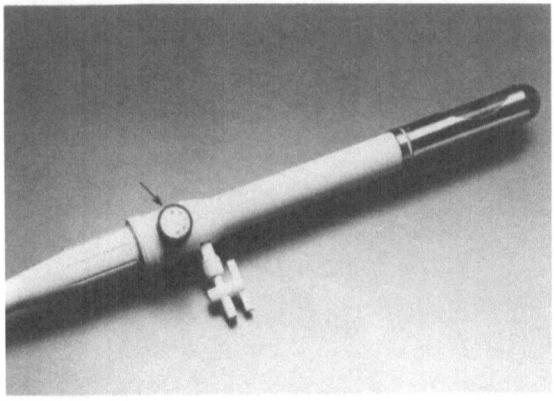

a

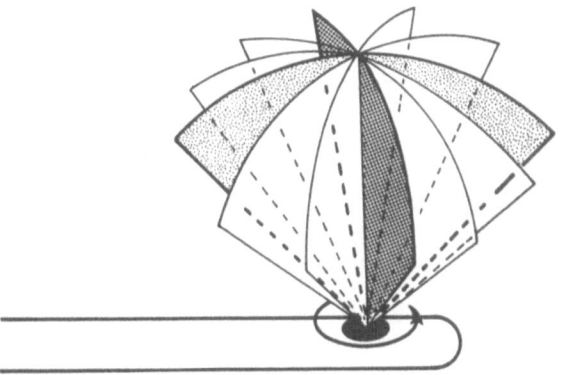

b

Figure 6.6. (a) Multiplane endorectal probe based on a mechanical sector transducer that can swivel around its ultrasound axis. The scan plane can be oriented by using the external knob (arrow). (b) Diagram showing the sagittal, transverse, and oblique scans available with this system.

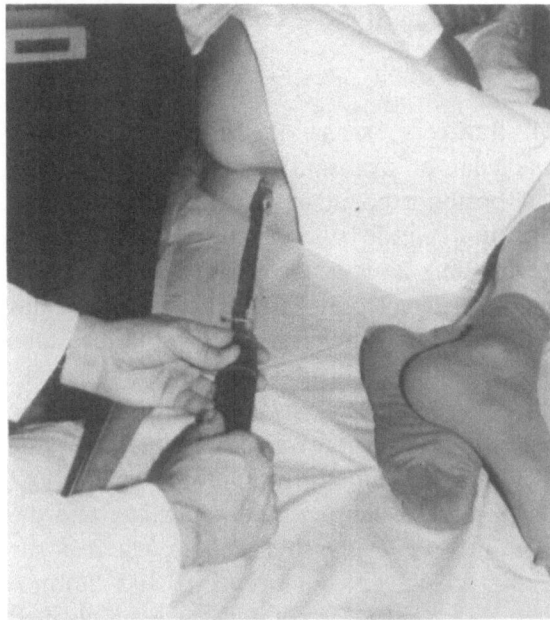

Figure 6.7. Transrectal examination is performed with the patient in the left lateral decubitus position with hips and knees flexed.

scanner and generously lubricated with acoustic coupling jelly. As it is gradually inserted in the rectum, the anterior pelvis is displayed on the video monitor. When separate probes are used to obtain the transverse and sagittal scans, the prostate is examined by progressive axial advancement of the radial probe and clockwise and counterclockwise axial rotation of the linear-array probe. A biplane (or multiplane) probe, however, as mentioned above, produces transverse and longitudinal views of the prostate *during the one examination*, enabling the operator to compare these views during the examination. The use of biplane probe also shortens the duration of the examination and thus greatly improves patient tolerance.

Most investigators advocate videotaping the whole examination, with the probe for transverse images scanning the prostate slowly and continuously from its base to its apex and with the probe for longitudinal images scanning from the midsagittal plane to the patient's left and right sides. Hard copies of frozen images should be taken at intervals of about 5 mm and 5° for transverse and longitudinal scans, respectively.

There are great variations in the display orientation of the prostatic scans according to ultrasound equipment, and the problem of standardization will probably soon be addressed.

Our protocol for ultrasound examination of the prostate is summarized in Table 6.1.

Table 6.1. Protocol for sonographic examination of the prostate.

---

1. Abdominal scanning, including a survey of the kidneys and suprapubic examination of bladder and prostate
2. Digital rectal examination
3. Transrectal examination using a biplane (or multiplane) probe (or a radial, then a linear-array probe)
4. Transrectal sonoscopic voiding study
5. Postvoid suprapubic examination to evaluate residual urine
6. Ultrasound-guided biopsy of suspicious lesions

Normal ultrasound anatomy

Transverse scans

On transverse scans, the prostate is grossly triangular or oval and symmetrical (Fig. 6.8). The posterior boundary becomes concave posteriorly when the balloon is fully distended. The surrounding fat is echogenic. A thin, echogenic margin is depicted by 7.5-MHz transducers; this margin is often referred to as the prostatic capsule, although histologic verification is lacking. Anechoic cross sections of periprostatic veins are well demonstrated in the periprostatic fat, particularly anteriorly (Santorini's plexus).

The area of the periurethral stroma and the prostatic sphincter is hypoechoic, whereas the acinar prostate is homogeneous and 'normo-echoic' (Fig. 6.9). Recently, it has been claimed that the transition zone can be separated from the adjacent peripheral and central zones and that the central zone has a greater echogenicity than the peripheral zone [26]. In our experience, McNeal's zones have not been separated sono-

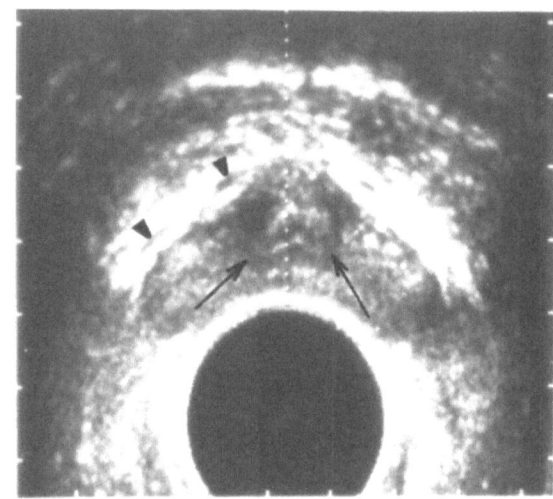

Figure 6.8. Normal prostate. Transverse scan shows a symmetrical prostate. The hypoechoic midline anterior area corresponds to the preprostatic region (arrows). Note the periprostatic veins (arrowheads).

graphically in normal subjects. The calcification of corpora amylacea with aging gives rise to minute (1 to 2 mm) prostatic calculi, which appear as small echogenic dots located virtually anywhere in the normal adult gland.

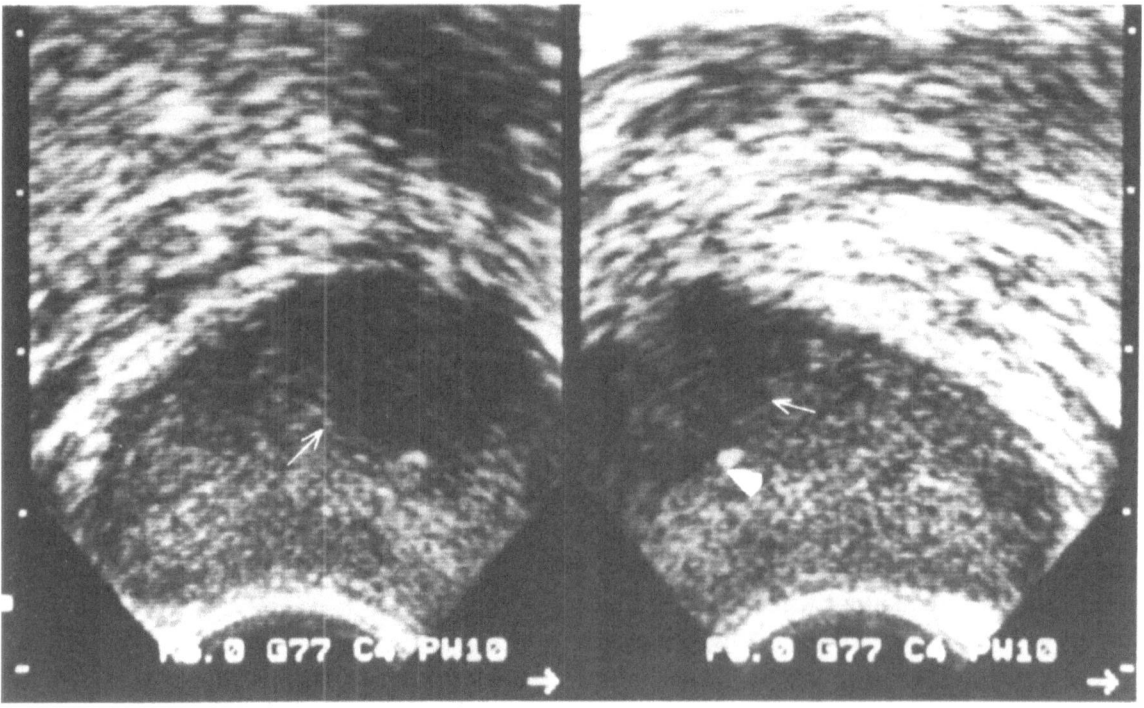

a   b

Figure 6.9. Normal prostate. Transverse sonograms of the right (a) and left (b) lobes show a homogeneous acinar echo pattern. Note the hypoechoic preprostatic region (arrow) and a minute calcification (arrowhead).

The seminal vesicles are hypoechoic with low-level echoes and occasionally internal septation. Transverse scans provide symmetrical views of the vesicles. The ampullae of the vasa deferentia are seen medially as two small, rounded hypoechoic areas a few millimeters in diameter (Fig. 6.10).

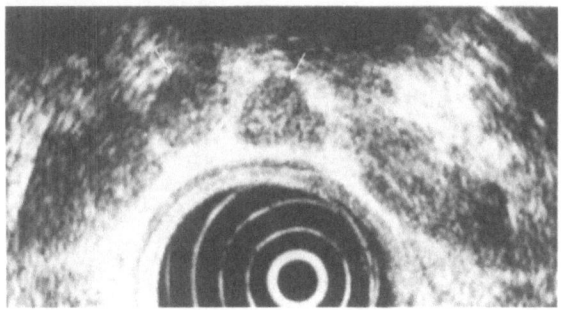

Figure 6.10. Transverse scan shows symmetrical hypoechoic seminal vesicles. The ampullae of the vasa deferentia are seen medially as two rounded hypoechoic structures (arrows).

Longitudinal scans

On longitudinal scans, the prostate tapers from its base to its apex. Midsagittal scans show the hypoechoic prostatic sphincter ensheathing the proximal urethra and continuous with the bladder neck (Fig. 6.11). These scans clearly show the bladder neck and prostatic apex, which are not well depicted on radial scans because of the tangential orientation of the scanning plane. A hypoechoic triangular zone is sometimes seen at the apex, representing the external sphincter. Posteriorly, the 2—3-mm rectal wall is well defined when the balloon is distended. A five-layer pattern is routinely depicted with the use of 7.5-MHz transducers. The rectal wall continues inferiorly with a hypoechoic area posterior to the prostatic apex, representing the anal sphincter [27]. Anteriorly, periprostatic venous plexuses can be visualized in the echogenic preprostatic fat (Fig. 6.12). When the sagittal scan plane is tilted laterally, the levator ani muscles are seen running obliquely from the posterior aspects of the pubic bones toward the hypoechoic anal sphincter (Fig.6.13) [28].

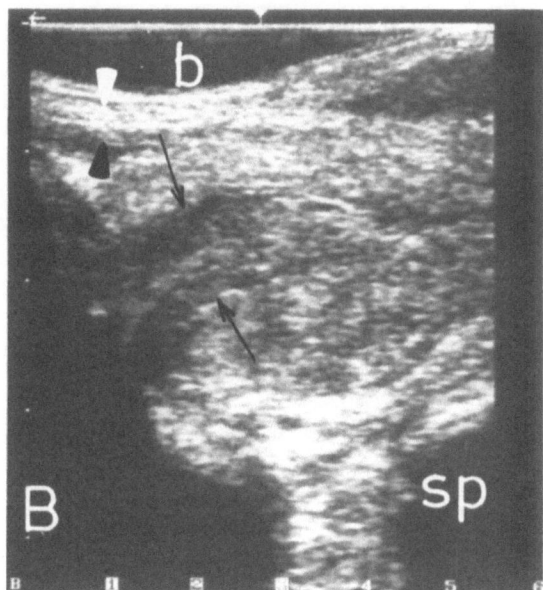

Figure 6.11. Normal prostate. Midsagittal scan performed with a 7.5-MHz linear-array transducer shows the hypoechoic prostatic sphincter (arrows), which surrounds the proximal urethra and which is continuous with the bladder neck. The acinar prostate is homogeneous. Also visualized is the rectal wall (arrowheads). B = bladder; b = intrarectal water-distended balloon; sp = symphysis pubis.

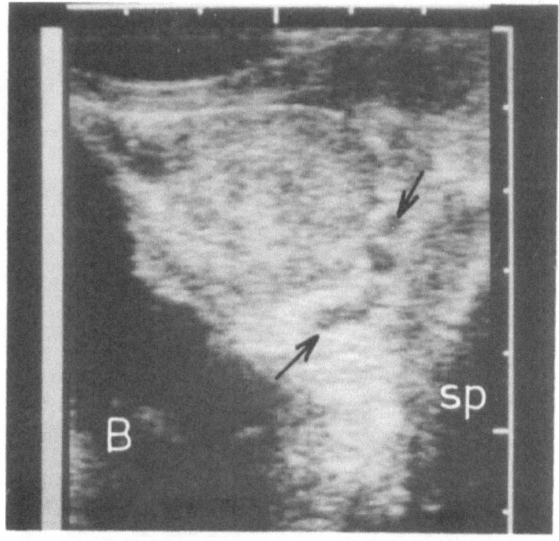

Figure 6.12. Longitudinal section of the prostate shows the hypoechoic cross sections of the anterior venous plexus (arrows) in the Retzius space. B = bladder; sp = symphysis pubis.

78

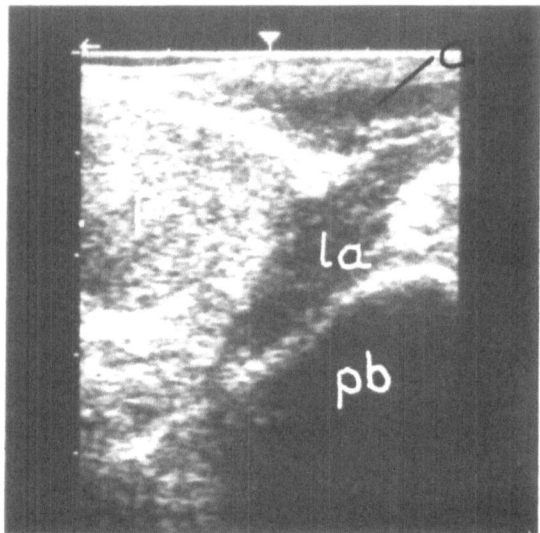

Figure 6.13. Laterally tilted, longitudinal section of the prostate shows the hypoechoic levator ani muscle originating from the posterior aspect of the pubic bone and merging with the hypoechoic anal sphincter. a = anal sphincter; la = levator ani muscle; P = prostate; pb = pubic bone.

With the use of high-resolution transducers, the collapsed urethra and the ejaculatory ducts can be seen as fine echogenic lines (Fig. 6.14) [27].

As on transverse scans, scattered tiny calculi are seen as echogenic foci (Fig. 6.15).

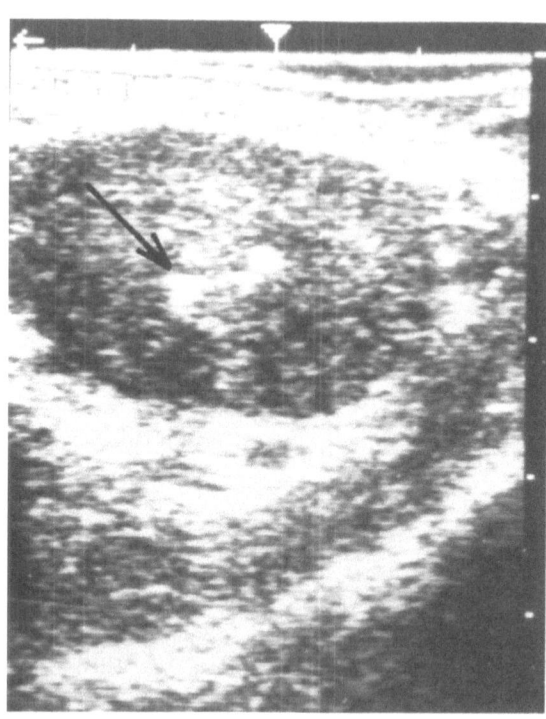

Figure 6.15. Longitudinal section of the prostate shows two bright, 2-mm foci thought to represent calcified corpora amylacea. One focus (arrow) is associated with a subtle shadow and comet-tail artifact.

Longitudinal scans show the seminal vesicles tapering and joining the base of the prostate (Fig. 6.16).

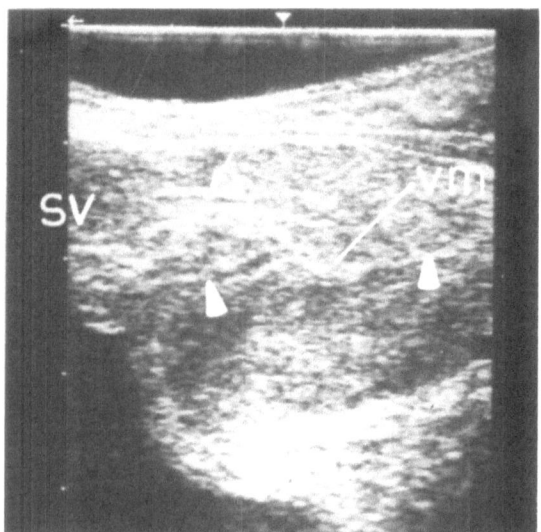

Figure 6.14. Midsagittal section shows the collapsed proximal urethra (arrowheads) and one ejaculatory duct (arrow). sv = seminal vesicle; vm = verumontanum.

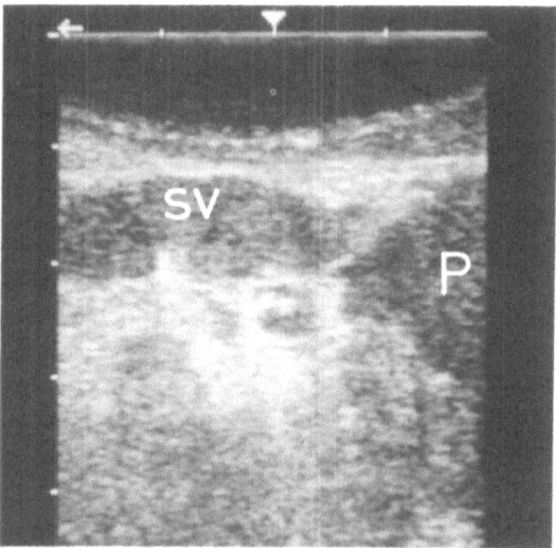

Figure 6.16. Longitudinal scan of a normal seminal vesicle. The vesicle is hypoechoic with fine low-level echoes. Note the sharp joining with the prostate. P = prostate; sv = seminal vesicle. (From ref. 27, with permission.)

Prostatic volume determination

Prostatic volume determination is instrumental in the selection of BPH patients for transurethral resection of the prostate (TURP) versus open prostatectomy and in the follow-up of patients with prostatic cancer treated conservatively. Two techniques are available. Planimetry of the prostatic area on serial parallel transverse transrectal scans has shown to be extremely accurate [29—31]. In daily practice, however, the volume is more rapidly obtained by using the volume formula for a prolate ellipsoid. Given the greatest width w as determined on transverse scans, and the greatest length l and thickness t as measured on the midsagittal scan (Fig. 6.17), the volume is:

$$V = 4/3\,\pi \left(\frac{w}{2} \times \frac{h}{2} \times \frac{t}{2} \right)$$

$$= 4/3\,\pi \left(\frac{w \times h \times t}{8} \right)$$

$$= 0.52\,(w \times h \times t) \approx \frac{w \times h \times t}{2}$$

Normal values for maximum width, length, and thickness of the adult prostate are approximately 4.5, 3.5, and 2.5 cm, which accounts for a volume of 20 cm^3.

Benign prostatic diseases

Benign prostatic hypertrophy

Benign prostatic hypertrophy (BPH) is common after the age of 50 and is associated with voiding dysfunction. It is generally accepted that as many as 80% of men over 70 have an enlarged prostate and that BPH grows slowly and continuously. However, Watanabe has shown that the prevalence of BPH in Japan may be less than 25% and that the enlargement progresses in these cases rather rapidly and is completed within a few years [32]. Digital rectal examination reveals a smooth, enlarged prostate with characteristic preservation of its softness and symmetry. Palpable benign nodules are very different in consistency from the stone-hard malignant nodules. It must be noted that the severity of clinical symptoms may not be directly related to the prostatic volume.

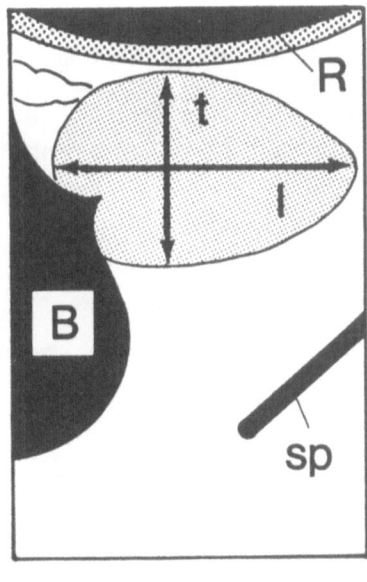

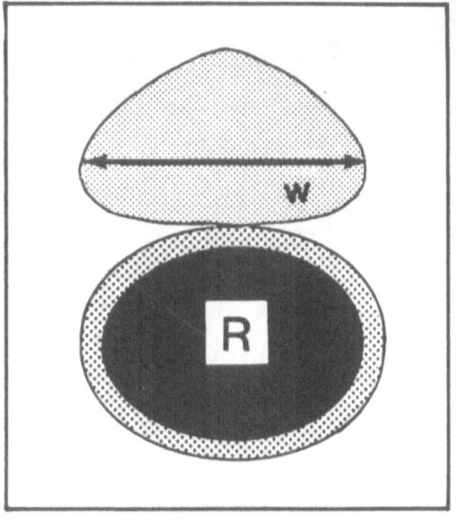

a   b

Figure 6.17. Prostatic volume determination using the formula for a prolate ellipsoid (see text for details). (a) Midsagittal section allows measurement of the maximum length l and thickness t of the prostate. (b) Transverse sonogram allows measurement of the maximum width w. B = bladder; R = rectum; sp = symphysis pubis.

80

Pathology

BPH develops from the transition zone. Bilateral anterolateral hyperplasia is most common. Hyperplastic nodules are mostly lateral to the urethra in early disease, whereas anterior nodules are predominant in massive enlargement. Except in subcervical hyperplasia, which results in the so-called enlarged median lobe, no nodules are found posterior to the urethra.

Hyperplastic nodules develop and coalesce into a single, often bilobed mass, which is separated by a more or less distinct cleavage plane from the rest of the prostate. The compressed, frequently atrophied, prostatic parenchyma represents the so-called prostatic shell or surgical (or false) capsule (Fig. 6.18). BPH grows concentrically with a predominant increase in the anteroposterior diameter, so that the prostatic shape changes from semilunar to spherical.

Microscopically, nodules may result from the hyperplastic development of any or all histologic components of the transition zone and preprostatic area, that is, glandular, connective or muscle tissue. Occasionally, fibromuscular hyperplasia is diffuse, without nodules.

Transverse scans

On transverse scans the enlarged prostate is oval to round (Fig. 6.19). Infrequently, a subtle

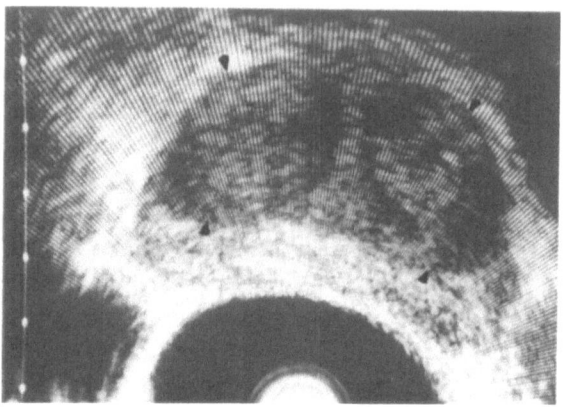

Figure 6.19. BPH. Transverse scan shows a rounded, symmetrical, enlarged prostate. The bilobar adenoma (arrowheads) is hypoechoic compared with the acinar prostate compressed posteriorly. (From ref. 27, with permission.)

asymmetry results from the anterolateral development of small subcapsular nodules. BPH usually shows a multinodular sonographic pattern; the nodules can be hypo-, iso-, or hyperechoic. A hypoechoic halo surrounding the nodules is sometimes demonstrated with the use of high-frequency transducers. In most cases the adenoma and the prostatic shell are clearly separated posteriorly. The general echogenicity of the adenoma varies from hypo- to hyperechoic compared with the rest of the prostate (Fig. 6.20). The texture of diffuse, nonnodular hyperplasia is slightly nonhomogeneous (Fig. 6.21) [27, 33].

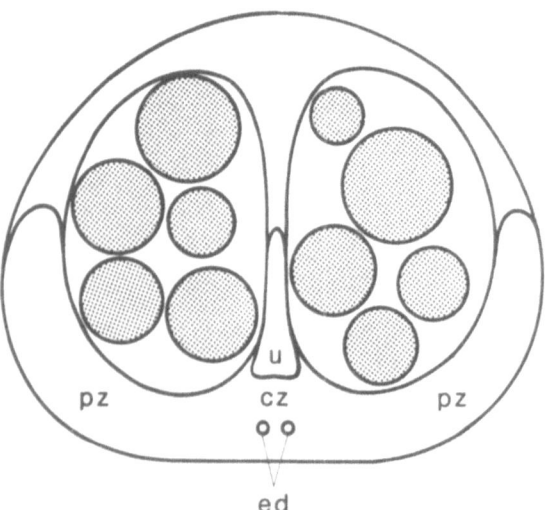

Figure 6.18. Diagram showing a multinodular, bilobar adenoma compressing the prostatic parenchyma peripherally. cz = central zone; ed = ejaculatory ducts; pz = peripheral zone; u = urethra.

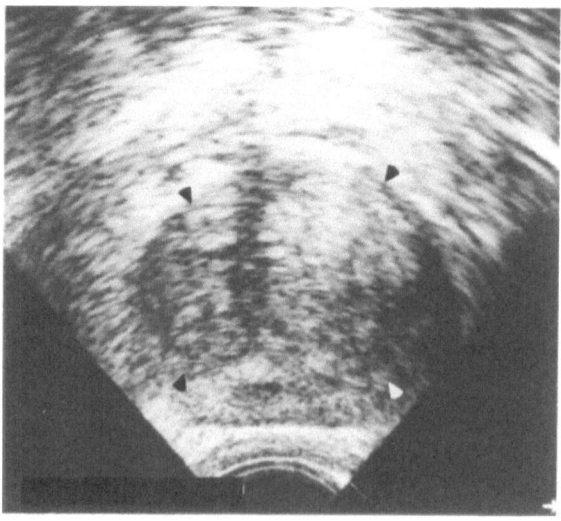

Figure 6.20. BPH. Transverse scan shows an adenoma (arrowheads) with markedly echogenic nodules.

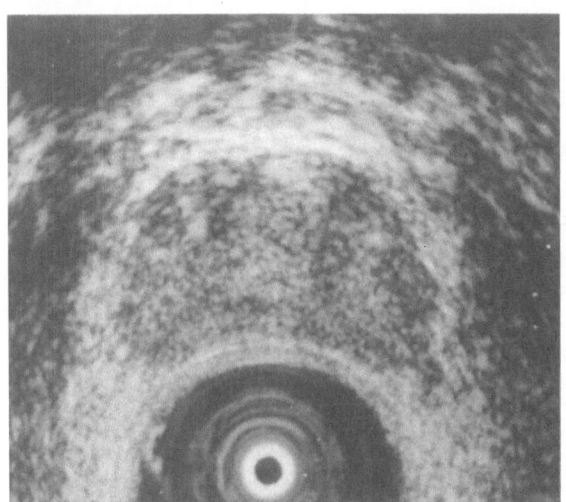

Figure 6.21. Diffuse BPH. Transverse scan shows a symmetrical, well-defined prostate. The whole prostate is diffusely involved with BPH and shows a diffusely nonhomogeneous texture.

Minute calculi (approximately 1 to 2 mm) often coexist with BPH. They lie along the urethra and ejaculatory ducts but are typically located posterior to the adenoma, in a chain-like arrangement (Fig. 6.22). They are only rarely found in the adenoma itself.

Longitudinal scans
Longitudinal scans better demonstrate the en-

larged median lobe protruding into the bladder and displacing the bladder neck (Fig. 6.23). As regards the echotexture, nodules are accurately demonstrated with the use of 7.5-MHz linear-array transducers (Fig. 6.24). The companion hypoechoic halo can also be demonstrated on longitudinal scans (Fig. 6.25) [34]. As on transverse scans, the separation between the adenoma and the homogeneous acinar prostate posteriorly is well seen (Fig. 6.26). Sagittal scans confirm the location of calculi along the urethra and the ejaculatory ducts and between the adenoma and the prostatic shell (Fig. 6.27).

When transverse and longitudinal scans are both performed, the volume of the adenoma can be accurately determined.

Prostatitis

Prostatitis is rarely confirmed pathologically; therefore, its sonographic appearance has rarely been evaluated in detail in the literature.

In *acute prostatitis*, the prostate is of normal size or moderately enlarged and its symmetry is usually maintained. Overall decreased echogenicity, an echo-free halo around an echogenic area

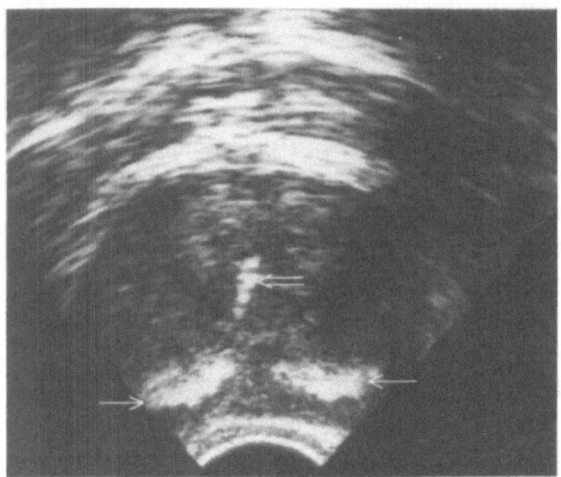

Figure 6.22. Calculi associated with BPH. Transverse scan shows the chain-like arrangement of small calculi (arrows) in the cleavage plane between the adenoma and the posterior prostate. Note some calculi along the urethra (open arrow).

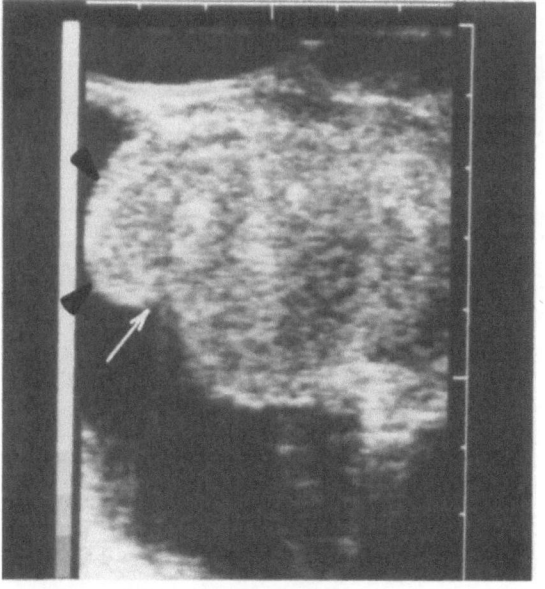

Figure 6.23. BPH with enlarged median lobe. Midsagittal section shows the enlarged median lobe (arrowheads) protruding in the bladder. The arrow points to the bladder neck. (From ref. 27, with permission.)

82

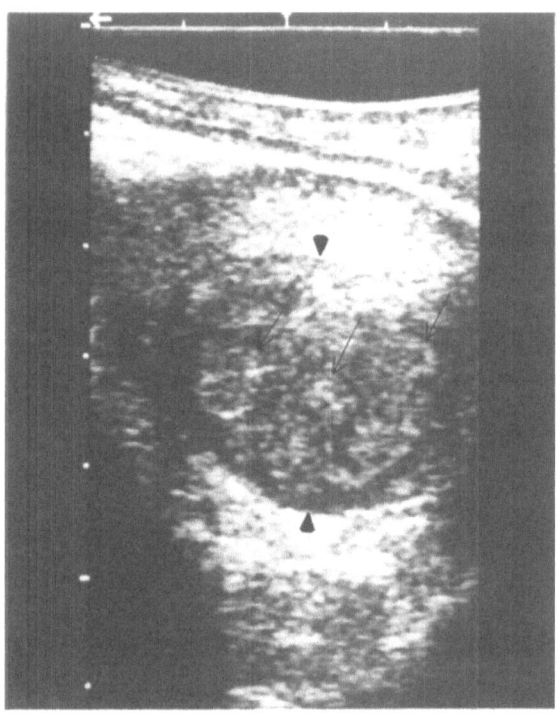

Figure 6.24. BPH. Longitudinal scan shows multiple iso-echoic nodules (arrows) within the adenoma (arrowheads). Note the homogeneous acinar prostate peripherally.

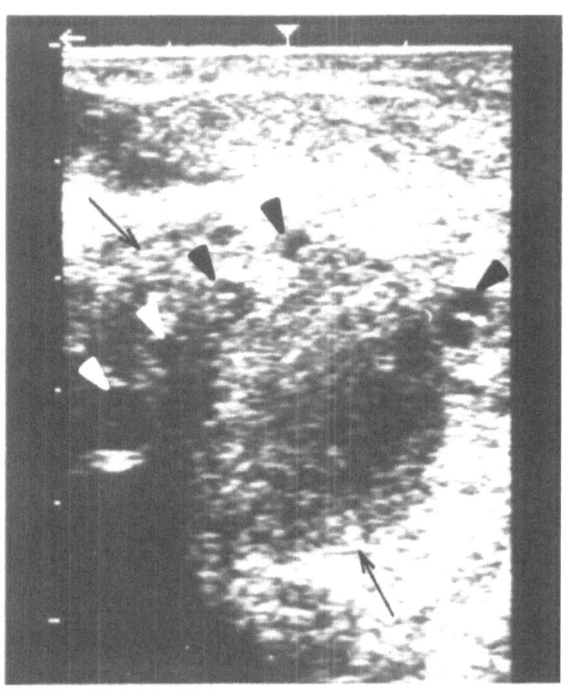

Figure 6.26. BPH. Longitudinal scan shows a hypoechoic adenoma (arrows), well demarcated from the peripheral prostate. Note minute cysts in the adenoma and in the peripheral prostate (arrowheads).

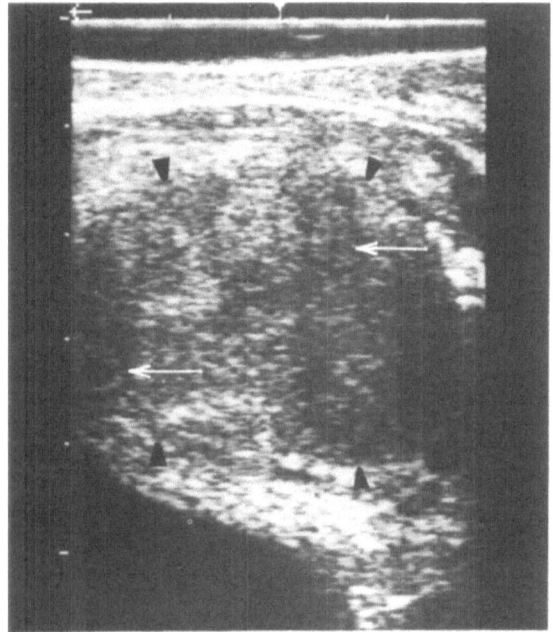

Figure 6.25. BPH. Midsagittal scan shows a multinodular adenoma (arrowheads), some nodules surrounded by a subtle hypoechoic halo (arrows).

in the periurethral zone of the prostate, multiple hypoechoic regions in the peripheral zone, and prominent periprostatic veins have been reported [35]. The seminal vesicles are occasionally swollen, deformed, or even involved by abscess formation.

In *chronic prostatitis*, the prostate is also of normal size or slightly enlarged. Deformity of the prostatic contours occasionally causes an asymmetrical pattern. The capsular continuity is usually maintained, although, exceptionally, blurring of the capsule has been found to mimic malignant infiltration (Fig. 6.28). Focal hypoechoic areas may be demonstrated in the peripheral gland, mimicking carcinoma (Fig. 6.29); however, areas of increased echogenicity, which probably represent fibrosis, can be found as well. Calculi secondary to previous episodes of acute inflammation may add to texture nonhomogeneity.

In patients over the age of 50, the major concern is the differentiation between chronic prostatitis and a cancer confined to the gland

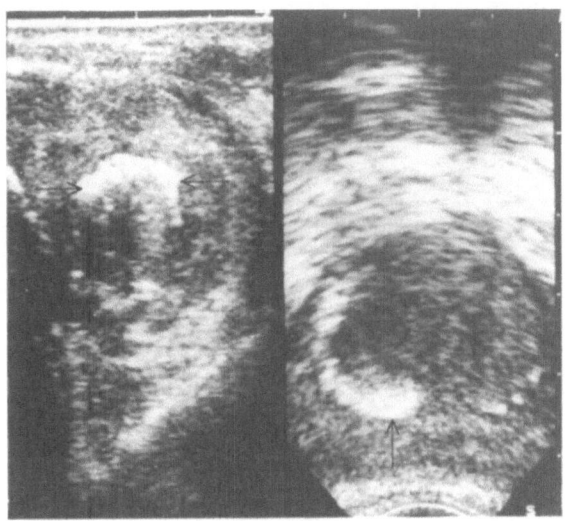

Figure 6.27. Calculi associated with BPH. Longitudinal (a) and transverse (b) scans obtained with a biplane probe show calculi (arrow) at the periphery of the adenoma.

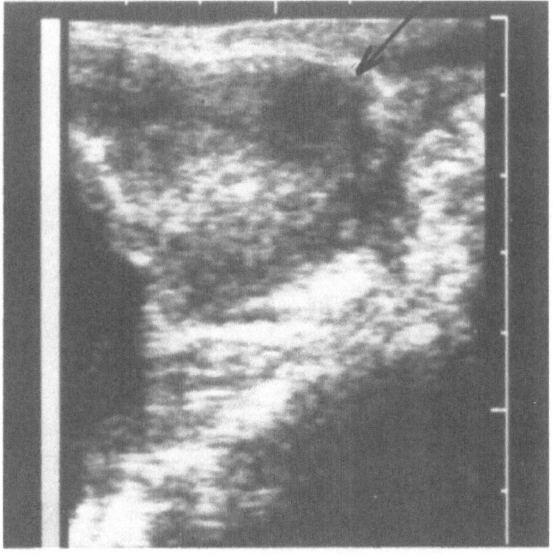

Figure 6.29. Chronic prostatitis. Longitudinal scan shows a hypoechoic area posterior to the apex (arrow) in a 32-year-old patient with a history of chronic prostatitis.

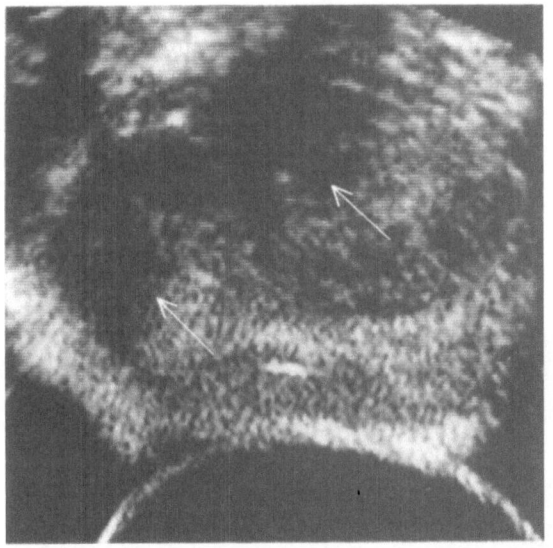

Figure 6.28. Chronic prostatitis. In vitro transverse scan of a cystoprostatectomy specimen shows a nonhomogeneous, multifocal hypoechoic area (arrows) involving the right lobe. Note the blurred capsule. Pathologic analysis confirmed granulomatous prostatitis and the absence of malignancy.

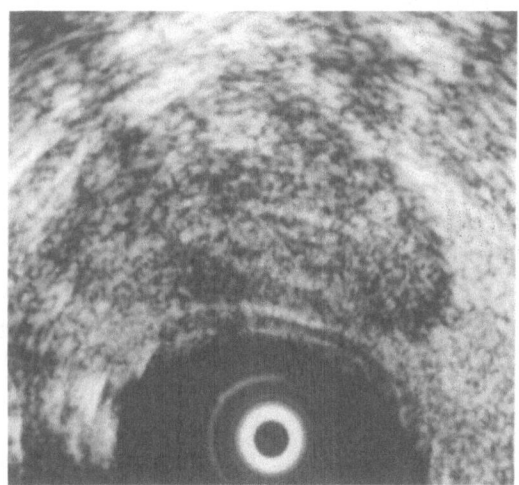

Figure 6.30. Chronic prostatitis. Transverse scan shows a nonhomogeneous prostate with slightly irregular and asymmetrical contours. This sonographic pattern could also represent a stage B2 carcinoma.

Prostatic calculi

(stage A or B cancer) (Fig. 6.30). When a hypoechoic focal area has been demonstrated, only ultrasonically guided biopsy can differentiate between focal prostatitis and early carcinoma. Transrectal sonography can also demonstrate concomitant seminal vesiculitis (Fig. 6.31).

Large stone clusters are seen as brightly echogenic foci clearly demarcated from the surrounding parenchyma, typically with an acoustic shadow (Fig. 6.32). They strongly support the diagnosis of chronic prostatitis in the appropriate clinical setting.

84

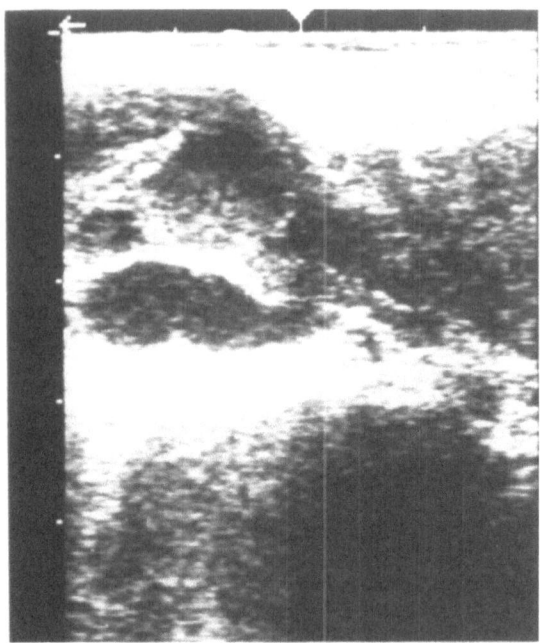

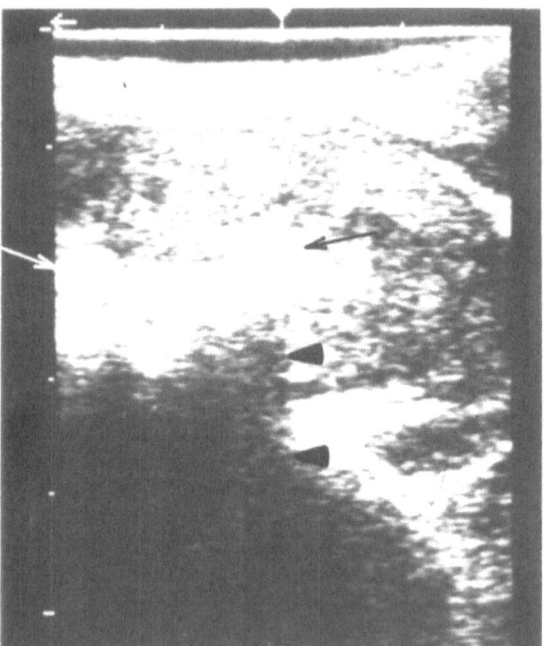

Figure 6.31. Chronic seminal vesiculitis. Longitudinal sonogram at 7.5 MHz shows a dilated, septated seminal vesicle (arrowheads). (From ref. 27, with permission.)

Figure 6.32. Chronic prostatitis with calculi. Longitudinal sonogram shows clustered calculi (arrows) with typical acoustic shadowing (arrowheads).

Small calculi (at most 2 to 3 mm in diameter) have been found in more than 50% of both normal and diseased prostates and are thought to represent calcifying corpora amylacea [36]. They appear as small echogenic dots and may cause a reverberating comet-tail artifact, instead of or in association with distal shadowing (Fig. 6.15). Minute calculi occasionally cluster and are seen as nonshadowing echogenic areas (Fig. 6.33).

Infrequently, transrectal sonograms demonstrate calculi or calcification in the seminal vesicles and along the vasa deferentia. In this situation, sequelae of previous infection should be considered. Whatever the size of the calcified material, acoustic shadowing is better seen with linear-array scanning than with radial or sector probes (Fig. 6.34) [20, 25, 37].

Abscess of prostate and seminal vesicles

Abscess formation may complicate an acute bacterial prostatitis, particularly in patients with diabetes mellitus. Prostatic abscesses appear as hypoechoic or sonolucent masses, usually with a thick wall, that may show septation or internal echoes (Fig. 6.35) [38—40]. Abscesses of the seminal vesicles are rare. They also have been described as thick-walled structures of complex echotexture [41, 42].

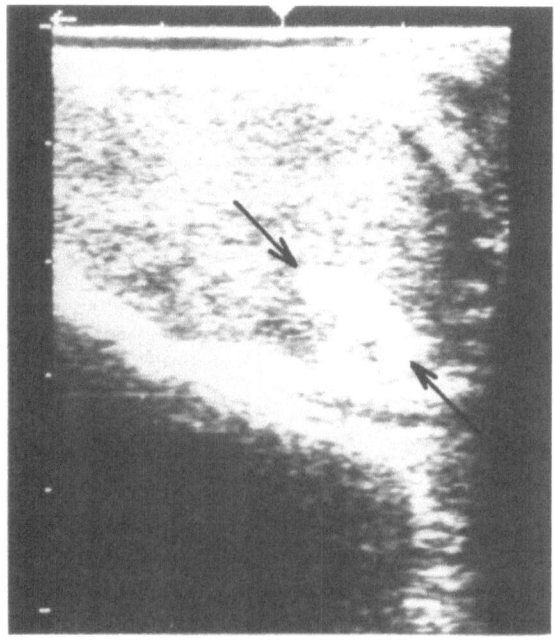

Figure 6.33. Chronic prostatitis. Longitudinal sonogram shows a nonshadowing cluster of minute calculi (arrows).

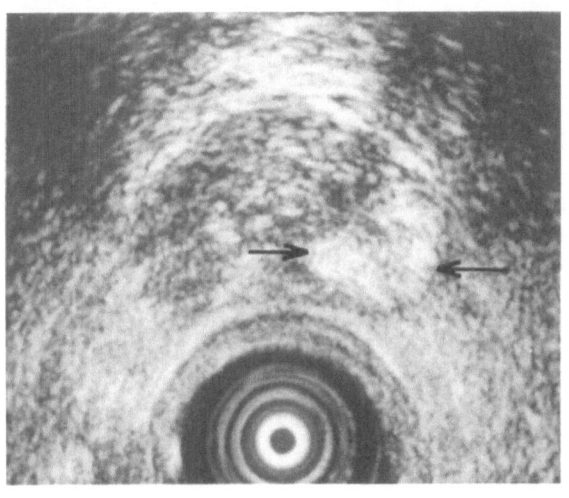
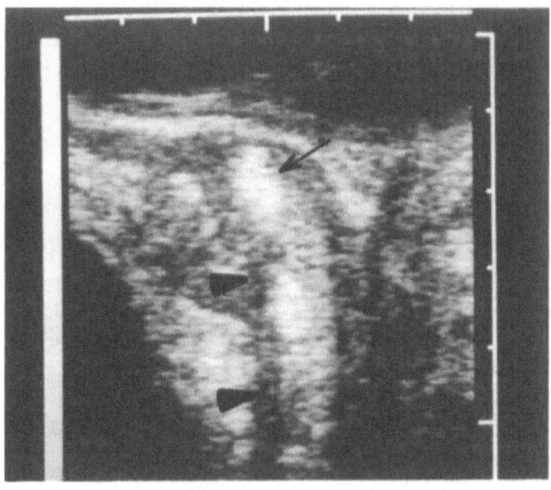

a　　　　　　　　　　　　　　　　b

Figure 6.34. Chronic prostatitis with calculi. (a) Transverse sonogram shows a markedly echogenic area in the left lobe (arrows). (b) Longitudinal sonogram of the left lobe confirms a densely echogenic focus (arrow) with a typical distal acoustic shadow (arrowheads).

Transperineal ultrasound-guided aspiration with culture of the aspirated fluid can readily confirm the abscess, and percutaneous drainage can be considered as an alternative to surgery in the case of unilocular abscess with nonviscous fluid.

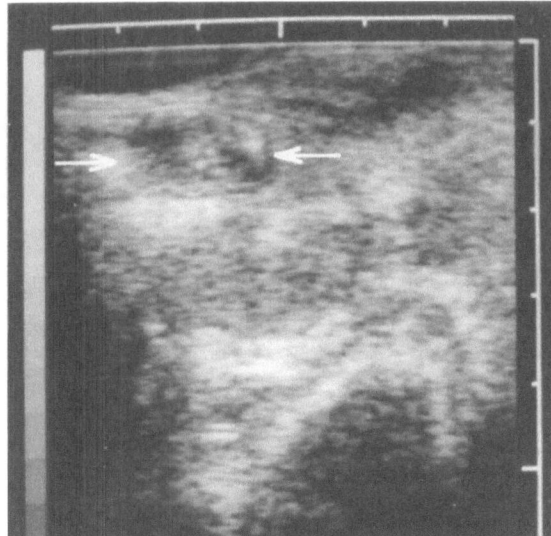

Figure 6.35. Asymptomatic prostatic abscess. Patient referred with lymph nodes involved by metastasis from an unknown primary. Digital rectal examination by the urologist was normal. Longitudinal scan shows a 15- × 10-mm area of mixed echogenicity in the posterior peripheral prostate (arrows). Ultrasound-guided transperineal biopsy yielded pus and a streptococcus was cultured. (From ref. 27, with permission.)

Prostatic cysts

Prostatic cysts that cause symptoms (e.g., urinary retention) are rare [43, 44]. However, cysts less than 1 cm in diameter (Fig. 6.36) have frequently been observed at necropsy [45]. Transrectal sonography can depict true retention cysts, most typically located in the peripheral prostate (Fig. 6.37). When a 7.5-MHz transducer is used, it is not uncommon to visualize dilated ducts and cysts as small as 2 or 3 mm (Fig. 6.38). Cysts

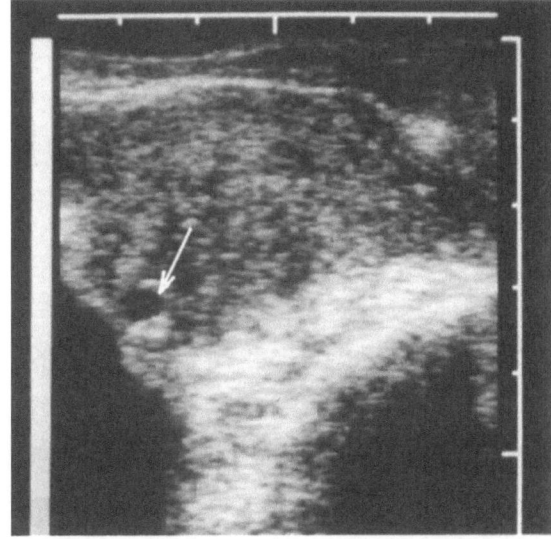

Figure 6.36. Small prostatic cyst. Longitudinal sonogram shows a well-defined, 5-mm cyst (arrow) in the vicinity of the bladder neck.

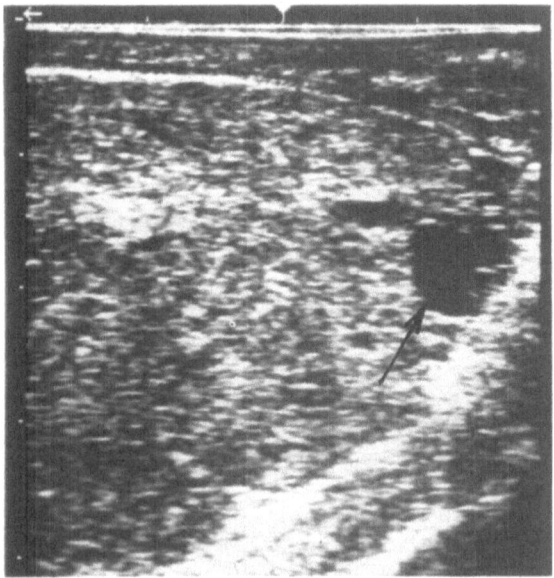

Figure 6.37. Small retention cyst. Magnified view of a longitudinal sonogram shows a well-defined, 7-mm cyst at the prostatic apex (arrow).

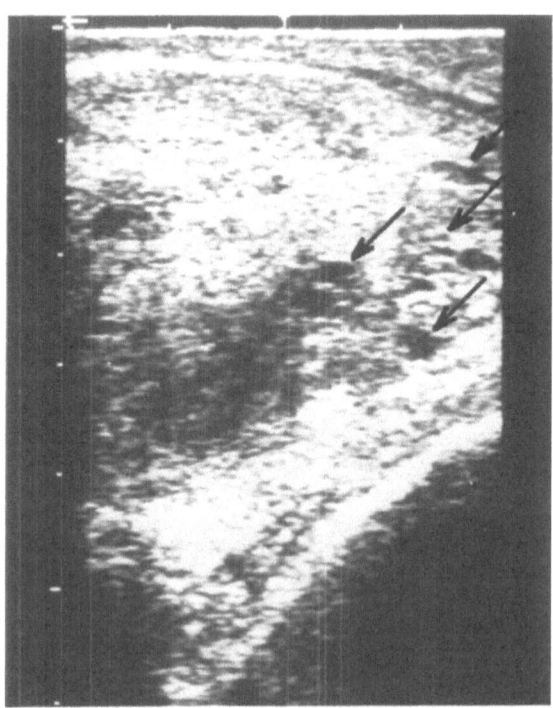

Figure 6.38. Dilated ducts and minute retention cysts. Longitudinal sonogram of the apex shows several 2- to 3-mm cystic structures (arrows), which represent dilated ducts and minute cysts.

smaller than 1 cm are frequently overlooked on suprapubic scans. Small cystic structures can also be seen within adenomas (Fig. 6.26).

The rare congenital cysts result from maldevelopment of the genitourinary tract. Utricular

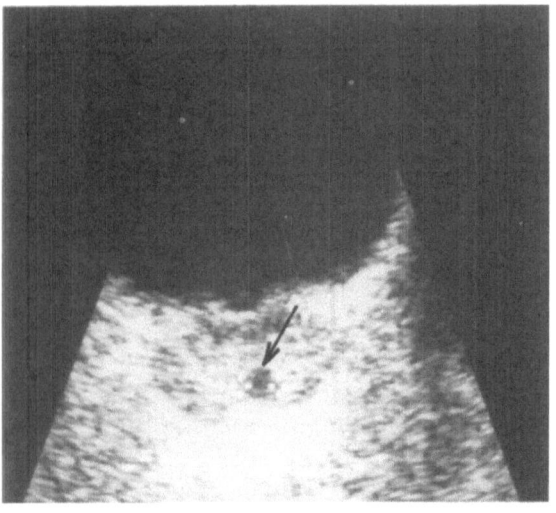

a

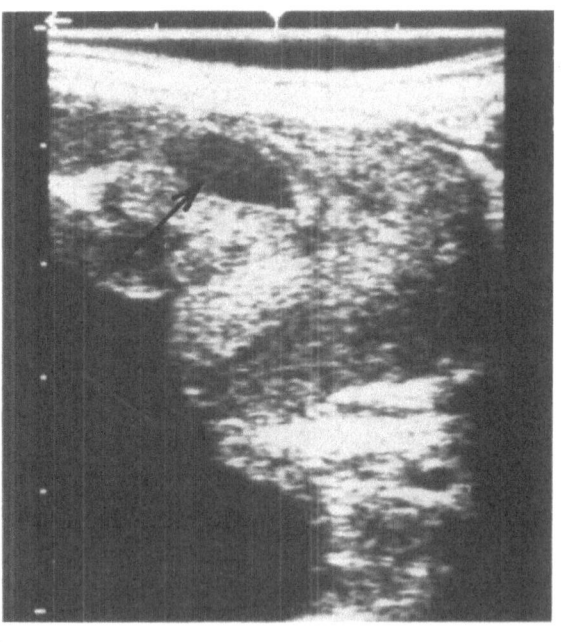

b

Figure 6.39. Small, nonpalpable utricular cyst. (a) Transverse suprapubic sonogram shows an ill-defined, midline posterior hypoechoic focus about 7 mm in diameter (arrow). (b) Midsagittal transrectal sonogram shows a well-defined utricular cyst (arrow).

and distal müllerian duct cysts are midline posterior structures [46, 47]. The utricular cyst is located close to the verumontanum (Fig. 6.39). It may not be possible to differentiate those cysts from ejaculatory ducts cysts without ultra-sound-guided aspiration and contrast medium injection. Seminal vesicle cysts are uncommon and usually congenital [48, 49]. Approximately two thirds are associated with ipsilateral renal agenesis.

Prostatic cancer

Prostatic cancer accounts for 21% of all cancers in men and now equals colorectal cancer as the second leading cause of cancer death in men. It is estimated that in 1989 there will be 103,000 new cases and 28,500 deaths from prostate cancer in the United States [50].

Pathology

Although the majority (70%) of prostatic adeno-carcinomas arise in the peripheral zone, approx-imately 20% are found in the transition zone and 10% in the central zone [26, 51].

In its classic presentation, early prostatic carcinoma is subcapsular, then it spreads cen-trally before penetrating the resistant capsule (Fig. 6.40) [52]. It is important to comprehend this progression to understand the sonographic patterns of prostatic cancer [53].

Clinical staging

Stage A
Stage A prostatic carcinoma is nonpalpable and confined to the gland. It is diagnosed incidentally by the pathologist in surgical material. Stage A1 refers to focal, well-differentiated lesions, whereas stage A2 designates multifocal or diffuse carcinomas, and any incidental lesions that are not well differentiated.

Stage B
In stage B, the tumor is palpable but still confined to the gland. Stage B1 tumors involve less than one lobe (including the discrete

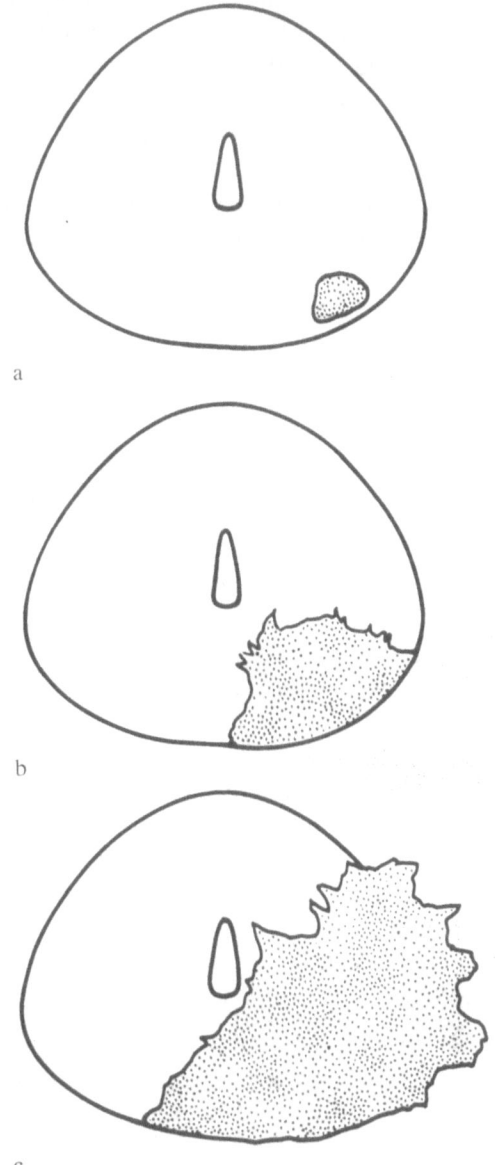

Figure 6.40. Diagram showing the patterns of progression of prostatic carcinoma. (a) Early cancer is subcapsular in location. (b) The carcinoma spreads centrally and causes the capsule to bulge slightly. (c) Finally, the tumor penetrates the capsule.

palpable nodule less than 1.5 cm in diameter). Stage B2 tumors involve more than one lobe.

Stage C
A stage C tumor extends beyond the capsule without metastases.

Stage D
In stage D, the primary tumor has produced distant metastases.

Some carcinomas may skip over stages. For example, a stage A2 carcinoma may produce metastases and turn directly into stage D [54]. But usually, prostatic cancer follows a predictable progression. It has been shown that the presence of metastasis is related to the volume of the tumor and the degree of capsule penetration [55]. Penetration through the capsule is the unequivocal criterion that separates the potentially curable stage A and B carcinomas from stage C tumors.

Sonographic patterns

Two points should be kept in mind when detection of early prostatic cancer is considered. First, there is obviously no chance of sonographically detecting malignant foci of microscopic size, and second, early cancer may be isoechoic, with 24% to 30% of early prostatic carcinomas going unrecognized on sonograms (Fig. 6.41) [56, 57].

Stage A carcinomas diagnosed on TURP are located in the vicinity of the urethra and include those arising in the transition zone. Stage B lesions often scan as subcapsular, more or less flattened hypoechoic areas (Figs. 6.42–6.44) [53, 56, 58]. Subcapsular nodules may also bulge locally and result in asymmetrical transverse scans. Stage B carcinomas that have spread

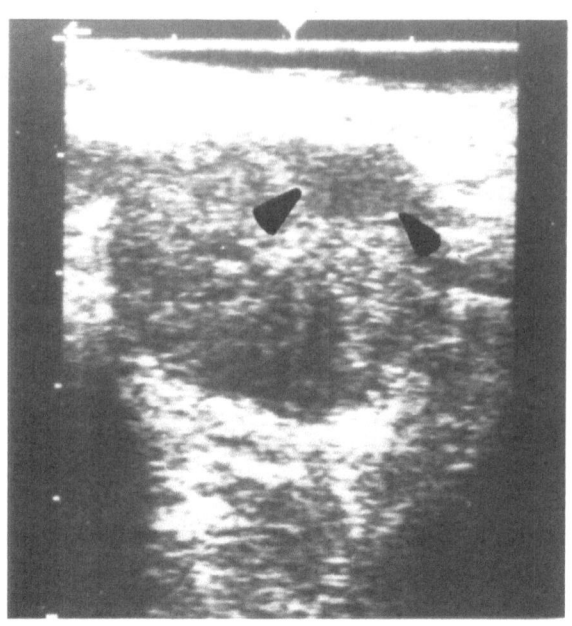

Figure 6.42. Early carcinoma. Longitudinal sonogram shows a small (about 1-cm), ill-defined, hypoechoic area (arrowheads) in the peripheral zone. The nodule bulges into the capsule and, although there is no overt penetration, microscopic invasion of the capsule cannot be totally excluded.

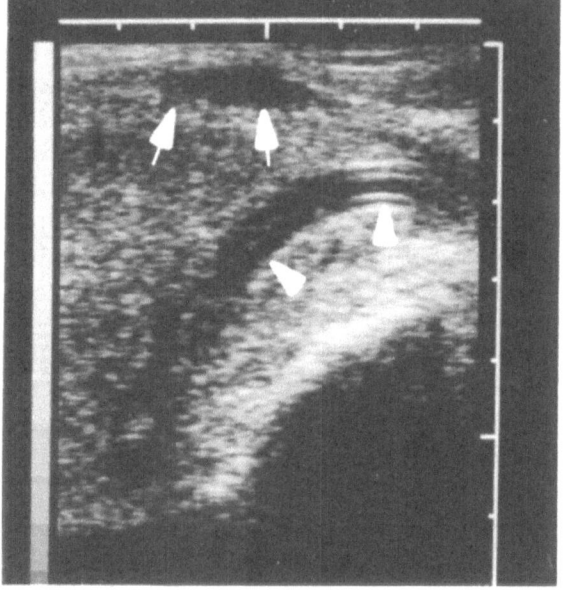

Figure 6.43. Nonpalpable prostate carcinoma associated with bulky BPH. Longitudinal scan shows a subcapsular, posterior, markedly hypoechoic carcinoma (arrows) that bulges into the capsule. Note also the bulky BPH and the Foley catheter (arrowheads). Microscopic invasion of the capsule was found at pathologic examination.

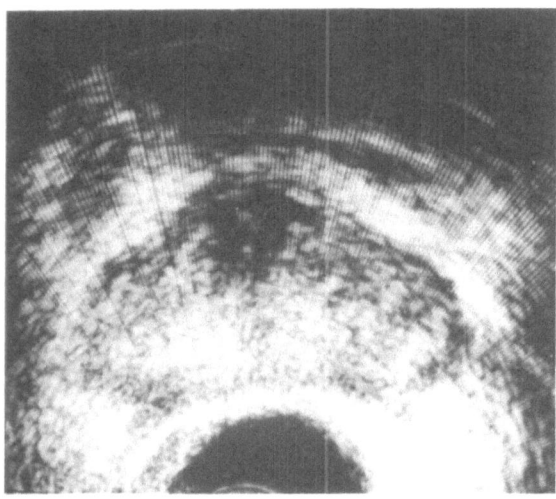

Figure 6.41. Isoechoic stage B1 cancer. Transverse sonogram in a patient with palpable, 1.5-cm malignant nodule in left lobe cannot delineate the tumor.

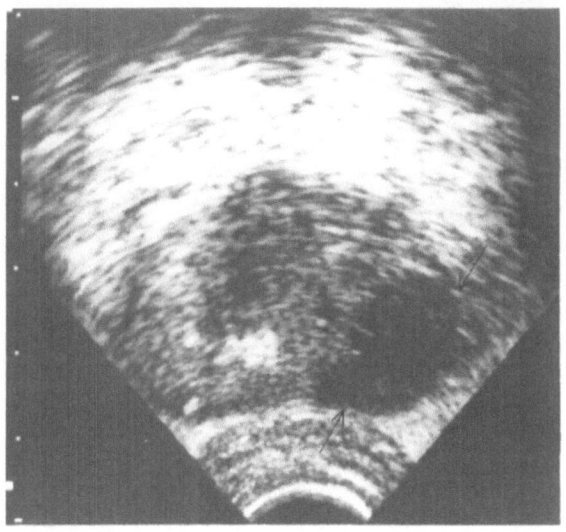

Figure 6.44. Prostatic carcinoma. Transverse scan shows a hypoechoic tumor (arrows) in the left peripheral zone.

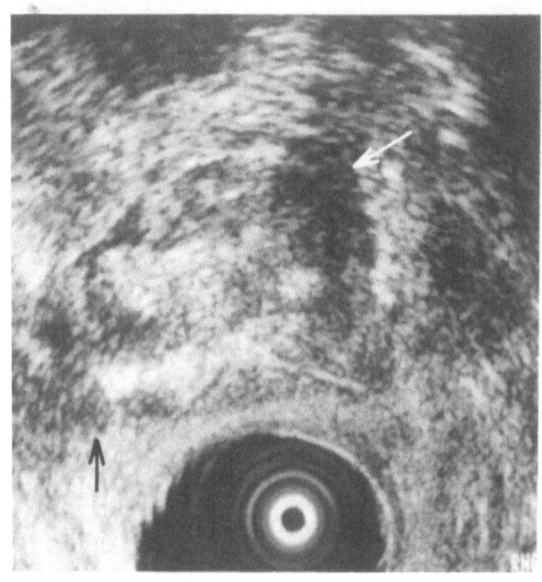

Figure 6.45. Stage C carcinoma. Transverse sonogram shows a markedly distorted prostate with mixed echotexture. Arrows point to capsular breaches.

through the gland (stage B2) often cause a diffusely nonhomogeneous mixed echo pattern, with areas of decreased or increased echogenicity; this is particularly the case when the hypoechoic carcinoma infiltrates into echogenic BPH areas. As a result, sonography can precisely delineate the malignant area only rarely.

Stage C carcinoma is often associated with a diffuse, primarily hypoechoic, nonhomogeneous echotexture and a poor delineation of the tumor itself. Contours are irregular and asymmetrical on transverse scans and capsular penetration is demonstrated (Figs. 6.45, 6.46). Involvement of the seminal vesicles may not be easily demonstrated. The obliteration of the sharp angle between the prostate and the vesicle is best seen on longitudinal scans (Fig. 6.47). Extension of prostatic cancer into the urinary bladder can be assessed on transrectal scans (Fig. 6.48) but is often demonstrated equally well and sometimes better using the suprapubic approach. Occasionally, prostatic carcinoma invades the rectal wall; this invasion is well demonstrated on transrectal scans (Fig. 6.49).

Most stage D cancers are locally advanced and present sonographically like stage C carcinomas. Occasionally, however, metastases may derive from a small, nonpalpable prostatic tumor.

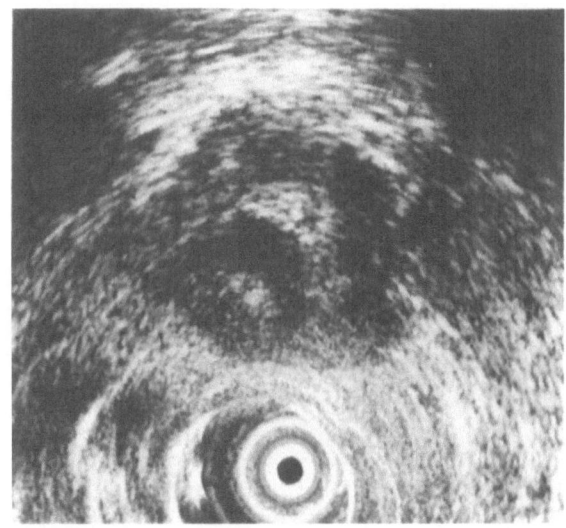

Figure 6.46. Stage C carcinoma. Transverse scan shows a markedly asymmetrical prostate with irregular contour. Note the central post-TURP defect.

Echogenicity of prostate cancer
The echogenicity of prostate cancer has been much debated. Early reports focused on echogenic tumors [13, 14, 16, 21–23]. These initial studies were performed using 3.5-MHz transducers and concerned large tumors. Recent studies with higher-frequency probes have indicated that the majority of early carcinomas

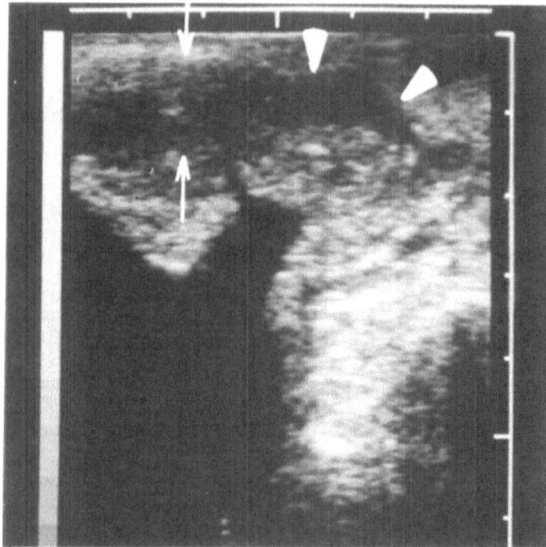

Figure 6.47. Stage C prostatic carcinoma invading the seminal vesicles. Midsagittal section shows a markedly hypoechoic carcinoma located in the posterior prostate (arrowheads), infiltrating into the seminal vesicles (arrows). Note the post-TURP defect.

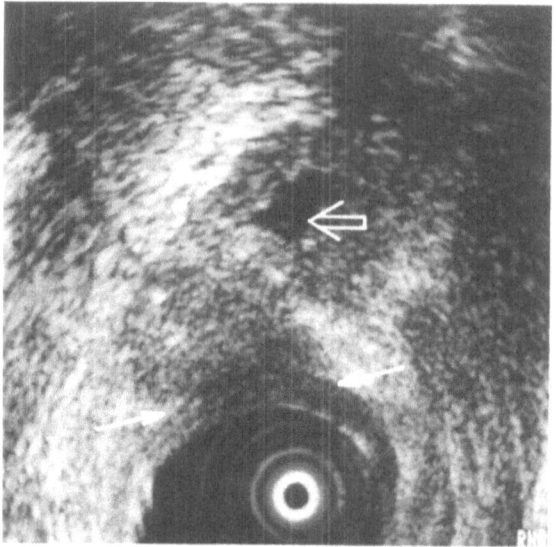

Figure 6.49. Stage C carcinoma infiltrating into the rectal wall. Transverse sonogram shows the hypoechoic malignant infiltration into the anterior rectal wall (arrows). Note the post-TURP defect (open arrow).

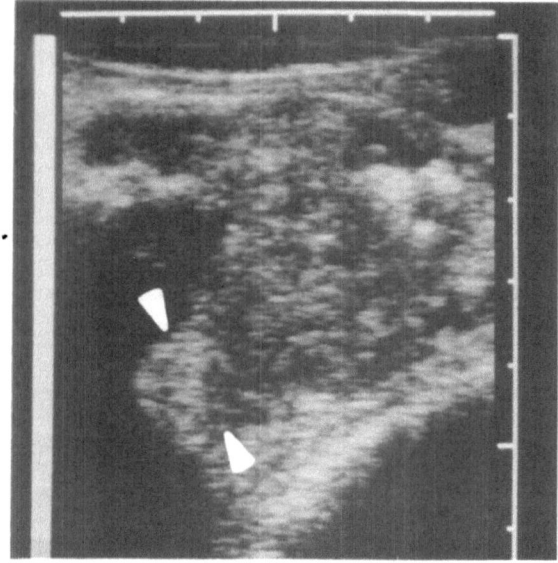

Figure 6.48. Stage C carcinoma. Sagittal section shows advanced prostatic carcinoma involving the whole prostate. The tumor extends anteriorly in the direction of the bladder (arrowheads). Note the post-TURP defect and the involvement of a seminal vesicle.

present as hypoechoic foci. As stated above, a significant number of small carcinomas are likely to be undetectable by ultrasound. The number of carcinomas that can be detected or missed when the presence of a small focal hypoechoic area in the peripheral prostate (and even more so in the whole gland) is used as the diagnostic criterion still needs to be evaluated. In a correlation between in vivo and in vitro sonograms and histopathologic mapping of whole-mounted prostates obtained at radical prostatectomy or cystoprostatectomy, (a) the sensitivity and specificity or ultrasound were as low as 50% and 52%, respectively, (b) all the early carcinomas correctly identified on the sonograms were hypoechoic, and (c) all incidental carcinomas less than 5 mm were isoechoic and could not be detected [59]. In the patients in this study whose diagnosis had been established by TURP rather than ultrasound-guided prostatic biopsy, it was not uncommon to find carcinoma *not* at the site of the hypoechoic area, but instead in a remote isoechoic area. This suggests further consideration of systematic additional random passes in contralateral, even normal-appearing areas during ultrasound-guided prostate biopsy.

The echogenicity of prostatic carcinoma may be related to tumor size. Small carcinomas tend to present as hypoechoic areas, while tumors that have grown and infiltrated into the normal (or more frequently, hyperplastic) central prostate result in patterns of mixed echogenicity [27, 33, 53, 60]. Although Lee *et al.* [53] and

Griffiths and associates [61] have reported no echogenic carcinomas, Salo *et al.* recently found 30% of carcinomas to be echogenic and 40% to be of mixed echogenicity in an in vitro study of radical prostatectomy specimens [57]. Therefore, the sonologist should be alert to any form of focal textural abnormality in the prostate.

Associated with the question of tumor echogenicity is the problem of the clear demarcation of the boundaries of the tumor on sonograms. Once again, extensive correlation between sonograms and pathologic mapping of radical prostatectomy specimens should provide objective data regarding the accuracy of sonography in the detection and measurement of prostate cancer.

Differential diagnosis

Although benign hyperplastic and malignant nodules are usually located in the internal or external prostate, respectively, it is now accepted that cancer can arise anywhere in the acinar prostate [26, 51].

The presence of a hypoechoic area in the prostate is routinely used as a diagnostic criterion for cancer. This finding is sensitive but has a low specificity; focal prostatitis, BPH, and even normal tissue may be associated with similar patterns [58]. Also, diffuse chronic prostatitis and a diffuse (stage B2) cancer confined to the gland may present with a similar overall non-homogeneous echotexture.

Postbiopsy changes may cause significant pitfalls [27] and therefore ultrasound, computed tomography (CT), or magnetic resonance (MR) examinations should always be performed prior to any prostatic needle biopsy.

Quantitative analysis of the prostatic geometry on transverse sonograms has been proposed [62] as a useful adjunct to the evaluation of textural changes in the differential diagnosis of prostatic diseases. This approach might be of great help when textural abnormalities are subtle, as is the case with isoechoic or diffuse carcinoma.

Accuracy of transrectal ultrasound versus digital rectal examination

In the diagnosis of palpable prostatic cancer, a very high sensitivity has been reported for both transrectal ultrasound and digital rectal examination, with a slight advantage for ultrasound [63]. However, the specificity of sonography in cases of palpable nodules is markedly superior to that of digital rectal examination, which barely exceeds 50% [63, 64].

Mass screening using transrectal ultrasound

Mass screening using ultrasound imaging should be geared toward the detection of subclinical (nonpalpable) lesions. Watanabe *et al.* have reported a 0.6% detection rate (6 cases in 1,071 examinations) of prostate cancer using a mobile screening unit [65]. Unfortunately, they provided no data about the size and clinical stage of those tumors detected with a chair-mounted, single-plane (transverse), 3.5-MHz scanner. In a recent series of 64 ultrasound-guided biopsies of suspicious abnormalities detected with state-of-the-art biplanar transrectal sonography in 784 self-referred men over 60 years, Lee *et al.* found 20 carcinomas, a detection rate of 2.6% twice as high as that of digital rectal examination [66]. Lesions detected with ultrasound had a mean size of 1.3 cm. However, there is no indication in this study of the location of the carcinoma, which is a crucial variable when comparing ultrasound and digital rectal examination. Also, because over twice as many patients were biopsied on the basis of ultrasound abnormalities versus digital examination findings, the superior detection rate of transrectal sonography might have been the result of chance alone [67].

The prevalence of stage A prostatic carcinoma and the proportion of these cancers that are amenable to sonographic detection are difficult to estimate. In mass screening, the low specificity of transrectal sonography (i.e., the high rate of false-positive results) would result in more ultrasound-guided biopsies of minute lesions, which may not be practical in many institutions. Also, the value of early detection of a biologically latent carcinoma has been questioned from a therapeutic viewpoint. However, well-controlled, experimental screening projects are needed to clarify all the uncertainties about this controversial topic [67].

Local staging

The distinction between stage B1 and stage B2 carcinomas is based on the extent of the tumor within the gland. Limitations of sonography in delineating tumor margins have already been noted above. The prostatic capsule is the frontier between stage A/B carcinomas, which are potentially curable, and stage C carcinomas, which are not. The capsule can be assessed with great accuracy when 7.5-MHz transducers are used.

Transrectal sonography can disclose a capsular breach in patients diagnosed by palpation alone to have carcinoma confined to the gland. Indeed, 28% to 44% of clinically stage B cancers are revealed as stage C tumors with transrectal sonography (Fig. 6.50) [16, 63, 68, 69]. Sonography can thus confirm candidates for radical surgery.

Pathologic evidence of malignant invasion of seminal vesicles is a well-known indicator of poor prognosis in patients with carcinoma clinically confined to the gland [70]. The accuracy of transrectal sonography in the detection of seminal vesicle invasion needs further evaluation.

Sonographic evaluation of response to therapy

Most prostate cancer ultrasound studies have focused on detection and diagnosis. However, sonography also plays a basic role in evaluating

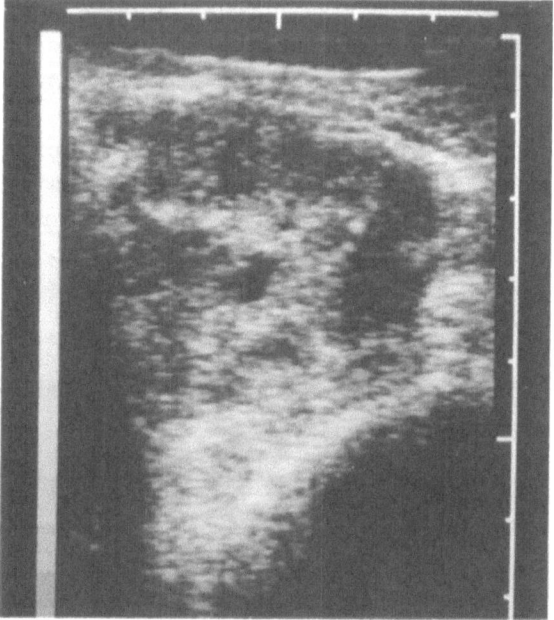

a

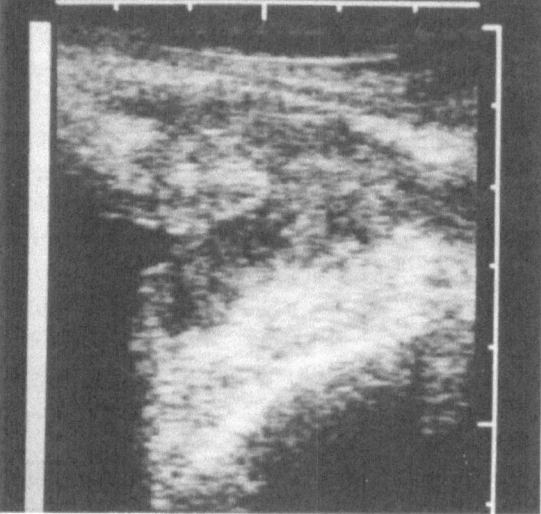

b

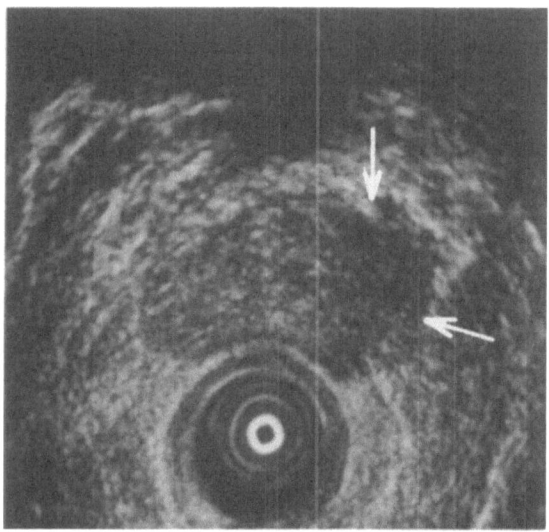

Figure 6.50. Prostate cancer. Transverse sonogram shows the left anterior transcapsular infiltration (arrows). This stage C carcinoma was classified stage B clinically.

Figure 6.51. Stage C carcinoma. Evaluation of response to treatment. (a) Pretreatment longitudinal sonogram shows a large, nonhomogeneous prostate. (b) Longitudinal sonogram performed 4 months after orchiectomy. There is marked shrinkage of the prostate, which is better demarcated. Also, the prostatic texture is more homogeneous.

the effects of endocrine therapy, radiation therapy, and chemotherapy. Carpentier *et al.* by transrectal ultrasound found mean volume decreases in prostatic volume following orchiectomy of 37% and 46% after periods of 3 and 9 months, respectively (Fig. 6.51) [71]. More recently, Kojima *et al.* used transrectal ultrasound to document the response of prostate cancer to the administration of a luteinizing hormone-releasing hormone (LHRH) analogue [72]. After radiotherapy, the volume decrease is less dramatic than after orchiectomy [73].

Textural alterations are associated with prostate shrinkage. For example, focal lesions tend to homogenize with the rest of the gland. In responsive patients with stage C disease, reformation of the capsule is noted [73], although prostatic contours usually remain more or less blurred. It has also been reported that invaded seminal vesicles are revisualized as discrete structures in some patients who respond to therapy [74].

After the prostatic volume has decreased and stabilized, any focal abnormality or increase in overall prostatic volume is a strong indicator of local recurrence. Nonpalpable local recurrence after radiation therapy or when the lesion develops anteriorly can be diagnosed by transrectal sonography.

In summary, the roles of transrectal sonography in patients with prostate cancer are: (a) early diagnosis through guided biopsies, (b) improved local staging as a result of the accurate demonstration of capsule penetration, (c) evaluation of the local response to treatment, and (d) follow-up of patients in clinical remission with early detection of local recurrence [75].

Intra- and postoperative endosonographic patterns

Transurethral ultrasound can be used to monitor TURP. Transverse scans are obtained by replacing the resector with the transurethral radial probe through the same sheath. The scans provide a direct view of the resection cavity and of the prostatic tissue that remains to be resected (see Chapter 7). Transrectal ultrasound has also

been used to monitor the extent of the frozen volume during transurethral cryosurgery. The iceball is characterized by a strong reflection from its proximal surface, trailed by a marked acoustic shadow [27].

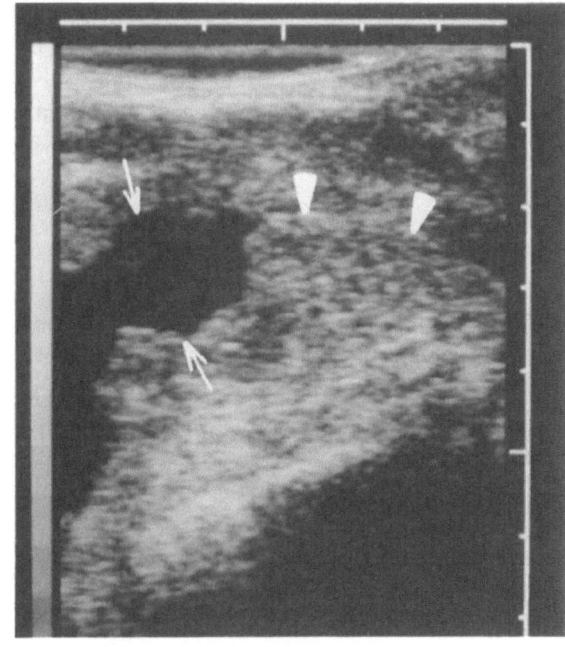

Figure 6.52. Sonographic pattern after TURP. Midsagittal scan shows the cavity from a recent resection (arrows) in communication with the bladder. Note also the collapsed remaining prostatic urethra (arrowheads).

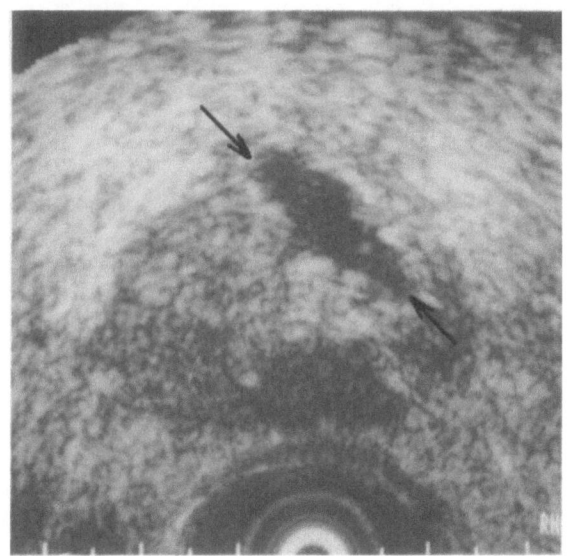

Figure 6.53. Post-TURP defect. Transverse sonogram shows an asymmetrical, irregular resection cavity (arrows). Note the echogenic margins of the cavity.

94

Sonography after open prostatectomy for BPH shows a rounded postoperative cavity corresponding to the excised adenoma, surrounded by the remaining surgical capsule. Post-TURP cavities show greater variability in shape (Fig. 6.52). Not infrequently, the margins of the defect are echogenic; this might represent post-traumatic granulomatous tissue (Fig. 6.53). The shape and size of the post-TURP defect also vary with time in a way that has yet to be quantified.

Ultrasound-guided biopsy of the prostate

Transrectal sonography has proved to be an accurate technique for guiding the biopsy of both palpable and nonpalpable prostatic lesions.

Transperineal biopsy

Technique using a radial probe
The technique of utilizing an endorectal radial probe to guide transperineal biopsy was first described by Holm and Gammelgaard in 1981 [76]. The patient is placed in the lithotomy position, and the probe is inserted in the rectum. The lesion to be sampled is visualized. A multichannel guide designed to maintain the needle parallel to the probe is attached to the shaft of the probe. After local anesthesia of the perineum, the needle is inserted through the guide transperineally until it reaches the transverse scan plane, where its cross section is seen as a brightly echogenic focus, in most cases associated with a comet-tail artifact (Figs. 6.54, 6.55) [77, 78]. The major disadvantage of this technique is that the cross section of the needle is visualized, but *not* its extremity, which may lie beyond the scan plane and possibly outside the lesion.

Technique using a linear-array probe
In 1983, we developed the technique of transrectal guidance of transperineal biopsy using a linear-array probe [19]. With the patient in the lithotomy position, the needle is inserted transperineally, parallel to the probe. As it enters the

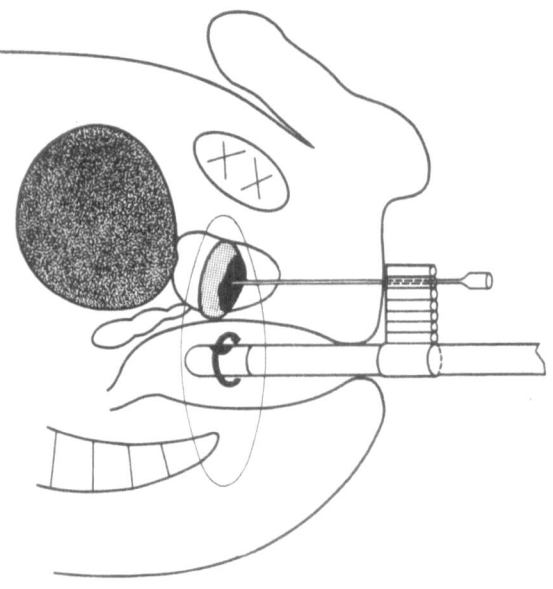
a

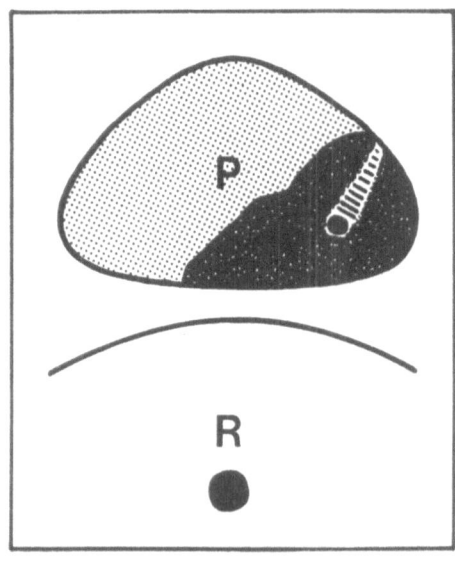
b

Figure 6.54. Technique of ultrasound-guided transperineal biopsy of the prostate using an endorectal radial transducer. (a) Diagram showing the transperineal needle penetrating the lesion displayed on the transverse scan plane. (b) Diagrammatic representation of the sonogram as displayed on the video monitor. The cross section of the needle is seen as a bright focus associated with a comet-tail artifact. P = prostate; R = rectum.

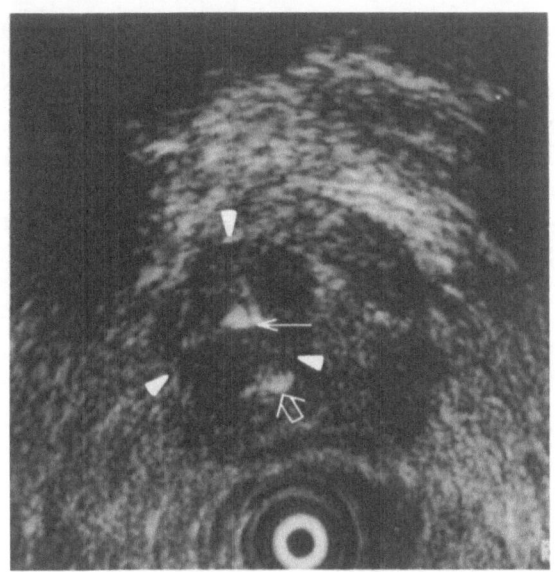

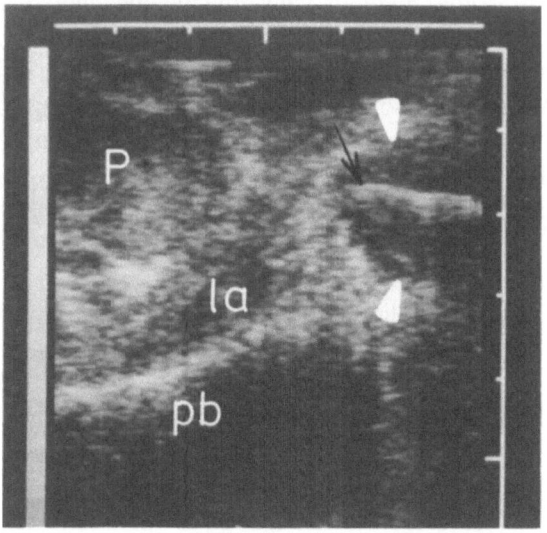

Figure 6.55. Ultrasound-guided transperineal biopsy of the prostate using an endorectal radial transducer. Transverse sonogram shows the echogenic cross section of the needle (arrow) in a hypoechoic mass (arrowheads). The needle can be differentiated from adjacent calculi (open arrow) because of the distal comet-tail artifact associated with it.

Figure 6.57. Ultrasound-guided transperineal biopsy using an endorectal linear-array transducer. The longitudinal sonogram allows continuous monitoring of the tip of the needle (arrow). Scan obtained during local anesthetization of the perineum shows the hypoechoic anesthetic fluid (arrowheads) around the tip of the needle. la = levator ani muscle; P = prostate; pb = pubic bone.

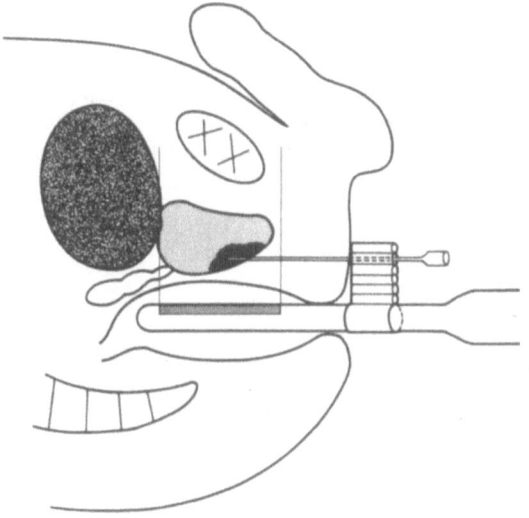

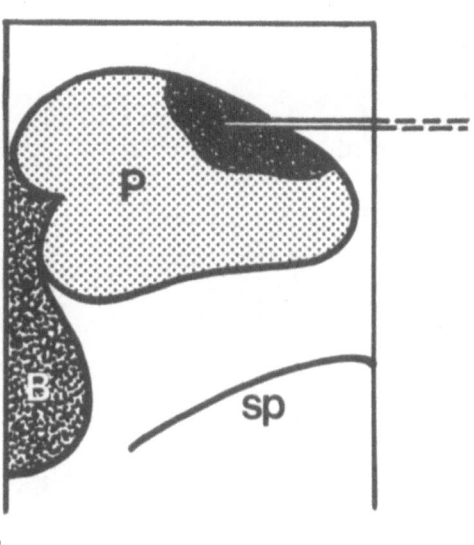

a

b

Figure 6.56. Technique of ultrasound-guided transperineal biopsy of the prostate using an endorectal linear-array transducer. (a) Diagram showing the transperineal needle penetrating the lesion as displayed on the longitudinal scan plane. (b) Diagrammatic representation of the sonogram as displayed on the video monitor. The image on the screen is reversed from top to bottom. The whole distal portion of the needle is visualized as an echogenic line. B = bladder; P = prostate; sp = symphysis pubis.

ultrasound field of view, the needle, which is perpendicular to the ultrasound beam, is seen as a highly reflective linear structure. Longitudinal scans allow continuous real-time monitoring of the tip of the needle, which makes the procedure accurate and safe (Figs. 6.56—6.59) [23, 24, 27, 34, 78, 79].

Technique using a biplane probe
Because it allows longitudinal and transverse scans to be displayed alternately, the biplane endorectal ultrasound probe provides optimal three-dimensional guidance for transperineal biopsies.

Needle guides designed to maintain the needle strictly parallel to the probe (Fig. 6.60) are useful when rigid large-bore needles are used. However, with fine needles, aspiration biopsy is best performed using the free-hand technique, by which it is easier to reposition the deviated flexible needle [27, 79].

Transrectal biopsy

Transrectal needle biopsy of the prostate can be guided by real-time transrectal sonography.

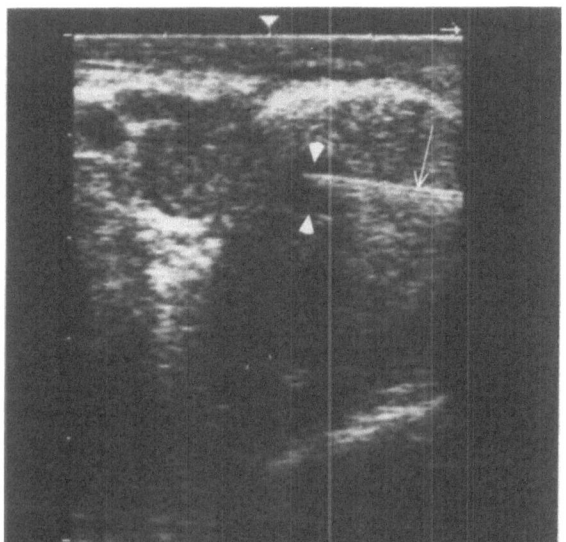

Figure 6.58. Ultrasound-guided transperineal fine-needle aspiration biopsy of the prostate using a linear-array transducer. The fine needle (arrow) penetrates a well-defined, 8-mm hypoechoic area in the peripheral zone (arrowheads). No malignancy was found on cytology.

Several probes — including linear-array (Fig. 6.61) and mechanical or phased-array sector (Fig. 6.62) transducers — are now available to provide this guidance in a longitudinal plane. End-firing endovaginal probes equipped with the needle guide for oocyte recovery can also be used for transrectal biopsy in either the sagittal or oblique transverse planes. Automatic spring-

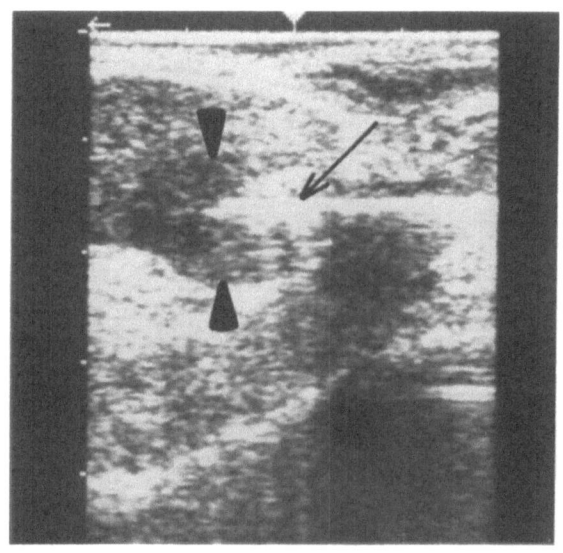

Figure 6.59. Ultrasound-guided transperineal biopsy of the prostate using a linear-array transducer and a 18-g Tru-Cut needle with a dedicated spring-loaded automatic biopsy device (Biopty instrument, Bard). The needle (arrow) is clearly visualized as a double-line pattern as it penetrates a hypoechoic area involving the anterior apex (arrowheads). No malignant tissue was found at pathologic analysis.

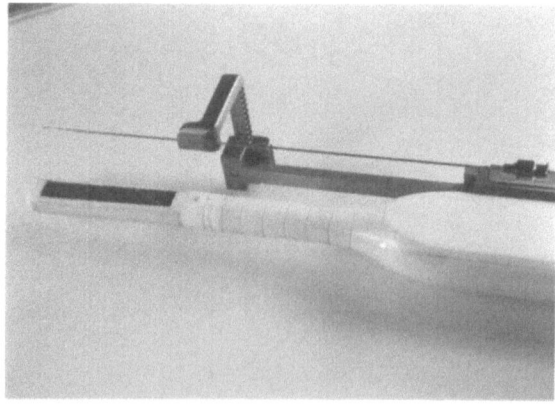

Figure 6.60. Adjustable needle guide for transperineal prostatic biopsy, attached to a linear-array transducer. Three channels of different size allow the use of a 22-, 18-, or 14- gauge needle. (From ref. 27, with permission.)

complications (including fatal sepsis) compared with the transperineal technique.

Indications for ultrasound-guided prostate biopsy

Indications for ultrasound-guided prostate needle biopsy include (a) diagnosis of masses whose nature is indeterminate on palpation, (b) characterization of nonpalpable sonographic focal abnormalities (other than typical cysts or calculi), which may indicate early-stage cancer, (c) pathologic confirmation of a clinically advanced cancer, prior to the initiation of therapy, and (d) early diagnosis of local recurrence. Because the incidence of hypoechoic focal areas in the prostatic parenchyma is high with the use of high-frequency transducers, ultrasound-guided biopsies are being used with increasing frequency to rule out early nonpalpable carcinoma. However, it has been shown that hypoechoic lesions smaller than 1.5 cm with normal digital rectal examination and prostate-specific antigen level are at low risk for cancer and therefore may not need to be biopsied [81].

Therapeutic applications of transperineal ultrasound-guided punctures of the prostate include (a) aspiration of symptomatic cysts, (b) percutaneous large-bore needle drainage of abscesses of the prostate and seminal vesicles (with the possible direct instillation of antibiotics into the abscess cavity) as an alternative to surgical drainage, and (c) percutaneous implantation of radioactive seeds in the prostatic tumor [82].

Transrectal voiding cystourethrosonography

With the patient in the lateral decubitus or the erect position, the endorectal linear-array probe is oriented so as to display the midsagittal section of the bladder neck and the prostate. The patient is then asked to urinate. Real-time examination monitors the entire micturition sequence, from bladder neck opening to urethral collapse [20, 28, 83]. Advantages of this procedure include real-time, cross-sectional imaging; visualization of surrounding soft tissues; and absence of irradiation and contrast medium. When the prostatic urethra is fully distended, the antero-

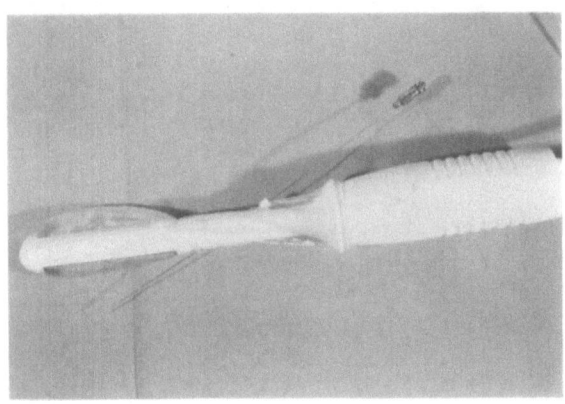

a

b

Figure 6.61. Transrectal fine-needle aspiration of the prostate using transrectal ultrasound guidance. (a) Endorectal linear-array transducer characterized by an oblique channel through the shaft of the probe, allowing passage of the transrectal biopsy needle. (b) Transrectal longitudinal sonogram. The transrectal biopsy needle enters the ultrasonic field of view obliquely and is seen as an echogenic line (arrows). Its tip has reached a hypoechoic carcinoma (arrowheads) that involves the posterior prostate and the seminal vesicles. (From ref. 27, with permission.)

loading biopsy instruments for transrectal cutting needle biopsy have recently been introduced (Fig. 6.62).

The transrectal technique offers the shortest path to the lesions — particularly to carcinomas, which often involve the posterior peripheral prostate [80]. However, transrectal biopsy of the prostate is associated with a greater risk of septic

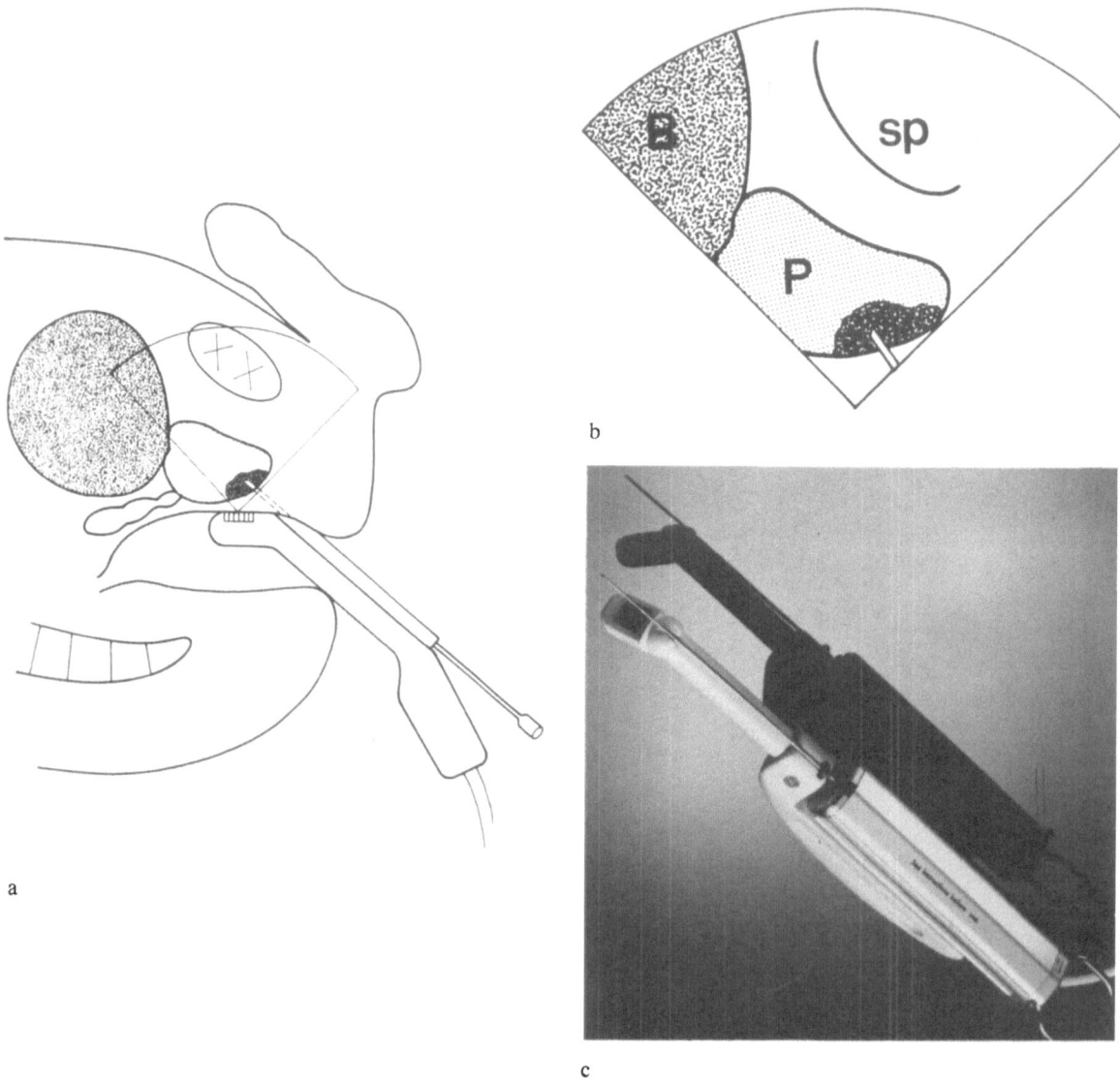

Figure 6.62. Transrectal prostate needle biopsy using transrectal ultrasound guidance. (a) Diagram showing the endorectal phased-array sector probe in place in the rectum and the path of the needle through the rectal wall, then into the prostate. (b) The biopsy needle enters the longitudinally oriented sector field of view obliquely and appears as an echogenic line. B = bladder; P = prostate; sp = symphysis pubis. (c) Endorectal phased-array sector probe equipped with an automatic device for large-bore cutting-needle prostatic biopsy. (Courtesy of General Electric Medical Systems.)

posterior diameter is about 5 to 7 mm; the verumontanum is seen as a bulge in the posterior urethral wall (Fig. 6.63).

In BPH, transrectal voiding sonography demonstrates the deviation and compression of the urethra by the adenomatous nodules (Fig. 6.64). The prostatic urethra infiltrated by cancer shows markedly irregular margins and an invariable stiffness during micturition. Bladder neck contracture, prostatic cysts, urethral stones and papillomas are less frequent causes of obstruction that can be evaluated by voiding cystourethrosonography [27]. In patients with neuromuscular bladder dysfunction, transrectal voiding sonography has proved useful in evaluating the response to various therapeutic agents. This in turn permits a precise calibration of dosages [84].

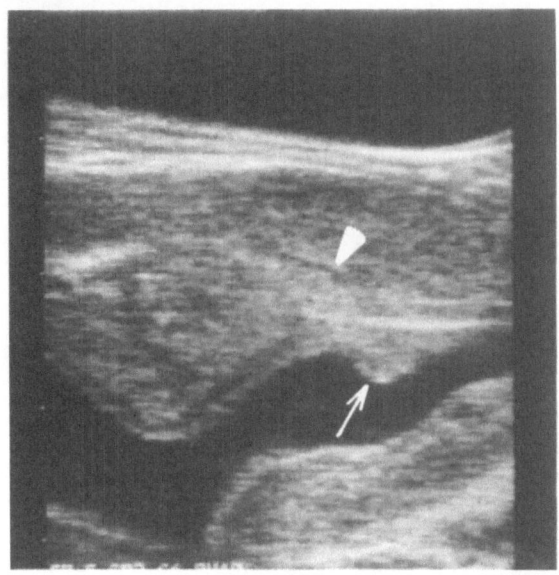

Figure 6.63. Normal transrectal voiding cystourethrosonography. Midsagittal sonogram obtained with a 7.5-MHz linear-array transducer shows the distended prostatic urethra. Note the course of an ejaculatory duct (arrowhead) and the verumontanum (arrow) on the posterior wall of the urethra.

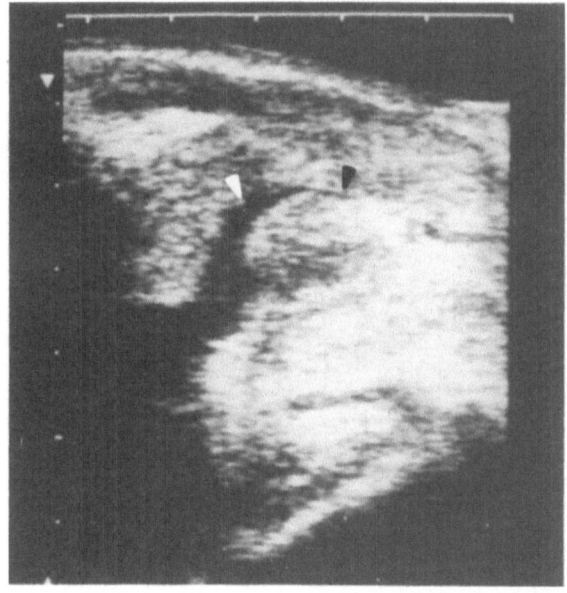

Figure 6.64. Transrectal voiding cystourethrosonography in a patient with BPH. A BPH nodule deviates the prostatic urethra posteriorly (arrowheads). (From ref. 27, with permission.)

Transrectal sonography *vis-à-vis* other imaging modalities for the prostate

Transrectal sonography is a highly accurate way to depict normal and pathologic prostatic anatomy. The axial resolution of the recently developed 7.5-MHz transducers is better than 0.5 mm. Fluid collections and stones are readily characterized. Ultrasound can detect the textural changes associated with carcinoma in lesions above a certain size (somewhat below 1 cm in diameter — i.e., 0.5 cm^3 in volume). Sonography, like other imaging modalities, cannot detect microscopic lesions. Sonography is the only real-time cross-sectional imaging technique and it can therefore be used for voiding studies and real-time guidance of biopsy needles. Biplane probes now allow immediate switching from a transverse view to a sagittal one. Transrectal sonography is harmless and, compared with CT and MR, quickly performed (particularly when biplane probes are used). The limitations of transrectal ultrasound include its restricted field of view, which precludes the evaluation of bulky tumors, its inability to detect lymphatic spread, and reliance on an experienced operator.

CT cannot differentiate between normal and malignant tissue within the prostate. A recent report has emphasized its inaccuracy in staging prostate carcinoma [85].

MR imaging of the prostate can depict the zonal anatomy of the prostate with great accuracy, separating McNeal's central and peripheral zones [86, 87]. However, no specific MR parameter enables differentiation between benign and malignant changes [88, 89], and a low sensitivity (67%) has been reported in the diagnosis of prostatic carcinoma in a series of stage B1 and B2 lesions [90]. The diagnostic accuracy of MR might be improved by the use of endorectal surface coils [91]. The capability of multiplanar imaging makes MR effective in staging prostatic carcinoma [92, 93]. While MR and CT are often compared, few comparisons have been made between MR and transrectal sonography.

100

Prospects

Clearly, there is a role for transrectal sonography in the diagnosis and local staging of palpable cancer, in guiding needle biopsies, and in monitoring the response of cancer to treatment. However, large-scale correlations between transrectal sonograms, ultrasound-guided needle biopsies, in vitro sonograms, and pathologic mapping of radical prostatectomy specimens (Fig. 6.65) are still needed to evaluate the accuracy of transrectal sonography in the detection of early nonpalpable prostatic carcinoma.

With 7.5-MHz biplane probes, endorectal sonographic equipment has probably come to maturity, and few advances in image processing that could result in greater diagnostic accuracy are expected in the near future. Thus, early diagnosis of cancer will undoubtedly rely more and more on the extensive application of ultrasound-guided biopsies of subtle textural abnormalities. However, a yet-to-be-determined percentage of small, purely isoechoic carcinomas will still be missed by transrectal ultrasound.

Transrectal probes with duplex Doppler capability have recently been commercialized and are currently in clinical evaluation. Preliminary results are encouraging, with the demonstration of high-velocity as well as low-impedance abnormal Doppler signals in malignant prostates (Figs. 6.66, 6.67). Transrectal color flow Doppler imaging should allow an easier and more accurate blood flow mapping of the prostate.

Voiding sonography should gain popularity as a new clinical application because it offers accurate real-time evaluation of bladder outlet obstruction.

As a real-time monitoring technique, transrectal prostatic sonography can be used to refine certain therapeutic procedures. Ultrasound guidance is already used for the transperineal placement of radioactive seeds in interstitial radiation therapy of prostatic carcinoma.

Urethroplasty with a balloon catheter has been developed to treat BPH [94]. We have recently used real-time transrectal sonography to place the balloon of the catheter in the

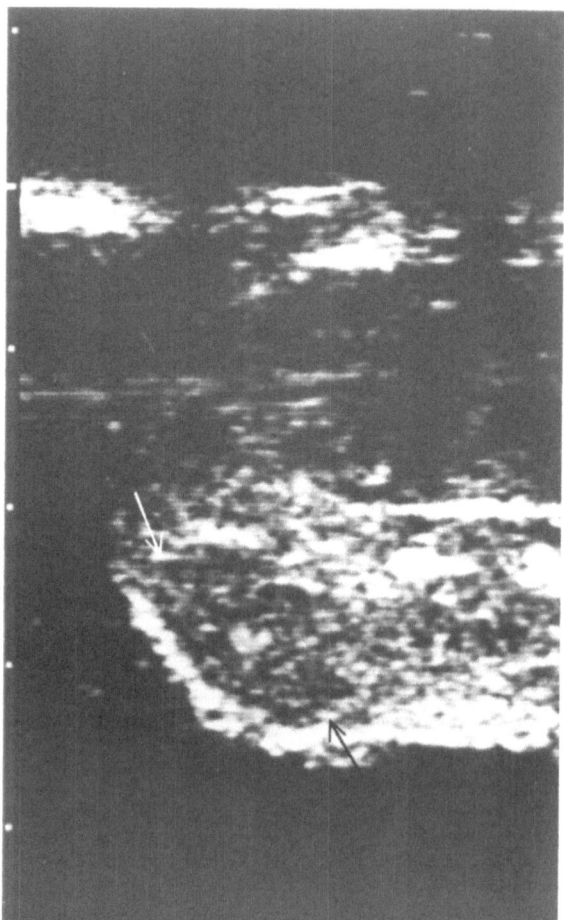

a

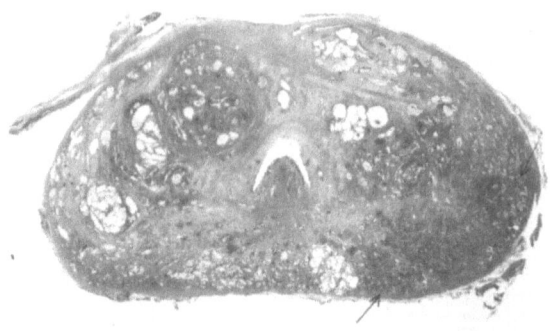

b

Figure 6.65. Correlation between in vitro·sonogram (a) and histopathologic section (b) of a radical prostatectomy specimen. Arrows point to the carcinoma.

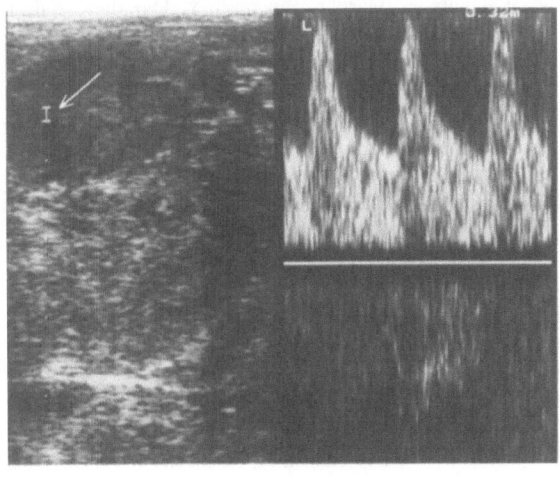

a   b

Figure 6.66. Prostatic carcinoma. Transrectal duplex sonography using a 7.5-MHz linear-array probe. (a) Longitudinal scan. The gate indicating the sample volume (arrow) has been placed in a hypoechoic area of the tumor. (b) Doppler study shows high-velocity signals.

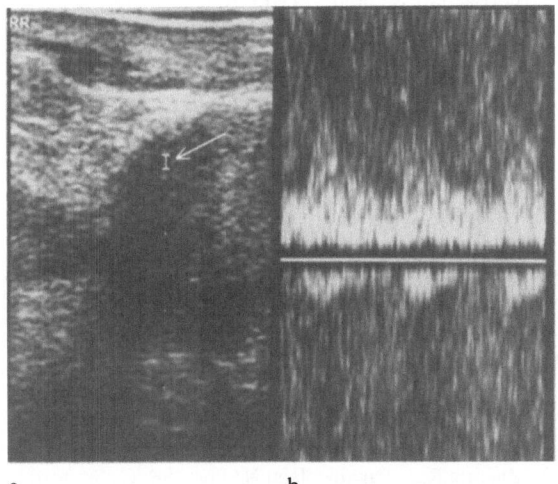

a   b

Figure 6.67. Transrectal duplex sonography of prostatic carcinoma. (a) The gate (arrow) has been placed in a hypoechoic area of the prostatic base. (b) Doppler study shows low-impedance waveform with continued flow through diastole.

stenosed area of the prostatic urethra and to monitor the urethral dilation (Fig. 6.68) [95].

The digital rectal examination and transrectal sonography are now the first two examinations that should be conducted in the evaluation of patients with symptomatic prostatic disease.

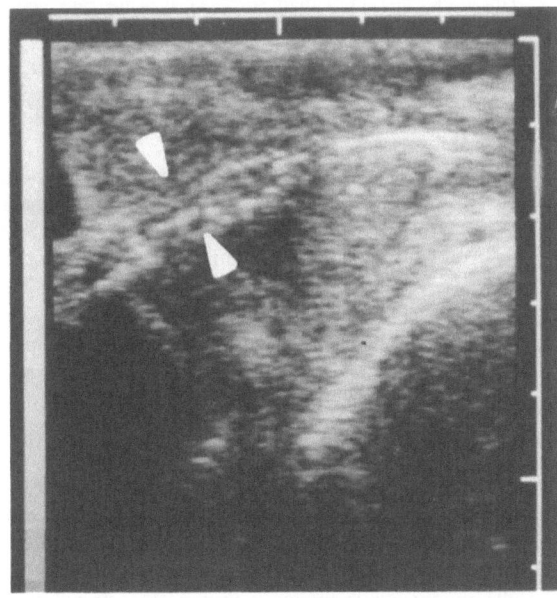

Figure 6.68. Transrectal sonographic monitoring of balloon catheter dilation of the prostatic urethra in a patient with BPH. Midsagittal sonogram shows the inflated dilatation balloon (arrowheads). (From ref. 95, with permission.)

References

1. Holm H. H., Northeved A.: A transurethral ultrasonic scanner. J. Urol., 1974, 111, 238—241.
2. Gammelgaard J., Holm H. H.: Transurethral and transrectal ultrasonic scanning in urology. J. Urol., 1980, 124, 863—868.
3. Komine Y., Kimura A., Niizuma M., Nakamura S., Kawabe K., Niijima T.: Transurethral ultrasonotomography of the prostate. Prostate, 1981, 1 (suppl.), 53—57.
4. McNeal J. E.: Normal and pathologic anatomy of prostate. Urology, 1981, 17 (suppl.), 11—16.
5. McNeal J. E.: The prostate gland: Morphology and pathobiology. Monogr. Urol., 1983, 4, 3—33.
6. Takahashi H., Ouchi T.: The ultrasonic diagnosis in the field of urology. On the diagnosis of prostate disease. Jpn. J. Med. Ultrason., 1963, Oct., 7—8.
7. Pell R. L.: Ultrasound for routine clinical investigations. Ultrasonics, 1964, 2, 87—89.
8. Gotoh K., Nishi M.: Ultrasonic diagnosis of prostatic cancer. Acta Urol. Jpn., 1965, 11, 87—90.
9. Watanabe H., Kato H., Kato T., Morita M., Tanaka M., Terasawa Y.: Diagnostic application of the ultrasonotomography for the prostate. Jpn. J. Urol., 1968, 59, 273—279.
10. Watanabe H., Kaiho H., Tanaka M., Terasawa Y.: Diagnostic application of ultrasonotomography to the prostate. Invest. Urol., 1971, 8, 548—559.

11. Harada K., Igari D., Tanahashi Y.: Gray scale transrectal ultrasonography of the prostate. J. Clin. Ultrasound, 1979, 7, 45—49.

12. Sekine H., Oka K., Takehara Y.: Transrectal longitudinal ultrasonotomography of the prostate by electronic linear scanning. J. Urol., 1982, 127, 62—65.

13. Resnick M. I., Willard J. W., Boyce W. H.: Recent progress in ultrasonography of the bladder and prostate. J. Urol., 1977, 117, 444—446.

14. Resnick M. I., Willard J. W., Boyce W. H.: Ultrasonic evaluation of the prostatic nodule. J. Urol., 1978, 120, 86—88.

15. Harada K., Tanahashi Y., Igari D., Numata I., Orikasa S.: Clinical evaluation of inside echo patterns in gray scale prostatic echography. J. Urol., 1980, 124, 216—220.

16. Brooman P. J. C., Peeling W. B., Griffiths G. J., Roberts E., Evans K.: A comparison between digital examination and per-rectal ultrasound in the evaluation of the prostate. Br. J. Urol., 1981, 53, 617—620.

17. Braeckman J., Denis L.: The practice and pitfalls of ultrasonography in the lower urinary tract. Eur. Urol., 1983, 9, 193—201.

18. Fornage B., Lardennois B.: Ultrasound imaging of the prostate: Recent developments using new equipment. Presented at the 67th Meeting of the Radiological Society of North America, Chicago, November 15—20, 1981.

19. Fornage B. D., Touche D. H., Deglaire M., Faroux M. J., Simatos A.: Real-time ultrasound guided prostatic biopsy using a new transrectal linear-array probe. Radiology, 1983, 146, 547—548.

20. Fornage B.: L'échographie endorectale de la prostate. Comparaison des sondes de types radial et linéaire. J. Radiol., 1984, 65, 375—384.

21. Rifkin M. D., Kurtz A. B.: Ultrasound of the prostate. In: Sanders R. C., Hill M. (eds.). Ultrasound annual 1983. New York, Raven Press, 1983, 95—132.

22. Rifkin M. D., Kurtz A. B., Choi H. Y., Goldberg B. B.: Endoscopic ultrasonic evaluation of the prostate using a transrectal probe: Prospective evaluation and acoustic characterization. Radiology, 1983, 149, 265—271.

23. Rifkin M. D., Kurtz A. B., Goldberg B. B.: Sonographically guided transperineal prostatic biopsy: Preliminary experience with a longitudinal linear-array transducer. AJR, 1983, 140, 745—747.

24. Fornage B.: Echographie de la prostate. Paris, Vigot, 1985.

25. Fornage B., Pourcelot L.: Improvement to endocavitary ultrasound probes. European Patent No. 0139574, 1988.

26. Lee F., Torp-Pedersen S. T., Siders D. B., Littrup P. J., McLeary R. D.: Transrectal ultrasound in the diagnosis and staging of prostatic carcinoma. Radiology, 1989, 170, 609—615.

27. Fornage B. D.: Ultrasound of the prostate. Chichester, John Wiley & Sons, 1988.

28. Fornage B. D.: Normal US anatomy of the prostate. Ultrasound Med. Biol., 1986, 12, 1011—1021.

29. Watanabe H., Igari D., Tanahashi Y., Harada K., Saitoh M.: Measurements of size and weight of prostate by means of transrectal ultrasonotomography. Tohoku J. Exp. Med., 1974, 114, 277—285.

30. Hastak S. M., Gammelgaard J., Holm H. H.: Transrectal ultrasonic volume determination of the prostate. A preoperative and postoperative study. J. Urol., 1982, 127, 1115—1118.

31. Bartsch G., Egender G., Hübscher H., Rohr H.: Sonometrics of the prostate. J. Urol., 1982, 127, 1119—1121.

32. Watanabe H.: Natural history of benign prostatic hypertrophy. Ultasound Med. Biol., 1986, 12, 567—571.

33. Rifkin M. D.: Endorectal sonography of the prostate: Clinical implications. AJR, 1987, 148, 1137—1142.

34. Burks D. D., Drolshagen L. F., Fleischer A. C. et al.: Transrectal sonography of benign and malignant prostatic lesions. AJR, 1986, 146, 1187—1191.

35. Griffiths G. J., Crooks A. J. R., Roberts E. E. et al.: Ultrasonic appearances associated with prostatic inflammation: A preliminary study. Clin. Radiol., 1984, 35, 343—345.

36. Dähnert W. F., Hamper U. M., Walsh P. C., Eggleston J. C., Sanders R. C.: The echogenic focus in prostatic sonograms, with xeroradiographic and histopathologic correlation. Radiology, 1986, 159, 95—100.

37. Rifkin M. D.: Transrectal prostatic ultrasonography: Comparison of linear array and radial scanners. J. Ultrasound Med., 1985, 4, 1—5.

38. Dana A., Cukier J.: Diagnostic échographique d'un cas d'abcès de la prostate. J. Urol. (Paris), 1981, 87, 255—257.

39. Lee F. Jr., Lee F., Solomon M. H., Straub W. H., McLeary R. D.: Sonographic demonstration of prostatic abscess. J. Ultrasound Med., 1986, 5, 101—102.

40. Thornhill B. A., Morehouse H. T., Coleman P., Hoffman-Tretin J. C.: Prostatic abscess: CT and sonographic findings. AJR, 1987, 148, 899—900.

41. Lee S. B., Lee F., Solomon M. H., Kumasaka G. H., Straub W. H., McLeary R. D.: Seminal vesicle abscess: Diagnosis by transrectal ultrasound. J. Clin. Ultrasound, 1986, 14, 546—549.

42. Zagoria R. J., Papanicolaou N., Pfister R. C., Stafford S. A., Young H. H. II: Seminal vesicle abscess after vasectomy: Evaluation by transrectal sonography and CT. AJR, 1987, 149, 137—138.

43. Hamilton S., Fitzpatrick J. M.: Ultrasound diagnosis of a prostatic cyst causing acute urinary retention. J. Ultrasound Med., 1987, 6, 385—387.

44. Sivaraman L., Sivasubramanian S. V.: Prostatic cysts. Ann. R. Coll. Surg. Engl., 1978, 60, 476—478.

45. Fischelovitch J., Meiraz D., Lazebnik J.: Cysts of the prostate. Br. J. Urol., 1975, 47, 687—689.

46. Van Poppel H., Vereecken R., De Geeter P., Verduyn H.: Hemospermia owing to utricular cyst: Embryological summary and surgical review. J. Urol., 1983, 129, 608—609.

47. Holm L., Forsberg L.: Computed tomography and

ultrasound studies of prostatic utricle cyst associated with unilateral renal agenesis. A case report. Scand. J. Urol. Nephrol., 1984, 18, 87—89.

48. Eisenberg D., Luis-Jorge J. C., Himmelfarb E. H., Kulkarni M. V., Shaff M. I.: Sonographic diagnosis of seminal vesicle cysts. J. Clin. Ultrasound, 1986, 14, 213—215.

49. Heaney J. A., Pfister R. C., Meares E. M. Jr.: Giant cyst of the seminal vesicle with renal agenesis. AJR, 1987, 149, 139—140.

50. Silverberg E., Lubera J.: Cancer statistics, 1989. CA, 1989, 39, 3—20.

51. McNeal J. E., Redwine E. A., Freiha F. S., Stamey T. A.: Zonal distribution of prostatic adenocarcinoma. Correlation with histologic pattern and direction of spread. Am. J. Surg. Pathol., 1988, 12, 897—906.

52. Mostofi F. K., Price E. B. Jr.: Tumors of the prostate. In: Mostofi F. K., Price E. B. Jr. (eds.). Tumors of the male genital system. Washington, D. C., Armed Forces Institute of Pathology, 1973, 177—258.

53. Lee F., Gray J. M., McLeary R. D. et al.: Transrectal ultrasound in the diagnosis of prostate cancer: Location, echogenicity, histopathology and staging. Prostate, 1985, 7, 117—129.

54. Whitmore W. F. Jr.: The natural history of prostatic cancer. Cancer, 1973, 32, 1104—1112.

55. McNeal J. E., Kindrachuk R. A., Freiha F. S., Bostwick D. G., Redwine E. A., Stamey T. A.: Patterns of progression in prostate cancer. Lancet, 1986, 1, 60—63.

56. Dähnert W. F., Hamper U. M., Eggleston J. C., Walsh P. C., Sanders R. C.: Prostatic evaluation by transrectal sonography with histopathologic correlation: The echopenic appearance of early carcinoma. Radiology, 1986, 158, 97—102.

57. Salo J. O., Rannikko S., Mäkinen J., Lehtonen T.: Echogenic structure of prostatic cancer imaged on radical prostatectomy specimens. Prostate, 1987, 10, 1—9.

58. Lee F., Gray J. M., McLeary R. D. et al.: Prostatic evaluation by transrectal sonography: Criteria for diagnosis of early carcinoma. Radiology, 1986, 158, 91—95.

59. Fornage B. D., Babaian R. J., Troncoso P.: Can transrectal sonography detect early prostatic carcinoma? Correlation with whole prostate pathologic mapping. Presented at the 5th Meeting of the World Federation for Ultrasound in Medicine and Biology, Washington, D.C., October 17—21, 1988.

60. Rifkin M. D., Friedland G. W., Shortliffe L.: Prostatic evaluation by transrectal endosonography: Detection of carcinoma. Radiology, 1986, 158, 85—90.

61. Griffiths G. J., Clements R., Jones D. R., Roberts E. E., Peeling W. B., Evans K. T.: The ultrasound appearances of prostatic cancer with histological correlation. Clin. Radiol., 1987, 38, 219—227.

62. Kimura A., Nakamura S., Niizuma M. et al.: Quantitative analysis of ultrasonogram of the prostate. J. Clin. Ultrasound, 1986, 14, 501—507.

63. Clements R., Griffiths G. J., Peeling W. B., Roberts E. E., Evans K. T.: How accurate is the index finger? A comparison of digital and ultrasound examination of the prostatic nodule. Clin. Radiol., 1988, 39, 87—89.

64. Jewett H. J.: Significance of the palpable prostatic nodule. JAMA, 1956, 160, 838—839.

65. Watanabe H., Ohe H., Inaba T., Itakura Y., Saitoh M., Nakao M.: A mobile mass screening unit for prostatic disease. Prostate, 1984, 5, 559—565.

66. Lee F., Littrup P. J., Torp-Pedersen S. T. et al.: Prostate cancer: Comparison of transrectal US and digital rectal examination for screening. Radiology, 1988, 168, 389—394.

67. McClennan B. L.: Transrectal US of the prostate: Is the technology leading the science? Radiology, 1988, 168, 571—575.

68. Fujino A., Scardino P. T.: Transrectal ultrasonography for prostatic cancer: Its value in staging and monitoring the response to radiotherapy and chemotherapy. J. Urol., 1985, 133, 806—810.

69. Sakamoto K., Tanaka F., Miyazaki Y., Ariyoshi A.: Diagnostic procedures for assessment of disease extent in prostatic carcinoma. Prostate, 1981, 1 (suppl.), 47—52.

70. Mukamel E., DeKernion J. B., Hannah J., Smith R. B., Skinner D. G., Goodwin W. E.: The incidence and significance of seminal vesicle invasion in patients with adenocarcinoma of the prostate. Cancer, 1987, 59, 1535—1538.

71. Carpentier P.J., Schröder F. H., Blom J. H. M.: Transrectal ultrasonotomography in the followup of prostatic carcinoma patients. J. Urol., 1982, 128, 742—746.

72. Kojima M., Watanabe H., Ohe H., Miyashita H., Inaba T.: Kinetic evaluation of the effect of LHRH analog on prostatic cancer using transrectal ultrasonotomography. Prostate, 1987, 10, 11—17.

73. Fujino A., Scardino P. T.: Transrectal ultrasonography for prostatic cancer. II. The response of the prostate to definitive radiotherapy. Cancer, 1986, 57, 935—940.

74. Braeckman J., Keuppens F., Chaban M., Denis L.: Ultrasound in urological oncology. Eur. J. Surg. Oncol., 1987, 13, 475—483.

75. Fornage B. D.: Ultrasound imaging of the prostate: Evaluation of prostate cancer. Cancer Bull., 1988, 40, 135—143.

76. Holm H. H., Gammelgaard J.: Ultrasonically guided precise needle placement in the prostate and the seminal vesicles. J. Urol., 1981, 125, 385—387.

77. Hastak S. M., Gammelgaard J., Holm H. H.: Ultrasonically guided transperineal biopsy in the diagnosis of prostatic carcinoma. J. Urol., 1982, 128, 69—71.

78. Lee F., Littrup P. J., McLeary R. D. et al.: Needle aspiration and core biopsy of prostate cancer: Comparative evaluation with biplanar transrectal US guidance. Radiology, 1987, 163, 515—520.

79. Fornage B. D.: Ultrasound-guided prostatic biopsy. Presented at the 72nd Meeting of the Radiological Society of North America, Chicago, November 30—December 5, 1986.

80. Torp-Pedersen S. T., Lee F., Lititrup P. J., *et al.*: Transrectal biopsy of the prostate guided with transrectal US: Longitudinal and multiplanar scanning. Radiology, 1989, 170, 23—27.

81. Lee F., Torp-Pedersen S. T., Littrup P. J., *et al.*: Hypoechoic lesions of the prostate: Clinical relevance of tumor size, digital rectal examination, and prostate-specific antigen. Radiology, 1989, 170, 29—32.

82. Holm H. H., Juul N., Pedersen J. F., Hansen H., Stroyer I.: Transperineal ^{125}iodine seed implantation in prostatic cancer guided by transrectal ultrasonography. J. Urol., 1983, 130, 283—286.

83. Rifkin M. D.: Sonourethrography: Technique for evaluation of prostatic urethra. Radiology, 1984, 153, 791—792.

84. Shapeero L. G., Friedland G. W., Perkash I.: Transrectal sonographic voiding cystourethrography: Studies in neuromuscular bladder dysfunction. AJR, 1983, 141, 83—90.

85. Platt J. F., Bree R. L., Schwab R. E.: The accuracy of CT in the staging of carcinoma of the prostate. AJR, 1987, 149, 315—318.

86. Phillips M. E., Kressel H. Y., Spritzer C. E. *et al.*: Normal prostate and adjacent structures: MR imaging at 1.5 T. Radiology, 1987, 164, 381—385.

87. Hricak H., Dooms G. C., McNeal J. E. *et al.*: MR imaging of the prostate gland: Normal anatomy. AJR, 1987, 148, 51—58.

88. Phillips M. E., Kressel H. Y., Spritzer C. E. *et al.*: Prostatic disorders: MR imaging at 1.5 T. Radiology, 1987, 164, 386—392.

89. Kjaer L., Thomsen C., Iversen P., Henriksen O.: In vivo estimation of relaxation processes in benign hyperplasia and carcinoma of the prostate gland by magnetic resonance imaging. Magn. Reson. Imaging, 1987, 5, 23—30.

90. Carrol C.L., Sommer F. G., McNeal J. E., Stamey T. A.: The abnormal prostate: MR imaging at 1.5 T with histopathologic correlation. Radiology, 1987, 163, 521—525.

91. Martin J. F., Hajek P., Baker L., Gylys-Morin V., Fitzmorris-Glass R., Mattrey R. R.: Inflatable surface coil for MR imaging of the prostate. Radiology, 1988, 167, 268—270.

92. Hricak H., Dooms G. C., Jeffrey R. B. *et al.*: Prostatic carcinoma: Staging by clinical assessment, CT, and MR imaging. Radiology, 1987, 162, 331—336.

93. Hricak H.: Urologic cancer. Methods of early detection and future developments. Cancer, 1987, 60, 677—685.

94. Castaneda F., Reddy P., Wasserman N. *et al.*: Benign prostatic hypertrophy: Retrograde transurethral dilation of the prostatic urethra in humans. Radiology, 1987, 163, 649—653.

95. Fornage B. D., Toubas O.: Transrectal sonographic monitoring of balloon dilatation of the prostatic urethra. J. Ultrasound Med., 1989, 8, 53—55.

7. Transurethral sonography

HANS H. HOLM, SOREN T. TORP-PEDERSEN, AND NIELS JUUL

In sonographic imaging of the urinary bladder and adjacent structures, a transurethral approach is theoretically superior to transabdominal scanning for several reasons. First, the abdominal wall is bypassed, as are other intervening structures that may degrade the image. Second, the amount of fluid in the bladder is controlled by the cystoscopist during the examination. Third, urine, which is echo free, allows the use of high-frequency transducers with optimal focusing.

The first ultrasonic transducer constructed to fit into a cystoscope was intended for scanning of the prostate during transurethral resection (TUR) [1]. The space required for the resector's loop only left room for a very small transducer and consequently, the bistable images obtained were suboptimal. Further, it soon became apparent that an ultrasound-guided TUR without the possibility of electrocoagulating bleeding vessels under visual control was associated with a high risk of problems related to hemostasis. The loop was then removed, which permitted larger transducers and improved images.

Since transurethral scanning requires the insertion of a cystoscope, it is clearly the urologist's tool. It may be used whenever the urologist wants to look behind the 'visual barrier' of optical cystoscopy. The main uses of transurethral sonography have proven to be the detection of bladder tumors when cystoscopic vision is poor, the staging of bladder tumors, and, rarely, the evaluation of the prostate and seminal vesicles during cystoscopic examination.

Instrumentation

The transurethral probe that we use consists of a motor-driven rotating steel tube with a transducer mounted on its distal end. Various cystoscope adaptors are available, and the probe fits into any 24-charriere (24 F, or 8-mm outer diameter) resectoscope (Fig. 7.1). The transducer, which is simply plugged in at the distal end of the probe, can be easily exchanged. Three different transurethral transducers are used in routine scanning: (a) an 8-MHz, 90° (i.e., side-viewing at a 90° angle to the rotating shaft of the probe) transducer with a focal range of 0—30 mm, (b) a 5-MHz, 90° transducer with a focal range of 10—40 mm, and (c) a 5-MHz, 45° 'retrograde'-viewing transducer. The 8-MHz transducer is sufficient in most cases, and only in cases of bulky tumors is the 5-MHz transducer necessary. The retrograde transducer is used for visualization of the bladder neck area.

Transurethral sonography is performed in the operating theater. The control panel of the ultrasound unit is smooth so that it can be fitted with a transparent sterile cover and so be manipulated under sterile conditions. The probe and its cable, excluding the plug, can be submerged in sterilizing fluid such as glutaraldehyde at 2% in 70% isopropanol (Cidex® or Korsolin®). The probe connected to the ultrasound unit is shown in Fig. 7.2.

As the transducer rotates inside the bladder, sectional transverse scans are obtained at a rate of 4 frames per second. The images are therefore

Bruno D. Fornage (ed.), *Endosonography*, pp. 105—119.
© 1989 *Kluwer Academic Publishers*.

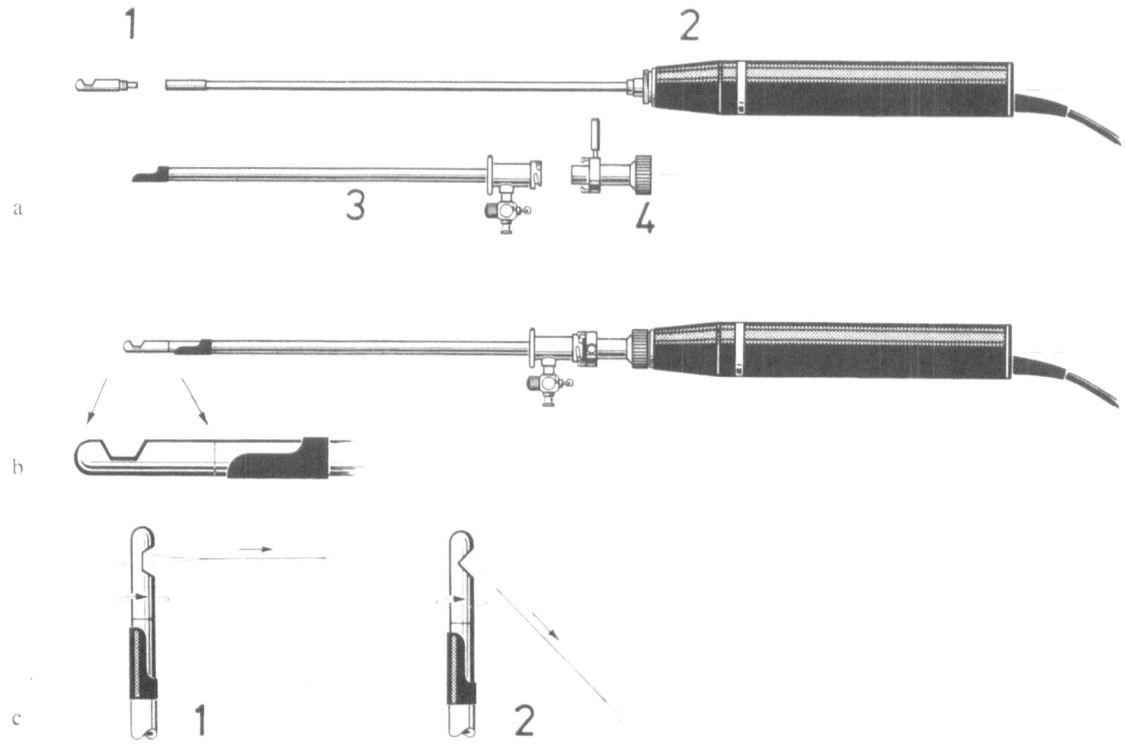

Figure 7.1. The transurethral radial probe. (a) The ultrasound transducer (1) is shown detached from the probe, whose motor unit is housed in the handle (2). The sheath of the resectoscope (3) and its adaptor (4) for the ultrasound probe are pictured as well. (b) System assembled. (c) Both 90° (1) and 45° retrograde-viewing (2) transducers are available.

not live, but this generally does not prove a disadvantage since the structures investigated by transurethral scanning do not move.

The whole procedure can be taped on a video recorder and subsequently reviewed, with selected still views hard-copied. Various photographic devices also allow hard copies of frozen images to be taken during the examination.

Technique of examination

The need for transurethral scanning arises during cystoscopy, so the transurethral probe should always be ready to use, submerged in sterilizing solution. When scanning is required, the ultrasound unit is wheeled into the room and the probe taken from the sterilization fluid and flushed with saline solution. The probe is plugged into the ultrasound unit by an assistant and then placed on a sterile tray. The optics of the 24-charriere resectoscope are removed and

the cystoscope sheath tilted so that its tip lies in the most anterior part of the bladder, enabling air to escape from the bladder. This is crucial because a large air bubble in the bladder will prevent the examination of a major portion of the anterior bladder wall. The probe is introduced and locked to the cystoscope sheath with the adaptor (Fig. 7.3). Since a completely empty bladder theoretically may be damaged by the rotating transducer, the bladder must be filled with fluid before scanning is started.

Transverse scans of the bladder are seen with the transducer in the center of the image. They are oriented according to the conventions for computed tomography and abdominal ultrasound (i.e., seen from below). The probe is gradually advanced, and the area of the transverse section of the bladder increases until an air bubble is seen at the top of the image (Fig. 7.4). That area then decreases as the probe approaches the dome.

The most common indication for trans-

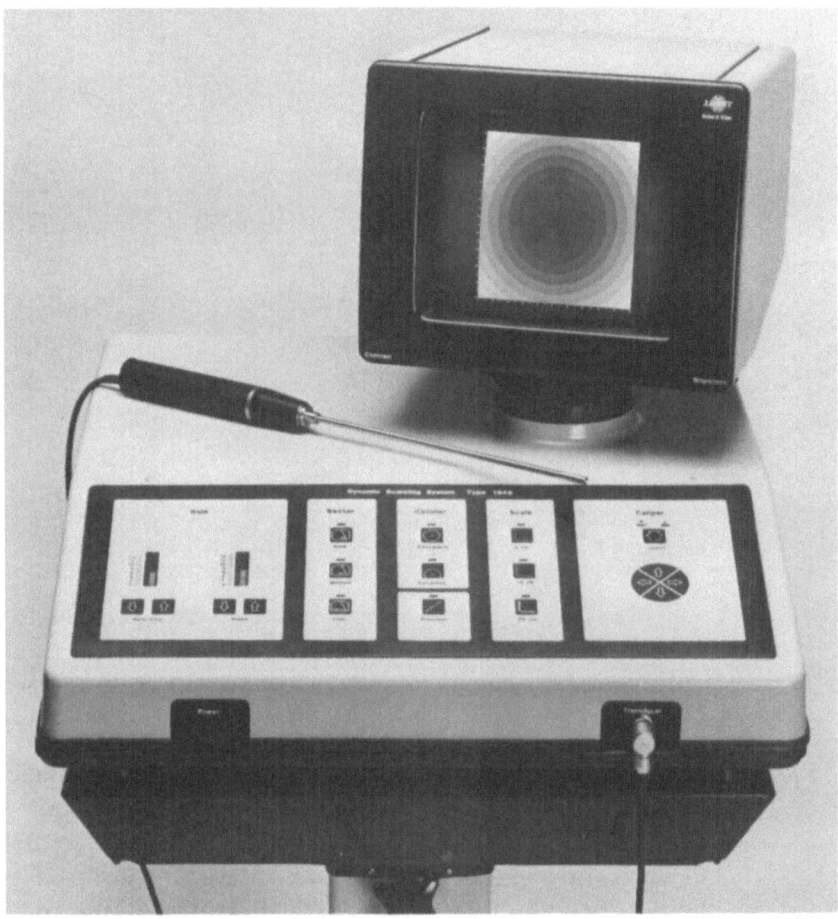

Figure 7.2. The ultrasound unit and the connected probe (equipment Brüel & Kjaër, type 1849).

urethral scanning is the visualization of a bladder tumor at cystoscopy. The technique is used in this context to evaluate deep tumor infiltration. However, the rest of the bladder is also searched for any additional tumor overlooked at cystoscopy. The tumor is scanned thoroughly by changing the position of the transducer to ensure that the bladder wall behind the tumor is in the focal zone. The gain settings may need to be adjusted as the distance between the transducer and the bladder wall changes or as the thickness of the tumor varies. Transurethral scanning should be performed prior to any biopsy and electrocoagulation since these often create a highly reflective superficial crust that can impair the visualization of the bladder wall.

When the 8-MHz transducer cannot define the bladder wall behind bulky tumor owing to sound attenuation, the probe is removed from the bladder and the 5-MHz transducer mounted instead.

The dome of the bladder is visualized by modifying the position of the transducer inside the bladder, whereas the examination of the region of the bladder neck requires, as mentioned above, the use of the retrograde-viewing transducer (Fig. 7.5). It must be noted that images obtained with the 45° transducer are distorted because the image displayed on the video monitor is a two-dimensional, planar representation of the surface of a cone.

During the examination, the distension of the bladder can be modified, in accordance with which the stretch of the detrusor will vary. Insufficient filling will result in mucosal folds that mimic tumor. However, it must be kept in

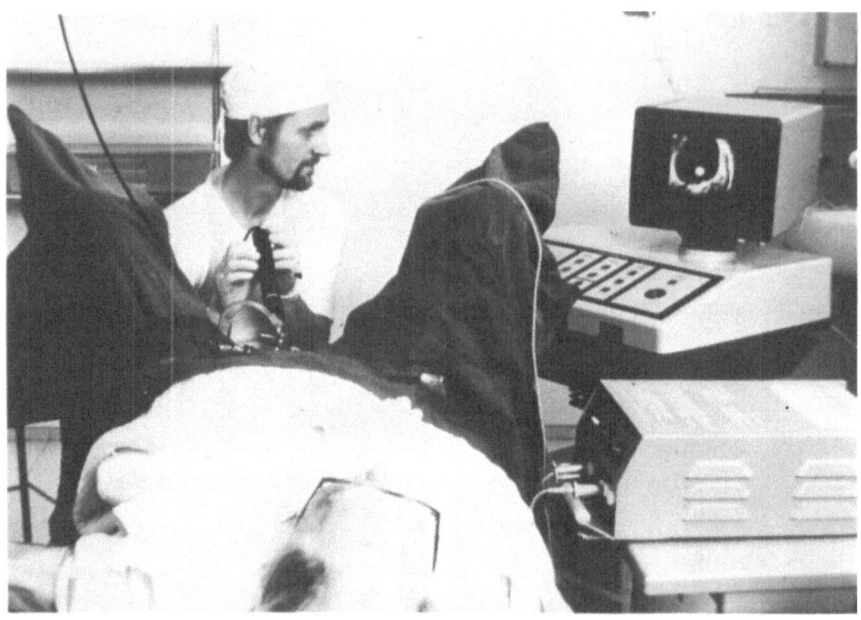

Figure 7.3. Transurethral scanning in theater. The images are displayed on the video monitor.

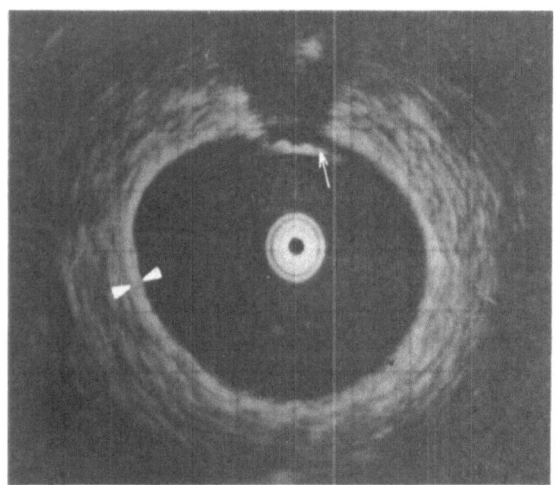

Figure 7.4. Transverse midsection of normal bladder. The rotating transducer is seen as a bright central ring. An air bubble at the top of bladder (arrow) is associated with acoustic shadowing. Arrowheads point to the bladder wall.

mind that transurethral scanning is an adjunct to cystoscopy and that interpretative errors due to artifacts or pitfalls are readily corrected when sonographic and cystoscopic findings are correlated.

Transurethral scanning of the prostate is performed by withdrawing the rotating trans-ducer and placing it in the prostatic urethra. The gain settings are adjusted to compensate for the higher attenuation of prostatic tissue compared with urine. Markedly enlarged prostates are better evaluated with a 5-MHz transducer.

Normal ultrasound anatomy

The urine is echo free. During retrograde fluid distension of the bladder, however, swirling echoes from microbubbles or turbulences are often seen. A ring in the center of the trans-urethral scan indicates the transducer. An air bubble is nearly always seen at the top of the image as a brightly echogenic horizontal line with acoustic shadowing (Fig. 7.4). The ureteral orifices are identified as two symmetric, hypo-echoic transmural slits in the bladder floor and serve as landmarks (Fig. 7.6). Occasionally, the interureteral ridge is depicted.

The most superficial layer of the bladder wall, the mucosa, which consists of transitional epithelium and a lamina propria of loose to dense connective tissue, may be seen as a thin, somewhat hypoechoic layer. In normal individuals, this layer does not exceed 1 mm and

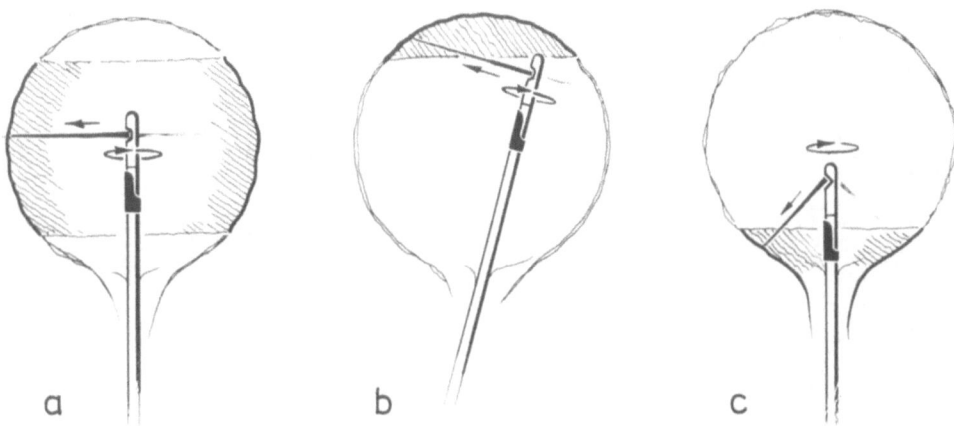

Figure 7.5. Technique of examination. (a) The 90° transducer visualizes the midportion of the bladder. (b) The 90° transducer is angled to visualize the dome. (c) The 45° retrograde-viewing transducer is dedicated to the examination of the bladder neck area.

consequently is not always visualized. Optimal depiction requires the wall to lie within the focal zone (Fig. 7.7). Beneath the mucosa, the muscular wall, or detrusor, which is made of smooth muscle fibers intermingled without distinct layers, appears as an echogenic structure. Its thickness depends on the degree of distension of the bladder. At the average filling for transurethral scanning (i.e., about 200 mL), it is approximately 4 mm thick. External to the detrusor, a poorly defined layer of varying thickness represents the perivesical fat.

Endovesical scanning can demonstrate the bony limits of the pelvis and most of the perivesical structures, including the obturator internus and levator ani muscles, the iliac vessels, and rectum (Fig. 7.8). In the female, the uterus and adnexal structures are seen (Fig. 7.9) provided there are not intervening gas-filled bowel loops. As the probe is withdrawn, the cervix and vagina are visualized. In the male, the seminal vesicles are seen as symmetric, hypoechoic, elongated, areolar structures posterior to the bladder. Also, the ampullae of the vasa deferentia are visualized proximal to their joining with the vesicles (Fig. 7.7). The prostate, scanned from the prostatic urethra, is seen as roughly semilunar or triangular. The internal gland is hypoechoic relative to the peripheral area. The prostatic capsule is well defined, as are the periprostatic venous plexuses (Fig. 7.10) [2–4].

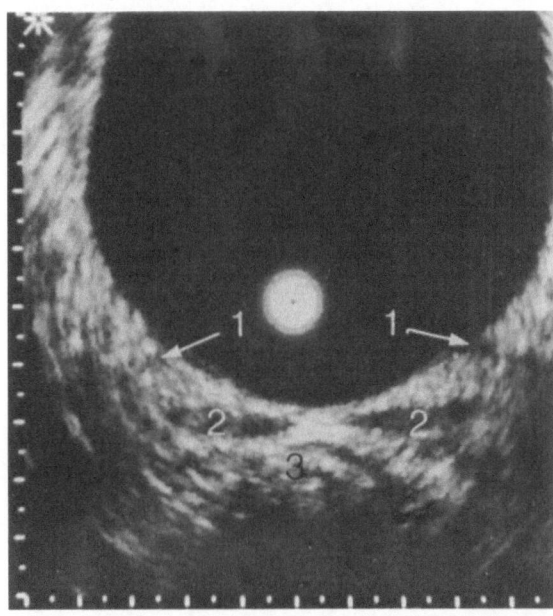

Figure 7.6. Lower transverse section of normal bladder in the male. 1 = ureteral orifices; 2 = seminal vesicles; 3 = rectum.

Bladder tumors

Papillomas as small as 2–3 millimeters can be detected by intravesical sonography (Fig. 7.11). However, it may not be easy to differentiate such lesions from localized trabeculation or fibrinous deposits, and the diagnosis of tumor is made at cystoscopy. In patients with papillomatosis

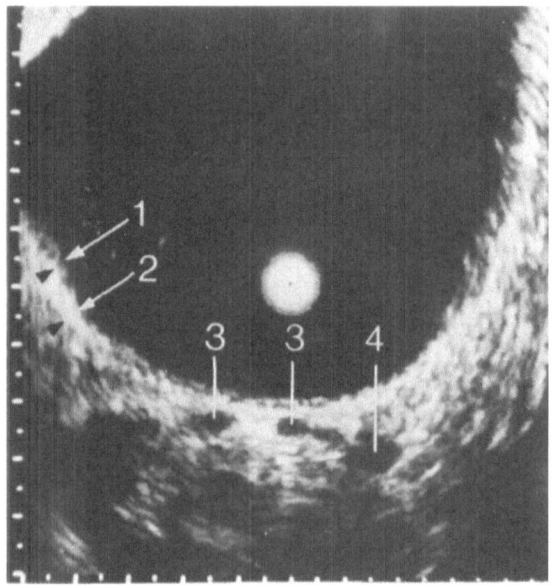

Figure 7.7. Lower transverse section of normal bladder in the male. 1 = mucosa; 2 = detrusor muscle; 3 = ampullae of vasa deferentia; 4 = left seminal vesicle.

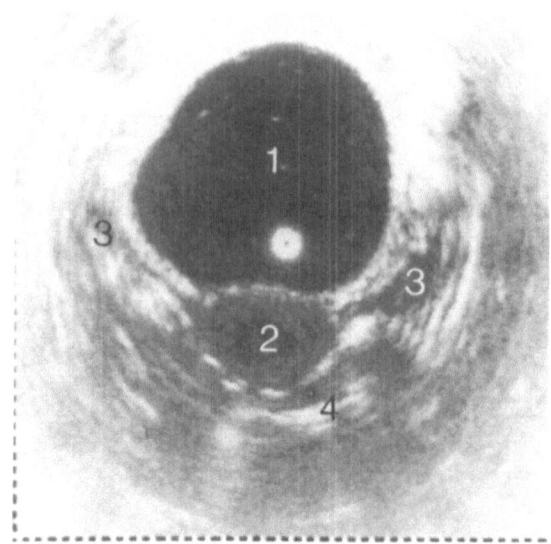

Figure 7.9. Normal bladder in the female. 1 = bladder; 2 = body of uterus; 3 = ovaries; 4 = rectosigmoid junction.

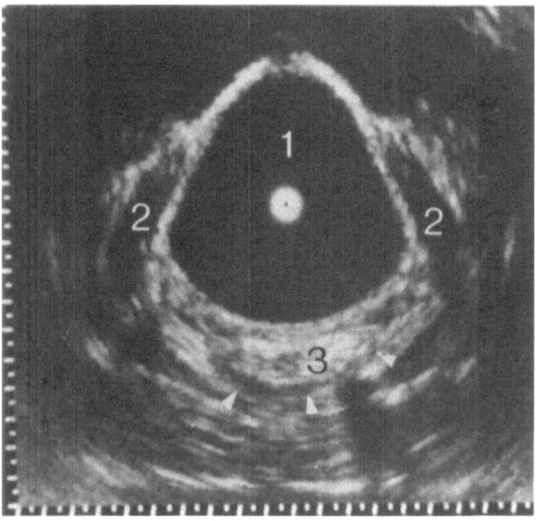

Figure 7.8. Normal bladder in the female. 1 = bladder; 2 = obturator internus muscles; 3 (and arrowheads) = vagina.

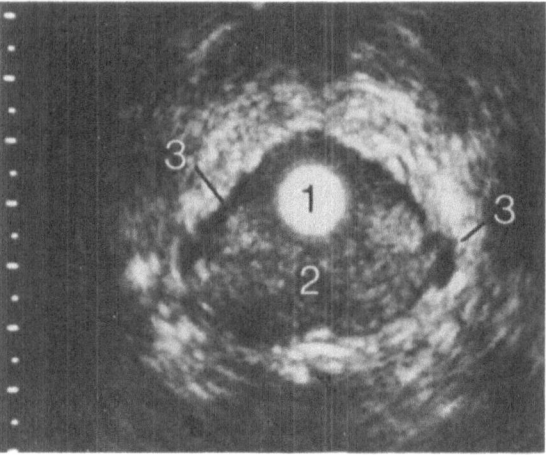

Figure 7.10. Normal prostate. The transducer (1) is seen in the prostatic urethra. The prostate (2) is roughly triangular in shape. Note anechoic periprostatic venous plexuses (3).

(Fig. 7.12), intravesical scanning is performed following electrocoagulation to exclude any small papilloma overlooked at cystoscopy.

Some papillomas are obviously pedunculated at both transurethral sonography and cystoscopy. In these cases, ultrasound does not provide additional information (Fig. 7.13). Other

papillomas, however, are so large that the stalk cannot be clearly demonstrated cystoscopically. This demonstration is possible in most cases with endovesical sonography. When the tumor lies in intimate contact with the bladder wall over a large area, mimicking a sessile tumor (Fig. 7.14), the rapid retrograde injection of fluid may displace the tumor from the wall and better demonstrate its stalk.

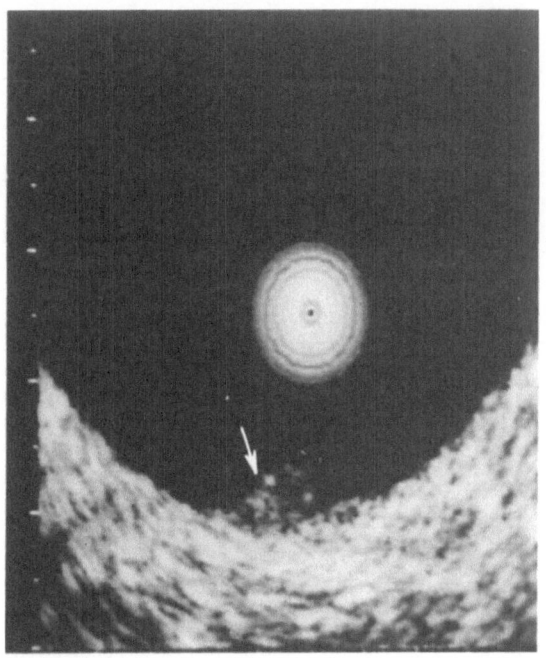

Figure 7.11. Transverse sonogram shows a minute (5-mm) superficial bladder tumor (arrow).

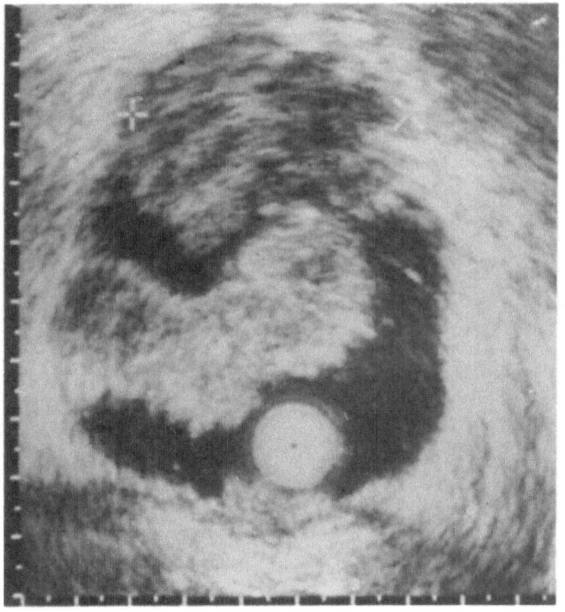

Figure 7.12. Transverse scan shows multiple papillary tumors filling the bladder lumen.

Ultrasound staging system

Because of resolution limitations, the ultrasound (U) staging system for bladder tumors is more

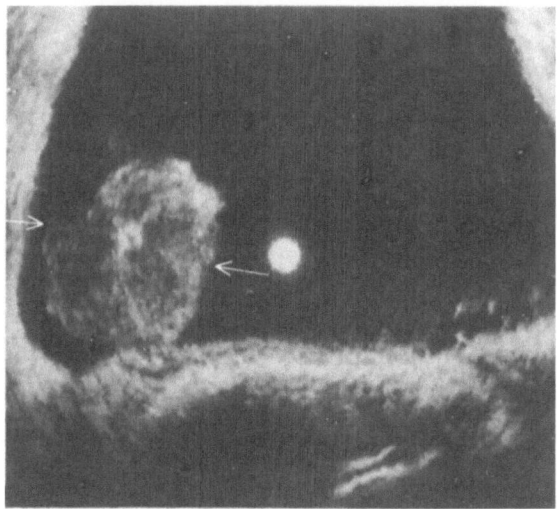

Figure 7.13. Pedunculated, noninfiltrating (stage U1) tumor (arrows).

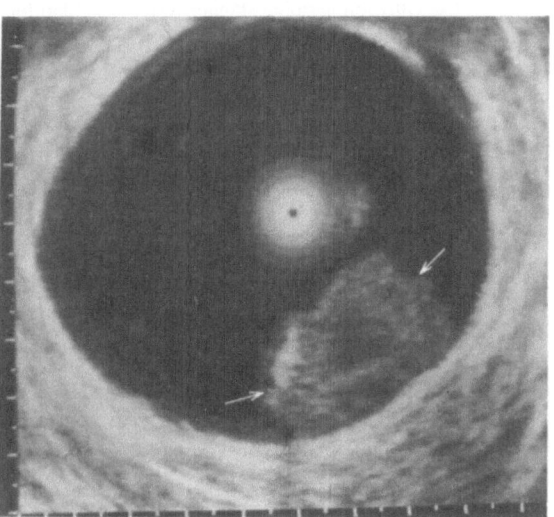

Figure 7.14. Apparently broad-based, stage U1 tumor (arrows). The tumor is actually pedunculated.

simple than either the tumor-node-metastasis (TNM) system or Jewett—Marshall system. The three staging systems are correlated in Fig. 7.15.

Stage U1

Stage U1 tumors are confined to the mucosa. They correspond to Ta and T1 tumors in the TNM classification, or to stage 0 and A tumors in the Jewett—Marshall system. Since normal mucosa is inconsistently visualized by ultrasound, the major criterion for U1 tumors is

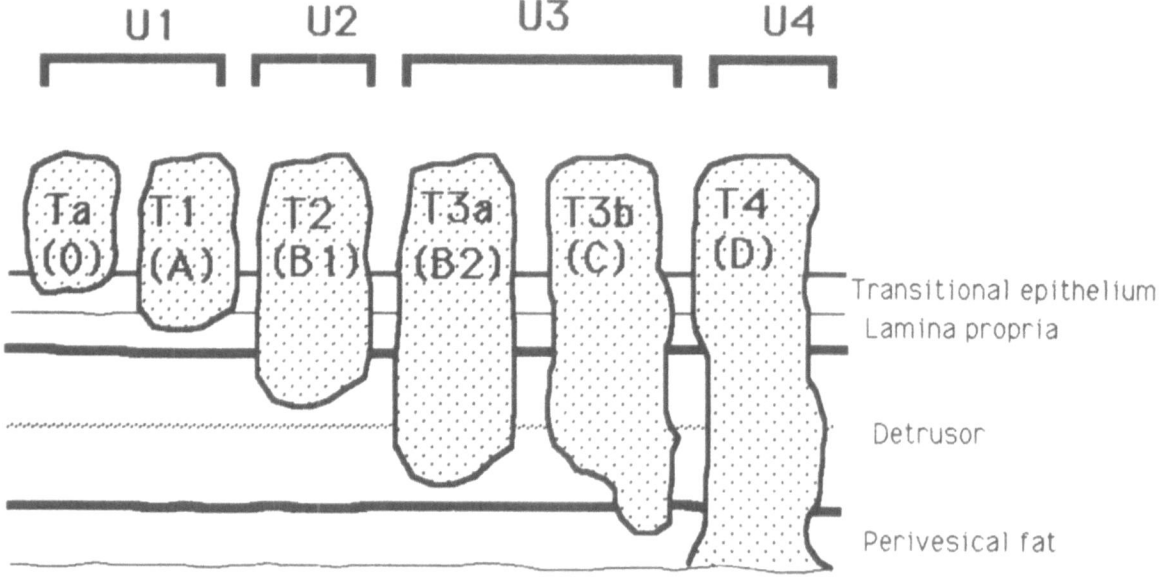

Figure 7.15. Ultrasonographic staging system for bladder carcinoma (U1-U4) correlated with TNM (Ta-T4) and Jewett—Marshall (0-D) classifications.

intactness of the echogenic detrusor muscle (Fig. 7.14).

Stage U2

In stage U2, tumor has infiltrated less than half of the thickness of the echogenic detrusor (Figs. 7.16, 7.17). This stage corresponds to TNM stage T2 or Jewett—Marshall stage B1. In some cases, a rigidity of the detrusor on dynamic examination (e.g., when the volume of intravesical fluid is modified) can be demonstrated, confirming the bladder wall infiltration.

Stage U3

Stage U3 tumors comprise tumors that infiltrate more than halfway through the detrusor muscle (stage T3a, or B2) and those that extend through the detrusor into the perivesical fat (stage T3b, or C) (Figs. 7.18, 7.19). These tumors may protrude slightly or dramatically into the lumen of the bladder, and rigidity of the wall is present.

Stage U4

Stage U4 tumors are characterized by infiltration into surrounding pelvic structures. They correspond to stage T4, or D, tumors. Occasionally, sonography demonstrates tumor extension

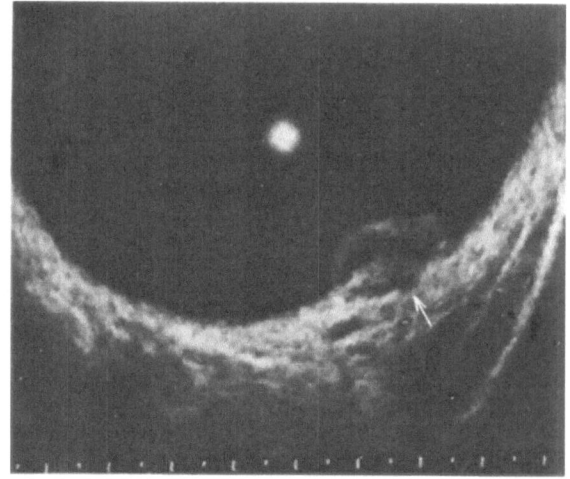

Figure 7.16. Broad-based, stage U2 tumor with infiltration of the superficial portion of the detrusor muscle (arrow).

to bony structures (Fig. 7.20). Tumor deposits (e.g., in the cul-de-sac) (Fig. 7.21) and metastasis to adjacent lymph nodes may also be demonstrated.

Limitations in detection and staging

Location of the tumor

The anterior, posterior, and lateral walls of the

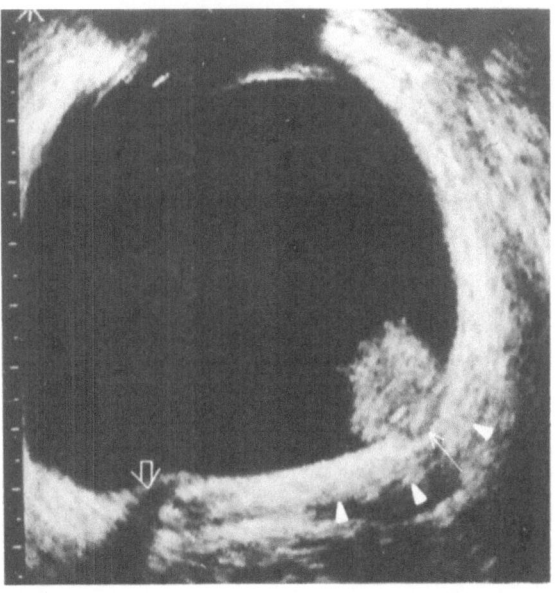

Figure 7.17. Stage U2 tumor infiltrating the superficial part of the detrusor muscle (arrow). Arrowheads point to the outer margin of the muscle. The right ureter is seen intramurally (open arrow).

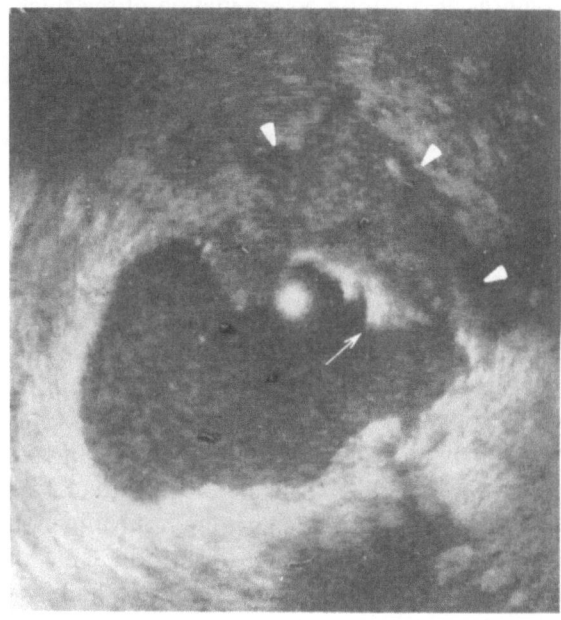

Figure 7.19. Stage U3 tumor. The arrow points to concretion at the surface of the tumor. The hypoechoic tumor infiltrates through the detrusor (arrowheads).

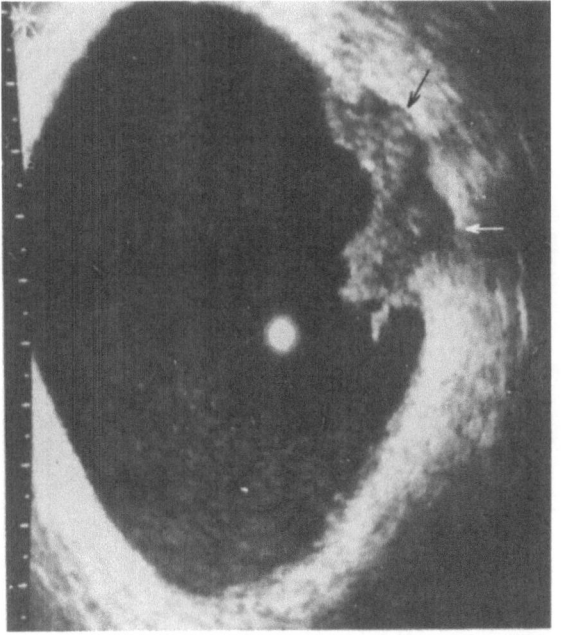

Figure 7.18. Broad-based, stage U3 tumor penetrating through the detrusor (arrows).

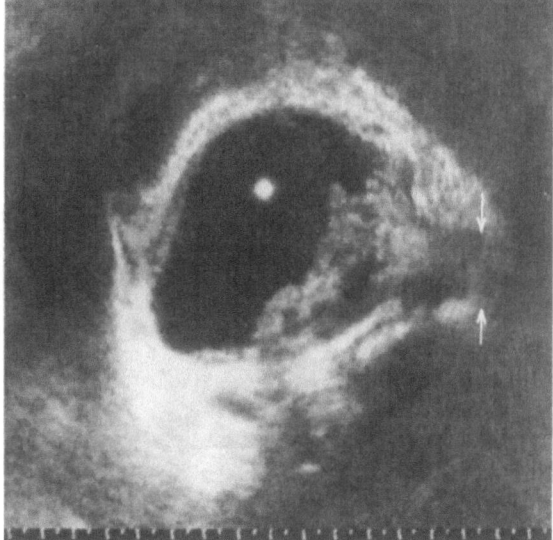

Figure 7.20. Stage U4 tumor. The large tumor has penetrated through the wall and reaches the pelvic sidewall (arrows).

located at the top of the bladder or in the vicinity of the bladder neck may not be adequately demonstrated.

Delineation of the outer border of the wall
Differentiation between U2 and U3 tumors

bladder are adequately evaluated because the beam is virtually perpendicular to the wall. Despite modified orientation of the probe or the use of the retrograde-viewing transducer, tumors

114

requires an accurate determination of the thickness of the bladder wall. However, in some cases the interface between the detrusor muscle and the perivesical fat is poorly defined (Fig. 7.22). The use of a transducer of higher frequency may improve the bladder wall delineation.

Sound wave absorption by the tumor

Bulky or calcified tumors are often associated with a marked distal attenuation of the ultrasound beam (Fig. 7.23). This obscures the detrusor distal to the tumor and tumor invasion may be simulated, resulting in overstaging. This pitfall may be avoided by carefully adjusting the gain settings and by changing the position of the transducer. A somewhat similar phenomenon can occur due to coagulated tissue after TUR of a bladder tumor (Fig. 7.24). It is therefore strongly recommended that transurethral sonographic examination be performed prior to TUR or biopsy.

Postirradiation changes

It has proven to be impossible to sonographically distinguish between postirradiation inflammatory changes in the bladder wall and diffuse tumor recurrence (Figs. 7.25, 7.26).

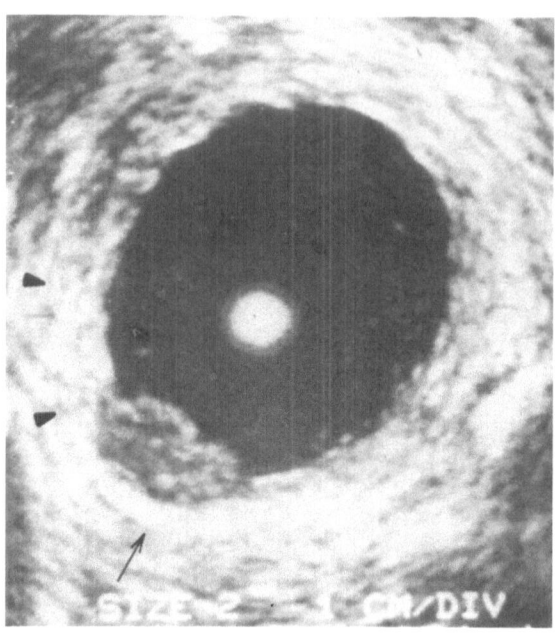

Figure 7.22. Poor delineation of the outer margin of the detrusor from the adjacent fat (arrowheads). The delineation is better (arrow) at the site of the tumor, which has not entirely penetrated the wall.

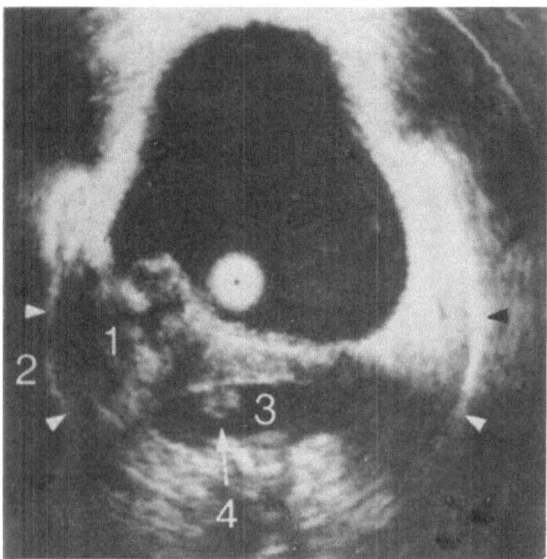

Figure 7.21. Stage U4 tumor. Endovesical sonogram shows a large tumor involving the posterior and right lateral aspect of the bladder and reaching the right pelvic sidewall. 1 = tumor; 2 (and arrowheads) = iliac bones; 3 = ascites in cul-de-sac; 4 = tumor deposit.

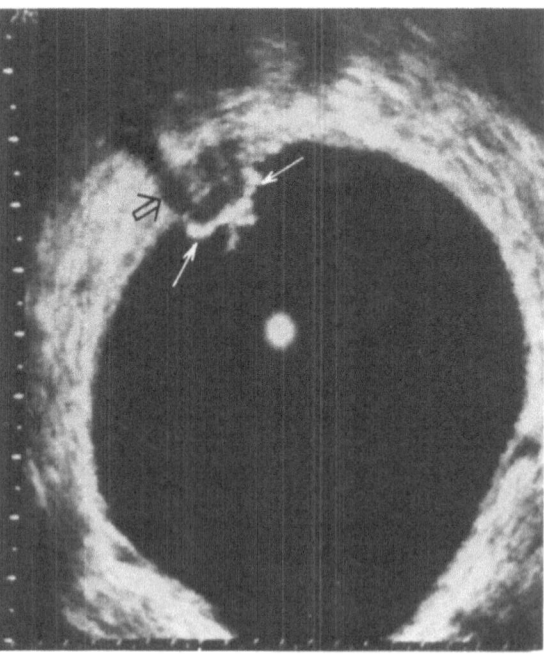

Figure 7.23. Calcified bladder tumor. The calcification (arrows) at the surface of the tumor is associated with acoustic shadowing (open arrow).

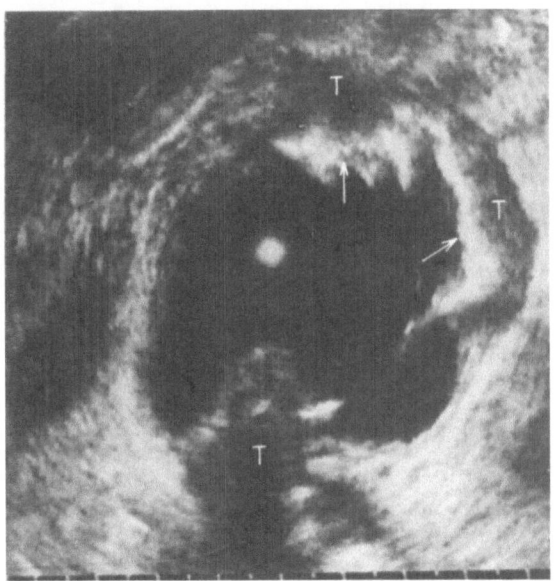

Figure 7.24. Large, multifocal bladder tumor (T) after TUR. Arrows point to the echogenic superficial layer of coagulated tissue.

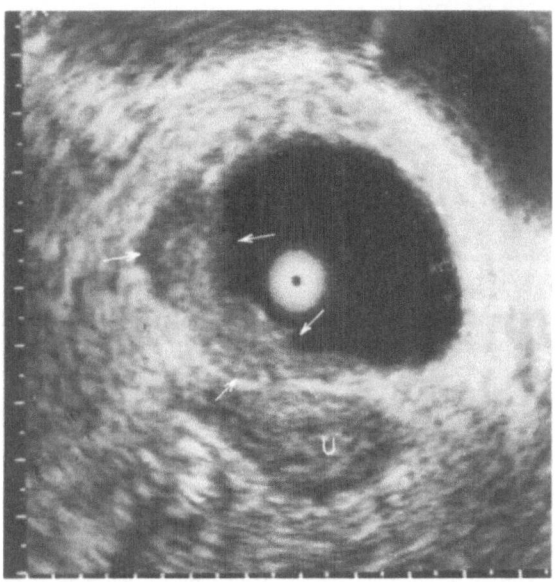

Figure 7.26. Chronic inflammatory changes in the bladder wall (arrows) after external-beam radiation therapy for cervical carcinoma. No bladder tumor was found at cystoscopy and biopsy. U = body of uterus.

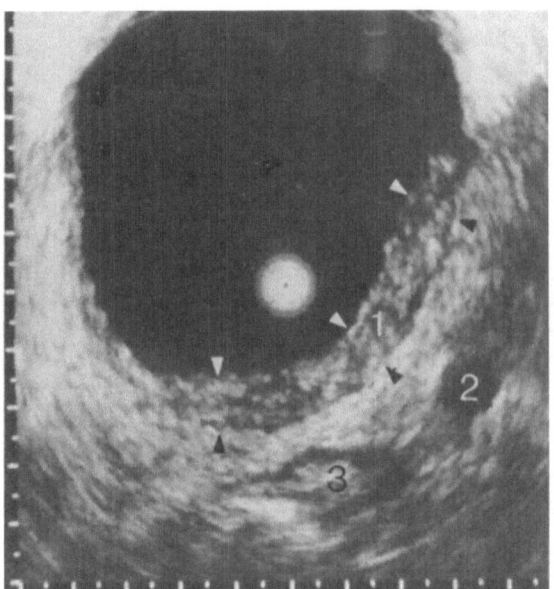

Figure 7.25. Submucosal tumor infiltration (1 and arrowheads). 2 = dilated left ureter; 3 = rectum.

Results

We have utilized transurethral scanning in 78 patients with bladder cancer in which local infiltration was suspected. A urologist and a sonologist were involved in the procedure, with cystoscopy carried out before the ultrasound examination. We excluded patients with tumors that were overtly superficial at cystoscopy because in such cases intravesical sonographic examination is superfluous. The ultrasound stage was registered and the histopathologic stage later obtained from TUR ($n = 67$) or bladder resection or cystectomy specimen ($n = 9$). It soon became obvious that intravesical sonography could not distinguish between an infiltrative bladder tumor and a situation of postirradiation sequelae without viable tumor. Therefore, 13 patients who had received radiation therapy were excluded from the series. Another five patients were excluded because of the absence of pathologic correlation or inconclusive ultrasound studies. Among the remaining 60 patients, ultrasound tumor staging was correct in 46 (77%), too high in 11 (18%), and too low in 3 (5%).

Since transurethral probes became commercially available, a number of investigators have reported their experience with the method [5–17] (Table 7.1). But most series have been small, and there has been marked variation in the distribution of tumors by clinical stage, making

Table 7.1. Results of bladder tumor staging by transurethral sonography (modified from ref. 17).

Author(s) [Ref.]	Pathologic staging						
	Ta/T1 tumors			T2/T3 tumors			
	No. of lesions	Accuracy (%)	Overstaging (%)	No. of lesions	Accuracy (%)	Understaging (%)	Overstaging (%)
Nakamura and Niijima [5]	15	93	7	5	100	0	0
Paoletti *et al.* [6]	Total number of lesions = 18; overall accuracy = 89%.						
Pfitzenmaier *et al.* [7]	16	31	69	15	100	0	0
Schüller *et al.* [8]	8	100	0	20	90	5	5
Alzin *et al.* [9]	48	100	0	142	84	13	3
Braeckman and Denis [10]	57	100	0	15	87	13	0
Greiner *et al.* [11]	6	83	17	19	58	21	21
Janetschek *et al.* [12]	24	79	21	17	95	ND	ND
Lopatkin *et al.* [13]	119	70	30		74—85	ND	ND
Schmidtbauer *et al.* [14]	14	93	7	30	83	17	0
Wenderoth *et al.* [15]	Total number of lesions = 19; accuracy = 37%; understaging = 42%; overstaging = 21%.						
Salo [16]	64	97	3	18*	83	11	6
Jaeger *et al.* [17]	341	71	29	230*	68	21	11

ND = no data available.   * lesions include T4 tumors.

comparisons difficult. Our series excluded tumors that were obviously superficial at cystoscopy. Taking these into account would have resulted in an increased overall accuracy. A major limitation of all the studies is the small number of cystectomies, the final diagnosis most often being obtained by TUR.

The largest series to date was published in 1986 by Jaeger *et al.* [17], comprising 571 patients with pathologically verified primary or recurrent bladder carcinoma. The staging by intravesical ultrasound was compared with the histopathologic category, determined by TUR in 523 patients and by partial bladder resection or cystectomy in the other 48. The authors found agreement in 70% of the cases, compared with an overall accuracy of 67% for conventional staging (consisting of physical examination with the patient under anesthesia). Ultrasound overstaged 29% of the superficial tumors (Ta and T1) and understaged 21% of the infiltrating carcinomas (T2, T3, and T4). Large superficial tumors were particularly likely to be overstaged. The sensitivity, specificity, and overall accuracy of transurethral sonography in identifying muscle invasion in this series were 90%, 71%, and

79%, respectively. This sensitivity was significantly higher than that of conventional staging (66%). In staging small broad-based papillary tumors (diameter of 1—3 cm), sonography had an accuracy of 76%, compared with 12% for conventional methods. The authors concluded that 'without doubt, diagnosis of bladder carcinoma has made a significant step forward with the introduction of transurethral sonography.'

Staging of bladder tumors, routinely accomplished by a combination of cystoscopy, bimanual palpation, and TUR or biopsy, is instrumental in the selection of therapy, prognostic evaluation, and also comparison of results from various institutions. It is generally accepted that cystoscopy and palpation are rather inaccurate [18]. Multiple biopsies indicate with a great degree of certainty the presence of tumor at the sites of biopsy. However, they cannot assess a large surface and may miss partial invasion in broad-based tumors, and it is at times difficult to determine with accuracy the depth of tumor infiltration from biopsy specimens.

Intravesical ultrasound can be expected to demonstrate early invasion of the detrusor and to differentiate between partial and complete infiltration. However, it must be borne in mind that endosonography, like other imaging modalities, cannot detect microscopic tumor infiltration. This doubtlessly accounts for some of the understaged cases. On the other hand, overstaging should be reduced with experience and improved equipment, since errors have often been due to misinterpretation of images.

Intravesical sonography is superior to computed tomography when tumor is confined to the bladder wall, while the latter is better at evaluating T4 tumors because of its better depiction of perivesical structures [16].

Other pathologic conditions in the bladder

Bladder trabeculation (Fig. 7.27) appears as a rough irregularity of the inner surface of the bladder, sometimes indistinguishable from papillomatosis.

Cystitis is characterized by a variable bladder wall thickening. In some cases, sonography is not able to differentiate between inflammatory changes and malignant infiltration confined to the bladder wall. Focal lesions of cystitis (which are rare) can mimic superficial tumors.

Blood clots, whose echogenicity vary with their age, appear as mobile intravesical masses.

But malignancy may be suggested when they adhere to the wall.

Bladder calculi are characterized by a bright acoustic reflection associated with distal shadowing (Fig. 7.28).

Bladder diverticula are seen as fluid-filled pouches adjacent to the bladder wall. The neck of the diverticulum is easily identified (Fig. 7.29).

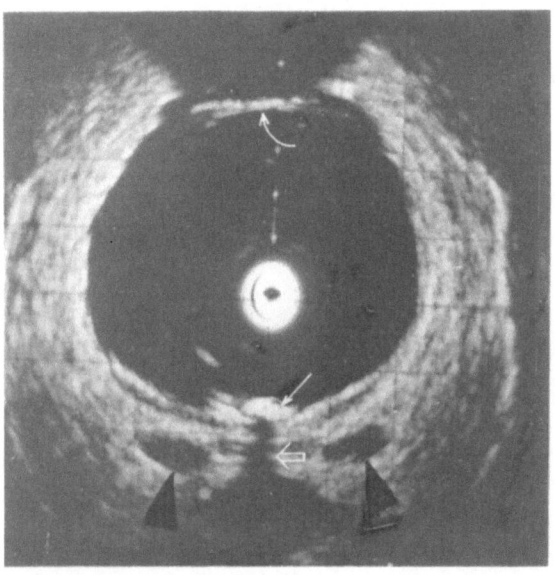

Figure 7.28. Bladder calculus. A brightly echogenic calculus (arrow) is seen in the dependent portion of the bladder with acoustic shadowing (open arrow). Arrowheads point to the seminal vesicles. Note the air bubble at the top of image (curved arrow), also followed by an acoustic shadow.

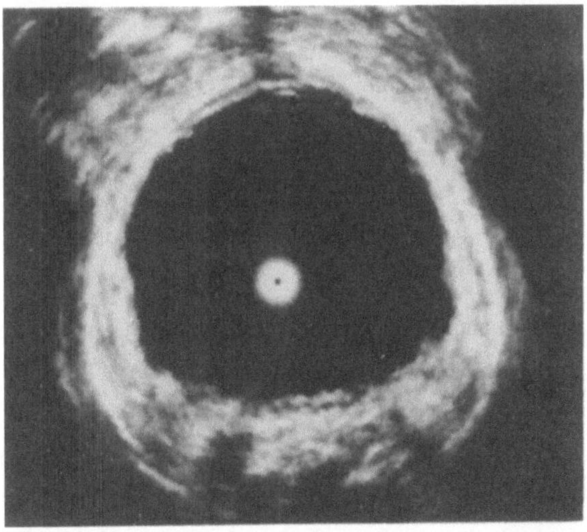

Figure 7.27. Bladder trabeculation. There is moderate thickening of the detrusor and irregularity of the mucosal surface.

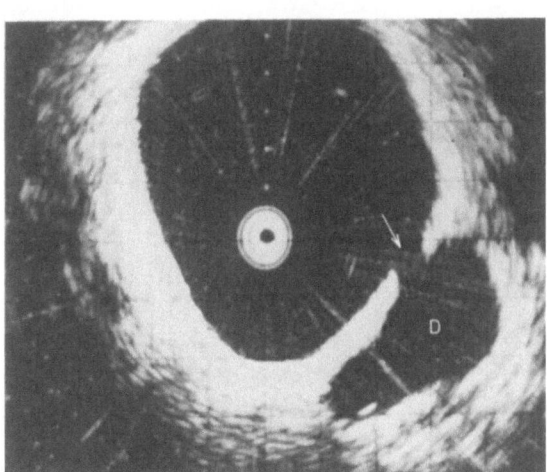

Figure 7.29. Bladder diverticulum. The diverticulum is seen as a sonolucent fluid-filled pocket (D). The neck is clearly visible (arrow).

Transurethral scanning is a useful adjunct to cystoscopy when an intradiverticular tumor is suspected.

Ureteroceles are seen as thin-walled, fluid-filled masses within the fluid-filled bladder at the site of a ureteral orifice or in an ectopic location.

Prostatic disorders

Transurethral scanning may be used during TUR for benign prostatic hypertrophy to visualize the amount of tissue still to be excised (Fig.

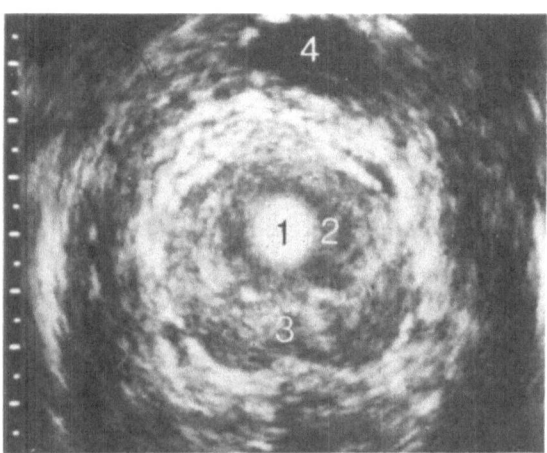

a

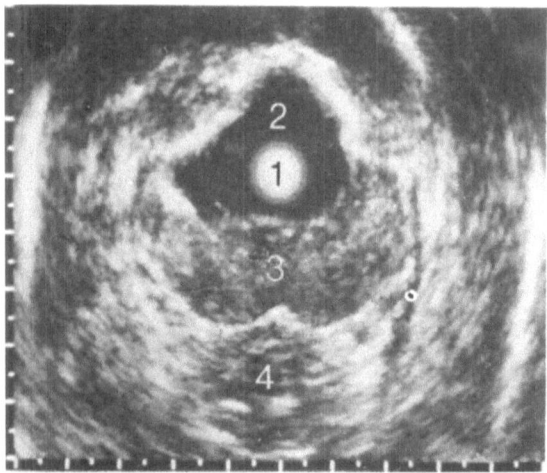

b

Figure 7.30. Scans of the prostate before (a) and after (b) transurethral prostatic resection. The transducer is in the prostatic urethra. (a) 1 = transducer; 2 = adenoma; 3 = peripheral prostate; 4 = bladder. (b) 1 = transducer; 2 = postresection cavity; 3 = peripheral prostate; 4 = rectum.

7.30). It is also useful for teaching purposes in this setting. In patients with prostatic carcinoma, a good impression of the capsular involvement, periprostatic tumor infiltration, and invasion of the seminal vesicles can be achieved. However, the routine approach for endosonography of the prostate and seminal vesicles remains the transrectal one since a larger transducer, yielding improved image quality, can be used and instrumentation of the urinary tract can be avoided.

References

1. Holm H. H., Northeved A.: A transurethral ultrasonic scanner. J. Urol., 1974, 111, 238–241.
2. Fornage B.: Echographie de la prostate. Paris, Vigot, 1985, pp 43–73.
3. Gammelgaard J., Holm H. H.: Transurethral and transrectal ultrasonic scanning in urology. J. Urol., 1980, 124, 863–868.
4. Komine Y., Kimura A., Niizuma M., Nakamura S., Kawabe K., Niijima T.: Transurethral ultrasonotomography of the prostate. Prostate, 1981, 1 (Suppl.), 53–57.
5. Nakamura S., Niijima T.: Staging of bladder cancer by ultrasonography: A new technique by transurethral intravesical scanning. J. Urol., 1980, 124, 341–344.
6. Paoletti P. P., Tenti S., Fiorelli C., Francalanci R., Paoletti M. C.: L'ecografia endocavitaria transurethrale. Urologia, 1982, 49, 648–654.
7. Pfitzenmaier N., Ikinger U., Möhring K.: Transurethrale Sonographie. Eine neue Methode zur Stadieneinteilung von Blasentumoren? 28. Tg. Nordrhein-Westf. Ges. Urol., 1982.
8. Schüller J., Walther V., Schmiedt E., Staehler G., Bauer H. W., Schilling A.: Intravesical ultrasound tomography in staging bladder carcinoma. J. Urol., 1982, 128, 264–266.
9. Alzin H. H., Braedel H. U., Schwaiger R., Kopper B.: Vergleich zwischen Computertomogramm und endovesikaler Sonographie bei der Diagnostik und Klassifikation grösserer Blasentumoren. Verh. Dtsch. Ges. Urol., 1983, 35, 231–233.
10. Braeckman J., Denis L.: The practice and pitfalls of ultrasonography in the lower urinary tract. Eur. Urol., 1983, 9, 193–201.
11. Greiner K. G., Jacob F., Klose K. C., Schwartz R.: Sicherung der T-Klassifikation von Harnblasentumoren durch transkutane Sonographie, intravesikale Sonographie und Computertomographie. ROFO, 1983, 139, 510–515.
12. Janetschek G., Jaske G., Egender G., zur Nedden D.: Der Stellenwert der endovesikalen Sonographie. Verh. Dtsch. Ges. Urol., 1983, 35, 221–222.
13. Lopatkin N. A., Darenkov A. F., Ignashin N. S.: [Ultra-

sonic diagnosis of vesical neoplasms]. Urol. Nefrol. (Mosk.), 1983, 4, 3—7.

14. Schmidtbauer C. P., Schramek P., Studler G.: Stadieneinteilung von Primärtumor und Rezidiv beim Blasenkarzinom durch endovesikale Sonographie. Verh. Dtsch. Ges. Urol., 1983, 35, 223—226.

15. Wenderoth U. K., Engelmann U., Walz P. H., Jacobi G. H.: Die intravesikale Sonographie in der Stadieneinteilung des Harnblasenkarzinoms. Verh. Dtsch. Ges. Urol., 1983, 35, 215—216.

16. Salo J.: Endo-ultrasonography and computed tomography in staging bladder and prostatic cancers. Thesis. Helsingfors Universitet, 1986.

17. Jaeger N., Radeke H. W., Adolphs H. D., Bertermann H., Vahlensieck W.: Value of intravesical sonography in tumor classification of bladder carcinoma. Eur. Urol., 1986, 12, 76— 84.

18. Kenny G. M., Hardner G. J., Murphy G. P.: Clinical staging of bladder tumors. J. Urol., 1970, 104, 720—723.

8. Transvaginal sonography of micturition and urinary incontinence

JACQUES L. BECO, MASEB S. SULU, AND JEAN-PIERRE J. SCHAAPS

Real-time sonography of micturition in the female using the transvaginal approach is a recent application of endosonography. It has recently been added to the tests used in evaluation of voiding abnormalities and urinary incontinence, augmenting physical, urodynamic, and radiographic studies. Ultrasound has a brief history in the assessment of female urinary incontinence. In the past decade, a few investigators have used transabdominal sonography to study the posterior bladder wall at rest [1] or to assess the mobility of the bladder neck localized by a urethral catheter during the bearing-down maneuver [2, 3]. A more accurate delineation of the bladder base, bladder neck, and urethra was obtained with transrectal sonography [4], and development of a small endorectal probe has enabled such imaging with excellent patient tolerance and no alteration of urethrovesical junction mobility [5]. The evaluation of female urinary incontinence by transvaginal sonography was first reported in 1985 by Debus-Thiede et al. [6]. These authors evaluated changes in the orientation of a urethral catheter depending on the hold and bear-down maneuvers in both normal women and patients with incontinence and measured the posterior vesicourethral angle and the postvoiding bladder residue. Jeny et al. in 1986 studied the lowering and opening of the bladder neck in patients with stress incontinence [7]. Similar to the combination of urodynamic studies with cinefluoroscopy, it is now possible to combine urodynamic manometric studies with real-time ultrasound imaging to obtain an accurate morphologic and dynamic picture of the urethra and bladder base [8].

Instrumentation

High-resolution linear-array intracavitary probes are preferred for the sonographic evaluation of micturition because of their high-quality near-field and wide field of view.

The urodynamic studies are performed using a standard four-channel instrument, one channel designated to record bladder pressure, one used for urethral pressure, and one reserved for intraabdominal pressure. The pressure profiles are displayed on a video monitor with memory capability. An electromyographic recorder with needle electrodes and a uroflowmeter can also be utilized.

Technique of examination

The uroflowmetric study is performed first. Upon its completion, the bladder is filled with normal saline solution via a transurethral catheter. The linear-array probe is then inserted in the vagina with the transducer placed in direct contact with the vesicourethral area. Care is taken not to exert any pressure on the urethra with the endovaginal probe; this factor is monitored by recording the urethral pressure. The accurate localization of the bladder neck and urethra is facilitated by the presence of the catheter (Böhler's catheter, 7F). The more

Bruno D. Fornage (ed.), *Endosonography*, pp. 121—128.
© 1989 *Kluwer Academic Publishers*.

proximal of the catheter's two pressure-recording transducers, which are 6 cm apart, is distinctly shaped and readily located sonographically.

Normal ultrasound anatomy

The *bladder* can only be visualized completely when it is virtually empty, that is, at the beginning of filling or at the end of voiding. Otherwise, only the bladder base is included in the field of view. The ureteral meatus are accurately localized by the echogenic turbulences ('jet phenomenon') caused by the ureteral ejections.

The *urethra* and *bladder neck* are localized by the cystometric catheter; the urethra is roughly parallel to the surface of the intravaginal probe (Fig. 8.1). A hypoechoic spindle-shaped area, the *sphincteric zone*, surrounds the urethra and corresponds to the functional profile length of the sphincteric unit, as indicated by the pressure recordings when the catheter is withdrawn under sonographic monitoring.

The posterior aspect of the *pubic bone* is visualized as a densely echogenic curved linear pattern associated with acoustic shadowing. The *symphysis pubis* is seen on the midsagittal scan as two convex lines. The line that is nearest the urethra corresponds to the subpubic ligament; the other represents the true posterior margin of the symphysis itself. The symphysis pubis attenuates the ultrasound beam less than the pubic bones.

The *space of Retzius* is delineated by the sphincteric zone posteriorly, the urinary bladder superiorly, and the pubis anteriorly. Sonographically, it appears as a slightly nonhomogeneous echogenic area. In some patients, large veins can be visualized.

In the area that extends from the clitoris to the external meatus, a thin, slightly hypoechoic, contractile layer a few millimeters thick, the *prepubic muscle*, can be depicted (Fig. 8.2). The detailed anatomy of this area is controversial. Rouvière described an extension of a deep layer of the bulbocavernosus muscle that terminates in Kobelt's pars intermedia [9]. According to Krantz, a significant number of fibers of the

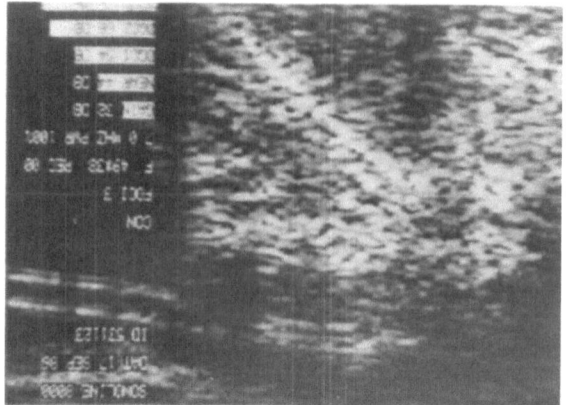

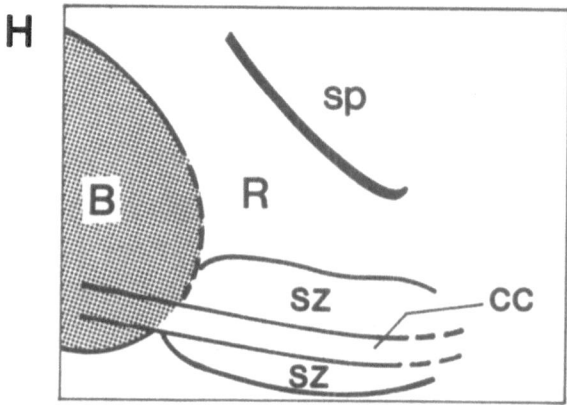

Figure 8.1. Midsagittal transvaginal scan of the periurethral structures. A cystometric catheter is in the urethra. It appears roughly parallel to the intravaginal ultrasound probe and has echogenic walls. The sphincteric zone is hypoechoic. B = bladder; cc = cystometric catheter; H = toward patient's head; R = Retzius space; sp = symphysis pubis; sz = sphincteric zone.

bulbocavernosus and ischiocavernosus muscles interlace in the interclitoromeatal area and terminate on the anterior and lateral aspects of the urethra [10]. According to Zacharin, this area would in fact represent a ligamentous structure extending from the pubis to the anterior periurethral area [11].

During micturition, the whole length of the female urethra can be visualized. Its course is that of a flattened sinusoidal curve whose general axis remains grossly parallel to the intravaginal ultrasound probe. Its caliber tapers from the bladder neck to the external meatus (Fig. 8.3). The bladder base comes progressively closer to the anterior vaginal wall, and at the

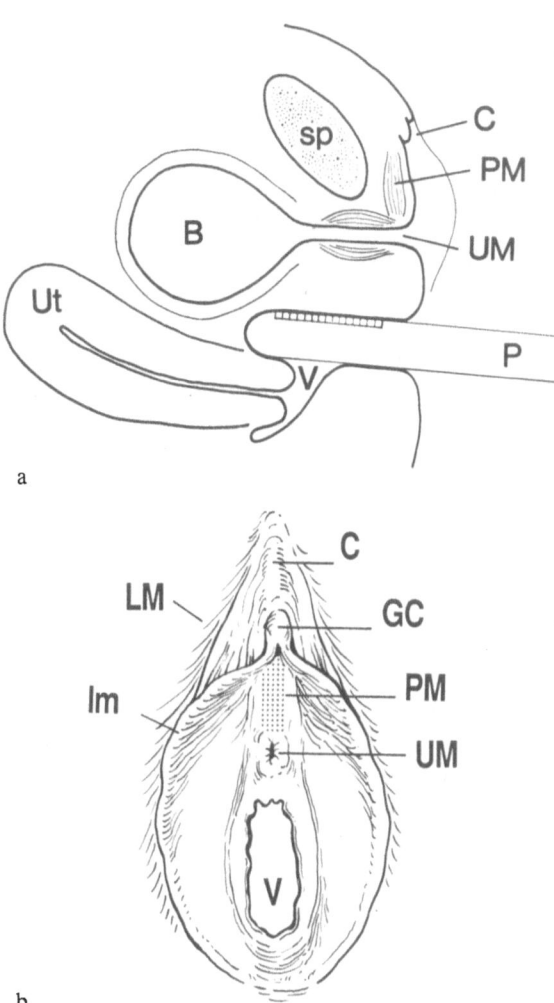

a

b

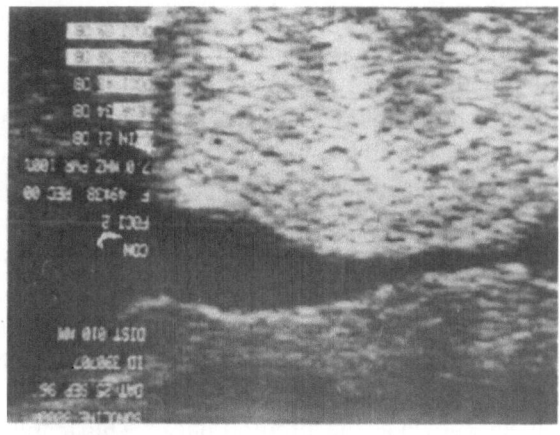

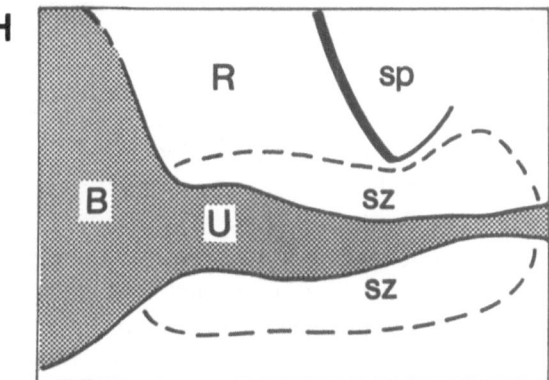

Figure 8.3. Midsagittal transvaginal scan. Normal voiding study. The distended urethra tapers from the bladder neck to the external meatus. B = bladder; H = toward patient's head; R = Retzius space; sp = symphysis pubis; sz = sphincteric zone; U = urethra.

Figure 8.2. The prepubic muscles (see text for details). (a) Diagrammatic midsagittal section shows the relationships of the prepubic muscle with the urethra and sphincteric zone. B = bladder; C = clitoris; P = intravaginal linear-array probe; PM = prepubic muscle; sp = symphysis pubis; UM = urethral meatus; Ut = uterus; V = vagina. (b) Diagrammatic representation of the vulva. C = clitoris; GC = glans of clitoris; LM = labium majus; lm = labium minus; PM = prepubic muscle; UM = urethral meatus; V = vagina.

cessation of micturition the traction by the prepubic muscle slackens and the urethral sphincter gently closes. Some contractions of the levator ani muscles may contribute to expel the last drops of urine by squeezing the urethra. These contractions, which are usually seen at the end of spontaneous micturition, are necessary to the hold maneuver required for the voluntary interruption of micturition.

Correlation between sonographic and urodynamic findings

Correlating sonographic and urodynamic findings requires the simultaneous display of the periurethral soft tissue structures and the localization of the manometric catheter transducers.

Normal findings

Static study
In a supine patient whose bladder has been filled with 250 mL of physiological saline, modifying the position of the manometric catheter allows determination of a simple pressure profile in the urethra. The urethral closure pressure is low at the level of the internal meatus and increases

gradually to reach a maximum value in the midurethra. The pressure then slowly drops as the manometric transducer comes out of the hypoechoic spindle-shaped periurethral area, which is thereby confirmed as the sphincteric unit. The length of the sphincteric unit as demonstrated on sonography roughly corresponds to the functional profile length described on urodynamic studies. In the sphincteric area, where the urethral closure pressure is greatest, the systolic blood flow results in a pulsation, which is transmitted to the urethral manometric transducer known as the 'urethral pulse.' This feature is more prominent in young women.

Dynamic study

Dynamic tests can be performed and their effects monitored both urodynamically and sonographically.

Stress from coughing or straining. No significant alteration of the position of the bladder neck in relation to the pubis is usually demonstrated in response to stress from coughing or bearing down. Occasionally, a slight decrease in the distance between the pubis and the anterior vaginal wall is noted. Urodynamic study shows a sustained or augmented urethral closure pressure during these stress maneuvers.

Hold maneuver. When the hold maneuver is performed, the action of pelvic floor muscles, particularly the levator ani muscles, results in back-to-front movement that brings the vagina closer to the pubis, squeezing the urethra. On the urodynamic recording from the manometric transducer placed at the area of maximum urethral pressure, this dynamic compression corresponds to an increase in closure pressure, namely, the maximum urethral pressure gain.

Voiding study. In our experience, 80% of normal volunteers could urinate during the combined sonographic-urodynamic examination. These studies have pointed out the major role of the prepubic muscle in micturition. At the initiation of micturition, the structure creates significant traction on the anterior aspect of the sphincteric zone and subsequently on the anterior lip of the bladder neck. The activity of the prepubic muscle results in a pressure drop in the urethra, sometimes associated with opening of the bladder neck. However, this opening will be followed by micturition only if bladder contractions are associated with a further drop in urethral pressure. This drop in pressure results from longitudinal contractile activity in the sphincteric zone and from the relaxation of the levator ani muscles, the latter represented on sonography by an increase in the distance between the anterior vaginal wall and the pubis. This significant role of the pelvic floor muscles can also be assessed using suprapubic sonography. In this case, the whole vagina moves away from the symphysis pubis in the prevoiding phase, whereas it is pushed anteriorly during the hold maneuver.

Pathologic results

Cystoceles and urethroceles

Cystoceles develop behind the urethra inferiorly and posteriorly. With straining, large cystoceles may compress the sphincteric zone with a 'molding' effect (Figs. 8.4, 8.5). *Urethroceles* are characterized by posterior sliding of the bladder

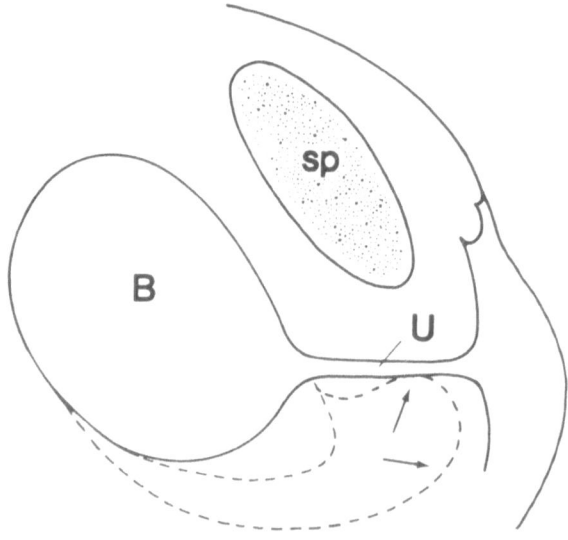

Figure 8.4. Diagrammatic midsagittal section shows the development of a cystocele (dotted lines). The cystocele may compress the urethra posteriorly. B = bladder; sp = symphysis pubis; U = urethra.

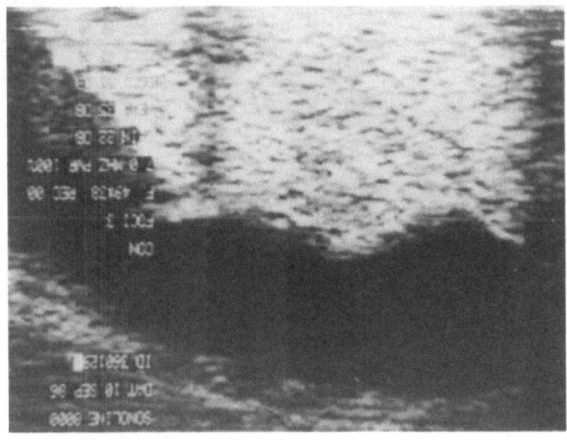

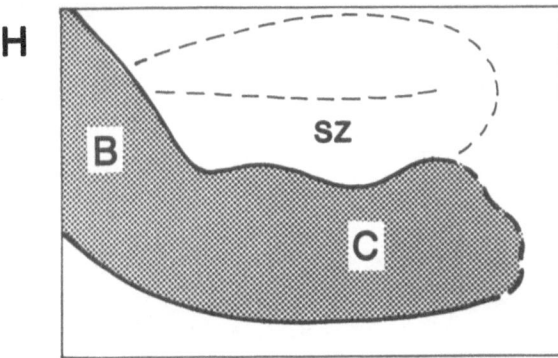

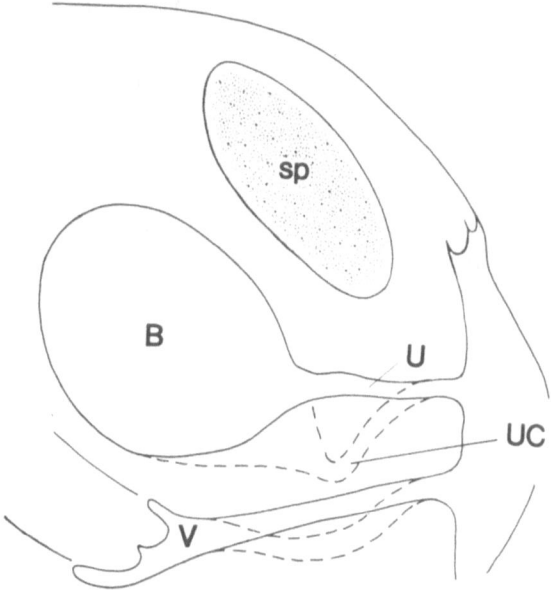

Figure 8.6. Diagrammatic midsagittal section shows the anatomic alterations in a case of urethrocele (dotted lines). Note the marked angle between the urethra and trigone. B = bladder; sp = symphysis pubis; U = urethra; UC = urethrocystocele; V = vagina.

Figure 8.5. Midsagittal transvaginal scan shows a cystocele between the collapsed urethra and the sphincteric zone anteriorly and the vagina posteriorly. B = bladder; C = cystocele; H = toward patient's head; sz = sphincteric zone.

neck, which results in an angle between the urethra and trigone (Fig. 8.6), best demonstrated at coughing.

Stress incontinence

Stress incontinence is the involuntary loss of urine from the urethra caused by an increase in intra-abdominal pressure, for example, with coughing, straining, laughing, or sneezing. Three factors influence the development of stress incontinence.

1. Defect in transmission (DT) of increased intra-abdominal pressure to the urethra. An increase in intra-abdominal pressure results in an increase in vesical pressure ($\varDelta VP$) greater than the increase in urethral pressure ($\varDelta UP$):

$$DT = \frac{\varDelta VP - \varDelta UP}{\varDelta VP}.$$

2. Urethral closure pressure (CP). This pressure represents the difference between the vesical and the urethral pressure and is directly responsible for continence.
3. Intra-abdominal peak pressure ($P_{\max}$). This pressure is obtained at coughing or straining. It varies by individual patient but is fairly constant in any given patient in follow-up studies.

Continence during stress maneuvers implies that the urethral pressure UP' remains greater than the vesical pressure VP', that is, that the residual closure pressure (residual CP) is positive:

$$\text{residual } CP = UP' - VP' = CP - (P_{\max} \times DT).$$

The better the transmission of intra-abdominal pressure to the urethra (or the smaller the DT), the higher the increase in urethral pressure and the residual CP.

For example, given a patient with a CP of 60 cm of water and a DT of 60%, the residual CP for a stress maneuver developing an increase in abdominal pressure of 80 cm of water would be:

residual $CP = 60 - (80 \times 0.6)$
$\qquad = 12$ cm of water,

and continence would be preserved.

If the same patient developed an increase in abdominal pressure of 120 cm of water, the residual CP would be:

residual $CP = 60 - (120 \times 0.6)$
$\qquad = -12$ cm of water,

and the patient would be incontinent.

Thus, patients who have a significant DT but develop only moderate peak stress pressures will remain continent, whereas those who have a moderate DT but are able to develop significant peak abdominal pressures will suffer from stress incontinence. The DT should always be related to the peak stress pressure in a given individual.

Stress incontinence can result from an isolated DT, isolated sphincteric weakness, or a combination of the two.

Origin in an isolated DT. Stress incontinence that develops from an isolated DT first occurs in the standing position. Later, it also appears in the supine position.

When stress incontinence occurs in the standing position, and not in the supine position, the most common sonographic finding is the sliding downward of the bladder neck posterior to the symphysis pubis (Fig. 8.7). The Retzius space behaves as a loose area, attached at its pubic and vesicourethral ends, and is subjected to a significant shear force. This results in the descent of the bladder neck obliquely downward and posteriorly. The descent can be quantified by measuring the displacement of the bladder neck in relation to a line drawn perpendicular to the urethral axis from the lower aspect of the symphysis pubis (Fig. 8.8). Infrequently, sonography can demonstrate the bladder neck opening when sagging is maximum.

When stress incontinence occurs in both the standing and supine positions, transvaginal sonography can usually demonstrate the passage of urine in the urethra at coughing.

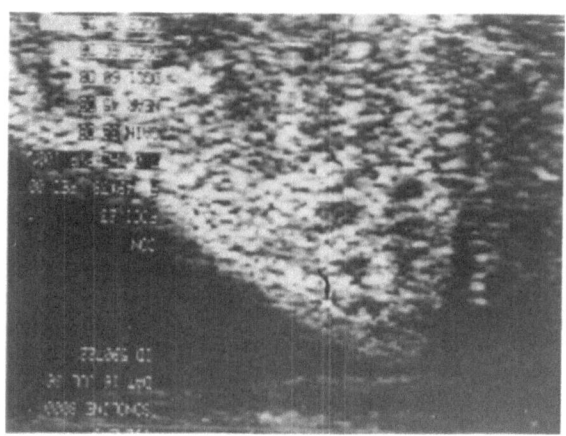

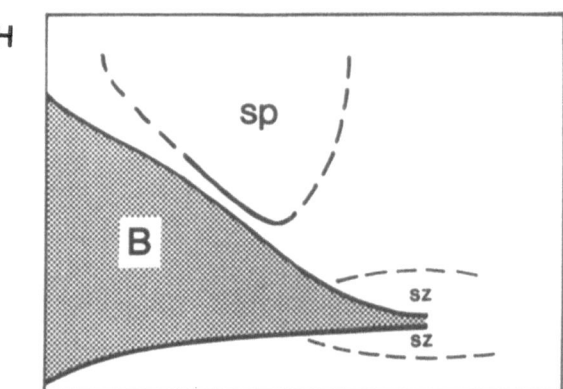

Figure 8.7. Midsagittal transvaginal scan. Stress incontinence due to defect in transmission (see text for details). The Retzius space slides below the symphysis. The bladder neck is dragged downward and opens. B = bladder; H = toward patient's head; sp = symphysis pubis; sz = sphincteric zone.

Origin in isolated impairment of sphincteric function. On the patient's coughing or bearing down, the bladder neck and the urethra open but no significant descent of the bladder neck can be seen.

Postoperative patterns. Various surgical techniques for the treatment of stress incontinence have been proposed. The Burch technique consists of anchoring the anterior vaginal wall to the Cooper's ligaments by three sutures on either side of the urethra and bladder neck.

On *static studies* performed after the Burch procedure, the urethra is no longer parallel to the ultrasound probe but parallel to the posterior aspect of the pubis. The thickness of the Retzius space is diminished.

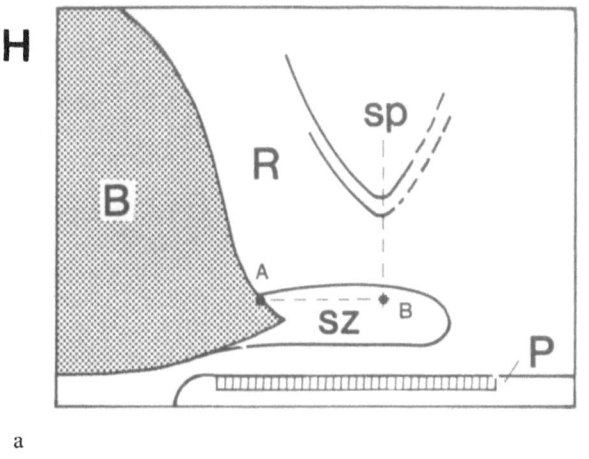

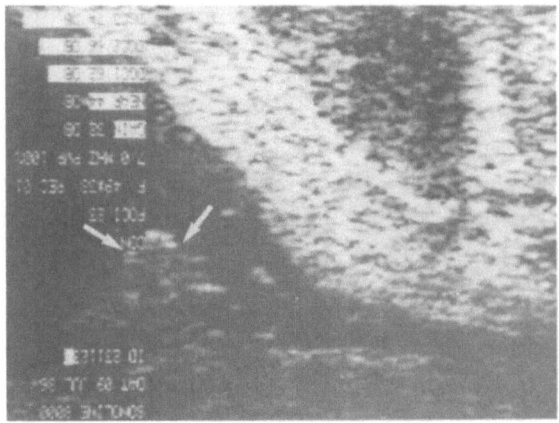

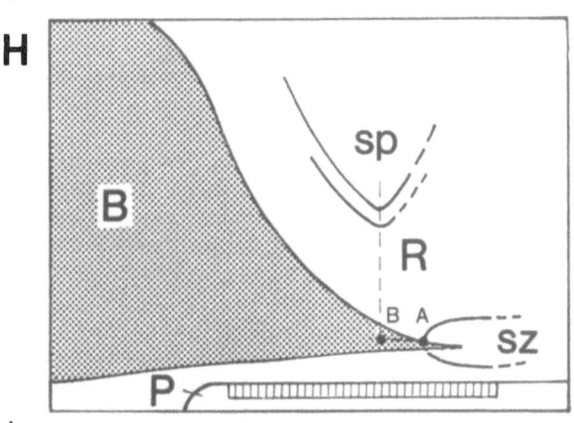

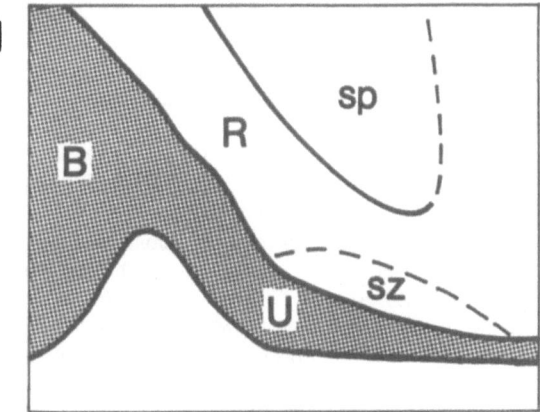

Figure 8.8. Measurement of the descent of the bladder neck. (a) At rest. (b) During stress maneuvers, the descent of the bladder neck can be quantified by the measurement of the distance AB. B = bladder; H = toward patient's head; P = intravaginal linear-array probe; R = Retzius space; sp = symphysis pubis; sz = sphincteric zone.

Figure 8.9. Midsagittal transvaginal scan. Postoperative pattern following colposuspension. Retzius space remains tightly attached to the pubis during coughing. The bulge from the suspension sutures is well depicted at the posterior aspect of the bladder neck (arrows). B = bladder; H = toward patient's head; R = Retzius space; sp = symphysis pubis; sz = sphincteric zone; U = urethra.

During coughing, there is a back transmission of the intra-abdominal peak pressure, with the force vector virtually perpendicular to the anterior vaginal wall [12].

In a *voiding study* after anterior colposuspension, a posterior ledge is frequently visualized at the bladder neck (Fig. 8.9). Distal to this ledge, echogenic turbulences are often depicted. Postoperative urodynamic studies confirm the decreased urinary flow rate that results from the posterior ledge at the bladder neck.

Urethral instability and urge incontinence
Urethral instability is characterized by repeated, involuntary drops in urethral pressure, during which it is possible to see the same activities as during the initiation of micturition. Relaxation of the levator ani muscles and contraction of the longitudinal fibers of the sphincteric zone and of the prepubic muscle can be seen independently or in combination. They may be followed by a bladder contraction that may result in incontinence.

Conclusion

Urodynamic studies are currently fundamental to the evaluation and management of urinary incontinence in women. Transvaginal sonography brings a new, morphologic dimension. A combination of real-time images and functional manometric data now allows a better understanding of the mechanisms of normal and pathological micturition.

Other potential benefits of transvaginal sonography of the female urethra include the evaluation of urethral tumors, diverticula, and strictures. Further investigation is needed in these applications.

References

1. Schaaps J. P., Romus M. A.: Ultrasonographic aspect of urinary incontinence in women (abstract). Proceedings of the 2nd Meeting of the World Federation for Ultrasound in Medicine and Biology, Miyazaki, July 1979, 345.
2. Bhatia N. N., McQuown D., Ostergard D. R.: Ultrasonography in the evaluation of urethrovesical dynamics of genuine stress incontinence and instability (abstract). Proceedings of the First Joint Meeting of the International Continence Society and the Urodynamic Society, Los Angeles, October 9—12, 1980, 303.
3. White R. D., McQuown D., McCarthy T. A., Ostergard D. R.: Real-time ultrasonography in the evaluation of urinary stress incontinence. Am. J. Obstet. Gynecol., 1980, 138, 235—237.
4. Nishizawa O., Harada T., Takada H., et al.: A new synchronous video urodynamics. Tohoku J. Exp. Med., 1982, 136, 349—350.
5. Bergman A., Ballard C. A., Platt L. D.: Ultrasonic evaluation of urethrovesical junction in women with stress urinary incontinence. J. Clin. Ultrasound, 1988, 16, 295—300.
6. Debus-Thiede G., Wagner U., Schurmann R., Christ F.: Erste Erfahrungen mit der transvaginalen Sonographie von Urethra und Blase in Rahmen der Inkontinenz Diagnostik. Geburtshilfe Frauenheilkd., 1985, 45, 891—894.
7. Jeny R., Corjon P., Leroy B.: Etude de la dynamique urétrale en échographie transvaginale. Journal d'Echographie et de Médecine Ultrasonore, 1986, 7, 278—284.
8. Beco J., Sulu M., Schaaps J.-P., Lambotte R.: Une nouvelle approche morphodynamique des troubles de la continence chez la femme: L'échographie urodynamique par voie vaginale. J. Gynécol. Obst. Biol. Reprod., 1987, 16, 987—998.
9. Rouvière H.: Anatomie humaine descriptive et topographique, ed. 6. Paris, Masson, 1948, 1077—1078.
10. Krantz K. E.: The anatomy of the urethra and anterior vaginal wall. Am. J. Obstet. Gynecol., 1951, 62, 374—386.
11. Zacharin R. F.: The anatomic supports of the female urethra. Obstet. Gynecol., 1968, 32, 754—759.
12. Hertogs K., Stanton S. L.: Mechanism of urinary continence after colposuspension: Barrier studies. Br. J. Obstet. Gynaecol., 1985, 92, 1184—1188.

9. Transvaginal sonography in gynecology

PATRICE M. BRET

The idea of using a transvaginal sonographic approach can be traced back to 1976 [1]. The technique was then developed in Europe [2], Japan [3], and North America [4, 5], mainly to monitor follicle maturation and as a proposed alternative to the transvesical or transurethral approach to follicle aspiration [6]. The interest in transvaginal sonography outside the field of in vitro fertilization began later, and since 1986 clinical studies have been reported in the evaluation of first-trimester pregnancy [7, 8] and gynecologic diseases [9].

Endosonographic technique places the transducer close to the organ of interest, enabling high-frequency scanning and an image quality significantly improved over that of conventional ultrasound. In gynecology, moreover, transvaginal sonography visualizes the pelvic organs without the full-bladder technique required in transabdominal scanning and, hence, without the patient discomfort and sound propagation artifacts associated with that technique.

This chapter highlights the contribution of transvaginal sonography in the evaluation of gynecologic diseases. Because the technique is fairly new, some applications are still under evaluation. A number of questions concerning its role *vis-à-vis* transabdominal sonography and the clinical significance of additional information it obtains have already been answered. Such other questions as the applicability of transvaginal sonography to screening for ovarian or endometrial carcinoma are still open.

Technical considerations

Sonographic equipment

Endovaginal probes are available with the four main scanning modes: mechanical sector, phased-array sector, linear-array, and convex-array (manufacturers usually offer the scanning mode that is available on their conventional ultrasound units). The main advantage of mechanical sector scanning is its simplicity, which means lower cost. Mechanical transducers are small enough for easy insertion into the vagina. The field of view of endovaginal mechanical sector transducers ranges from 90° to 240°. Most of the mechanical sector transducers with an oscillating or rotating crystal are end-firing (i.e., the main axis of the sector scan is aligned with the general axis of the probe). Phased- and convex-array transducers have no mechanically activated parts and scan at a higher frame rate than mechanical scanners. The major drawbacks of phased-array sector systems are the restricted field of view and poor resolution in the nearfield; the latter limitation is overcome by convex-array technology.

Endovaginal transducers now in use have frequencies of 5 to 7.5 MHz. A 7.5-MHz transducer optimizes visualization of the uterus and ovaries, up to a depth of 4 to 5 cm, but its sound penetration is insufficient for more deeply located structures, such as large fundal fibroids. Some manufacturers have therefore designed mechanical sector probes with dual-frequency transducers, operating at 5 and 7.5 MHz.

Some endovaginal probes have pulsed Doppler capability. Although only a few studies with

Bruno D. Fornage (ed.), *Endosonography*, pp. 129—147.
© 1989 *Kluwer Academic Publishers.*

transvaginal Doppler examination have been reported [10], duplex studies are expected to prove useful in evaluating both the physiologic and pathologic conditions of the uterus and ovaries. There are safety limitations to the use of pulsed Doppler transvaginal examinations during pregnancy.

Technique of examination

Although the use of a gynecologic table with supporting arms for the patient's legs is convenient, transvaginal sonography can be performed with the patient lying on a conventional examination table. In the latter setting, it may be helpful to place a foam cushion under the patient's buttocks.

To avoid contamination by the patient's flora, the probe is covered with a condom in which acoustic gel has been poured. A finger of a sterile surgical glove can also be used. Care must be taken to avoid trapping any air bubble at the surface of the transducer. Gel (K-Y jelly or standard acoustic gel) is also placed on the outside surface of the condom to facilitate probe insertion and to provide acoustic coupling. Between each case, the probe is soaked in glutaraldehyde (Cidex) solution for at least 10 minutes. If the condom breaks during the examination, more thorough sterilization is required. Commonly used acoustic coupling gels have been reported to affect sperm motility [11]; therefore, water or no lubricant should be used in patients evaluated for infertility.

The best results in transvaginal sonography are obtained with a completely empty bladder. It must be noted that when the patient has drunk a large amount of water for a preceding transabdominal examination, the bladder may refill very quickly, notably if the patient has had to wait for

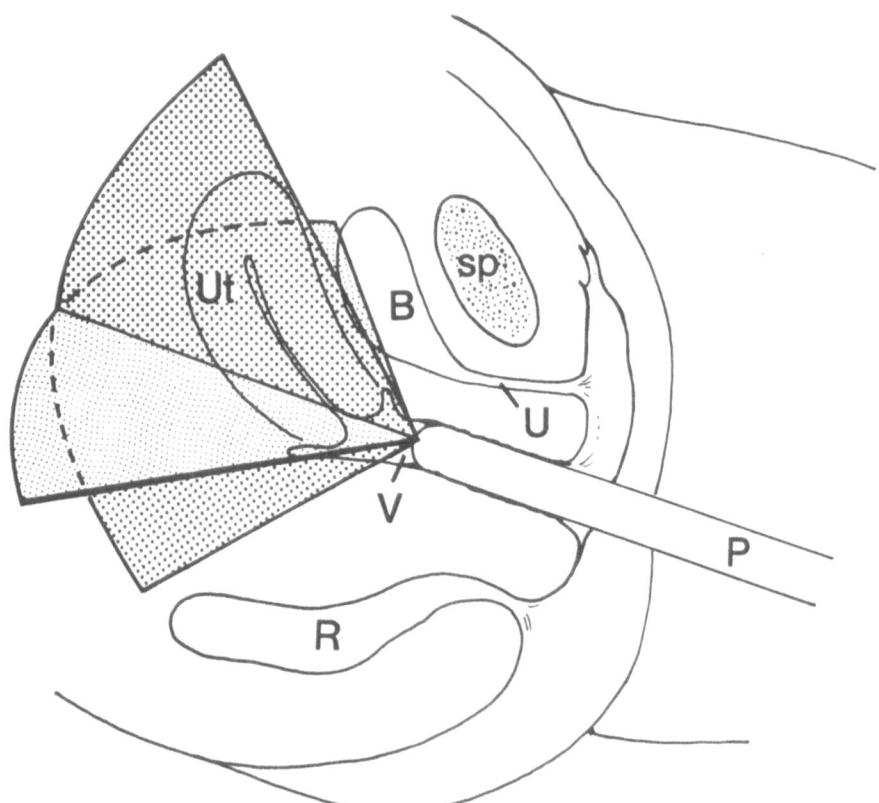

Figure 9.1. Diagrammatic representation of transvaginal sonography using an end-firing mechanical sector probe. Sagittal and coronal scan planes (and any intermediate plane, not shown here) are obtained through the axial rotation of the probe. B = bladder; P = intravaginal probe; R = rectum; sp = symphysis pubis; U = urethra; Ut = uterus; V = vagina.

some time between voiding and the transvaginal examination.

In our institution, when clinically indicated, transvaginal sonography is performed immediately after transabdominal examination. The reason for and the technique of the transvaginal study are explained to the patient, who is then asked to empty her bladder. Depending on the patient's wish, the sonographer, the physician, or the patient herself introduces the probe into the vagina. The examination is then carried out by the sonographer under the supervision of the radiologist, as in conventional ultrasound examinations. Sagittal and coronal scans are obtained by rotating the transducer 90° (Fig. 9.1); the probe can also be tilted upward, downward, or laterally, or partially pulled out, to visualize the different regions of the pelvis. First, the uterus is examined by scanning from back to front in the coronal plane, and from the midsection to the lateral aspects in the sagittal plane. Scanning the cervix is best performed by pulling the probe 2 to 3 cm back from the vaginal vault. Next, adnexal regions are examined. The internal iliac vessels are a crucial landmark in this exploration because the ovaries usually lie medial to them. Identification of follicles or cystic structures greatly helps in ovarian detection. After identification of the ovaries, the fallopian tubes should be searched for from the uterine horns to the ovaries.

During the examination, all possible placements of the probe and all possible orientations of the scan plane should be utilized. Abdominal palpation can be used to bring the pelvic organs, in particular the ovaries in large patients, into the ultrasonic field of view or to assess the mobility or adhesion of pelvic lesions. It is sometimes necessary for the patient to flex her hips or to lie in the left lateral decubitus position so that the transducer's handle can be tilted further posteriorly and a more complete image of the uterine fundus obtained.

Patient acceptance and tolerance, even in postmenopausal patients, are excellent provided the procedure has been thoroughly explained. A majority of patients who have had both transabdominal and transvaginal examinations would prefer the latter, primarily because the discomfort of an overdistended bladder is avoided [12]. Advantages and limitations of transvaginal sonography are listed in Table 9.1 and Table 9.2, respectively.

Table 9.1 Advantages of transvaginal sonography over transabdominal imaging.

- More detailed anatomy (high-frequency transducers)
- Lower risk of sound-propagation artifacts (e.g., from bowel gas)
- Does not require a full bladder
- Better tolerance by patients
- Original scanning planes (e.g., coronal)
- Better evaluation of retroverted uterus

Table 9.2. Limitations in transvaginal sonography.

- Not suitable for very young patients
- Evaluation of anteverted uterus sometimes limited
- Limited depth of field of view with high-frequency transducers

Transvaginal sonography should be performed when transabdominal scanning has failed because of obesity, bowel gas, or inability to distend the bladder, or when transabdominal findings are normal in a patient in whom a pelvic lesion was found at physical examination or strongly suspected clinically. The most common indications for transvaginal sonography in gynecology are listed in Table 9.3.

Uterus

Normal ultrasound anatomy

The normal uterus is well demonstrated on transvaginal sonograms. A wide field of view allows visualization of the entire uterus on a sagittal view and better depicts the cervix (Fig. 9.2). Anteverted and retroverted uterus can be easily differentiated: in an anteverted uterus, the endometrial line bulges downward, whereas in a retroverted uterus, the endometrial line bulges upward. Transvaginal sonography is of particular value in evaluating the fundus of a retroverted

Table 9.3. Indications for transvaginal ultrasound in gynecology.

Uterus
- Retroverted uterus
- Fibroids
- Depiction of normal endometrial cycling
- Suspicion of endometrial abnormalities
- Staging of endometrial carcinoma
- Cervical abnormalities (staging of cervical carcinoma)

Fallopian tubes
- Pelvic inflammatory disease (initial diagnosis and follow-up)
- Hydro-, pyosalpinx

Ovaries
- Visualization
- Origin of indeterminate mass
- Adnexal mass characterization
- Polycystic ovarian disease
- Follow-up after treatment for malignancy
- Screening for early diagnosis of cancer?

Cul-de-sac
- Detection and characterization of fluid
- Free fluid versus fluid-filled bowel loops

Infertility
- Diagnostic workup
- Ovulation monitoring

Ectopic pregnancy
- All patients in whom transabdominal ultrasound fails to demonstrate a live embryo

Monitoring of interventional procedures
- Transvaginal biopsy
- Pelvic abscess drainage

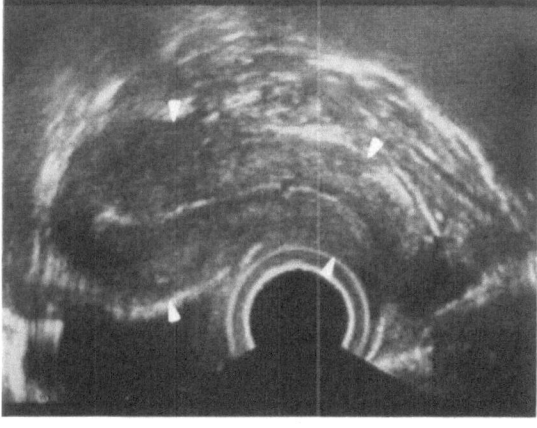

Figure 9.2. Normal uterus. Transvaginal midsagittal scan obtained with a 240° transducer (which gives the widest view available) provides a complete longitudinal section of the uterus (arrowheads).

uterus, which on transabdominal scanning is difficult to examine and may mimic a fibroid. The cervix is readily visualized, and the external and the internal os can be displayed.

Transvaginal sonography also provides unique information on the vascular supply of the uterus: large vessels are seen in the myometrium, usually at the junction between its inner two thirds and its outer third. Slow flow can be seen in these vessels on real-time images, and venous-type flow signals recorded on pulsed Doppler study. Although arteries are rarely well seen on real-time sonograms, arterial flow can be detected with pulsed Doppler. In some cases multiple calcifications are seen along these vessels; histologic correlation has shown that they represent deposits of calcium in the tunica media of uterine arteries (Mönckeberg's arteriosclerosis) (Fig. 9.3). Other vessels are also seen around the cervix, which are not commonly seen with transabdominal sonography: they usually present as multiple round structures connected with one another and represent veins and arteries.

The normal endometrium is visible on transabdominal sonography, and several authors have described the normal changes of the endometrium during the menstrual cycle [13–16]. In the proliferative phase, the total thickness (two layers) of the endometrium is 3 to 5 mm. A hypoechoic central lining between the two echogenic layers is seen around the time of ovulation. Next, a small amount of hypoechoic secretion can be seen. In the secretory phase, the endometrium is 5 to 8 mm thick and is surrounded by a hypoechoic layer of myometrial tissue (see also Chapter 11).

Transvaginal scanning has proved superior to transabdominal scanning in imaging the endometrium, particularly in those patients with a retroverted uterus [17]. In a comparative study in 179 patients [12], the endometrium was better seen on transvaginal scans in 146 (82%) (Fig. 9.4) and on transabdominal scans in 5 (3%); the techniques worked equally well in the remaining 28 patients (15%). A similar study found transvaginal sonography superior, inferior, and equal to transabdominal imaging of the endometrium in 85%, 5%, and 10% of cases, respectively [9].

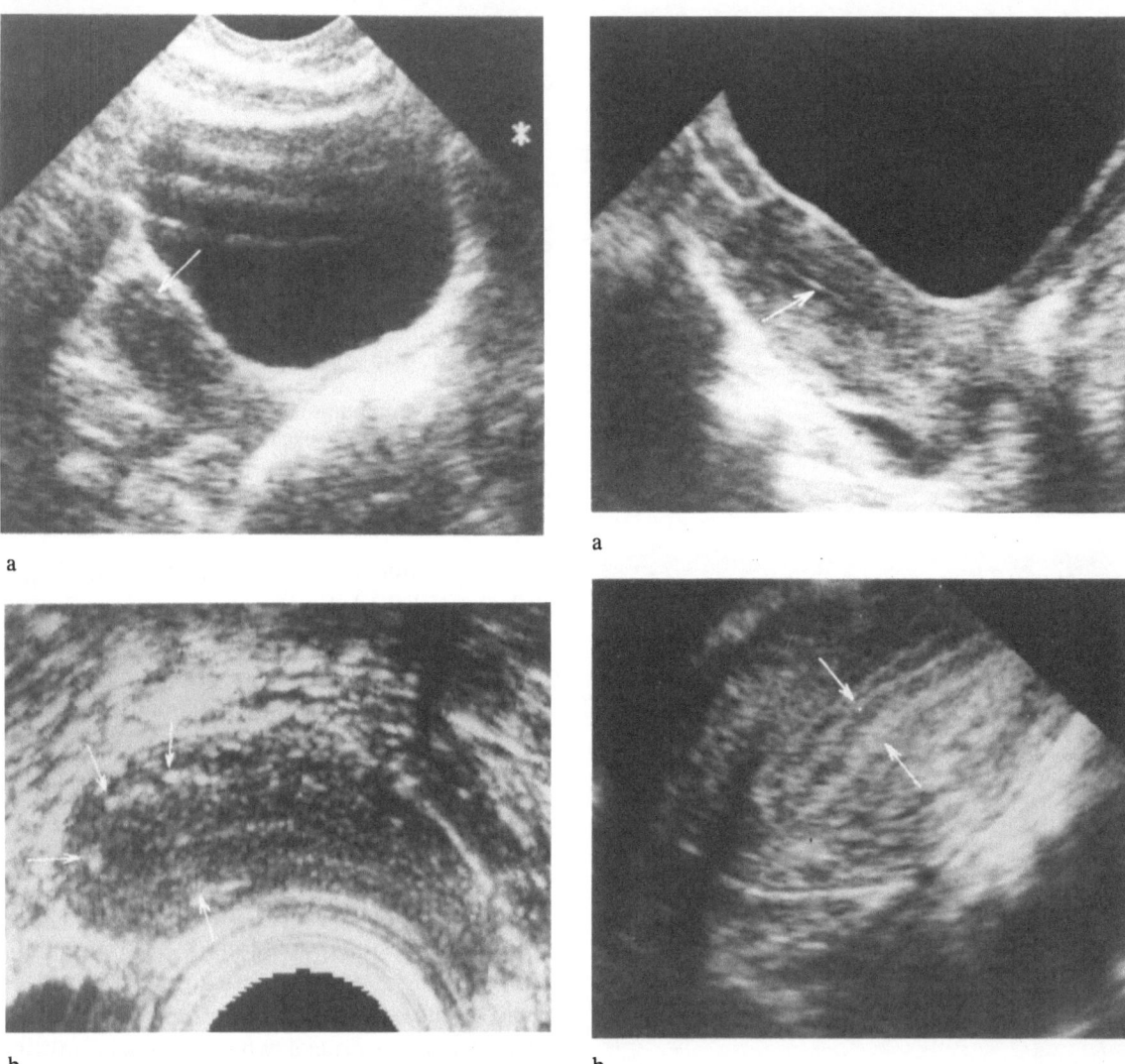

a

b

a

b

Figure 9.3. Calcification of the uterine arteries (Möncke-berg's syndrome). (a) Transabdominal sagittal scan. The uterus is atrophic, and some bright echoes (arrow) are seen at its periphery. (b) Transvaginal sagittal scan. Calcifications are visible along the uterine arteries (arrows); correlation with the surgical specimen showed these calcifications to lie in the tunica media.

Figure 9.4. Normal endometrium. (a) Transabdominal sagittal scan. The endometrium (arrow) is poorly demon-strated. A small amount of fluid is seen in the cul-de-sac. (b) Transvaginal sagittal scan clearly shows the two layers of the endometrium (arrows).

Pathologic findings

Congenital abnormalities

Congenital abnormalities, such as bicornuate or arcuate uterus, are better demonstrated with transvaginal than with transabdominal sonography (Fig. 9.5) (see also Chapter 11).

Endometrial pathology

In a series of 29 patients with endometrial abnormalities, Mendelson et al. [18] found that transvaginal sonography provided unique diagnostic information in 23% of cases.

Little has been written on the sonographic diagnosis of endometrial carcinoma. The common view is that the role of sonography is to define the extent of an already diagnosed tumor, rather than to provide early diagnosis. It is too early to know what improvements in diagnosis might be expected from transvaginal scanning. Correlation between in vitro sonography and pathologic examination has shown that early,

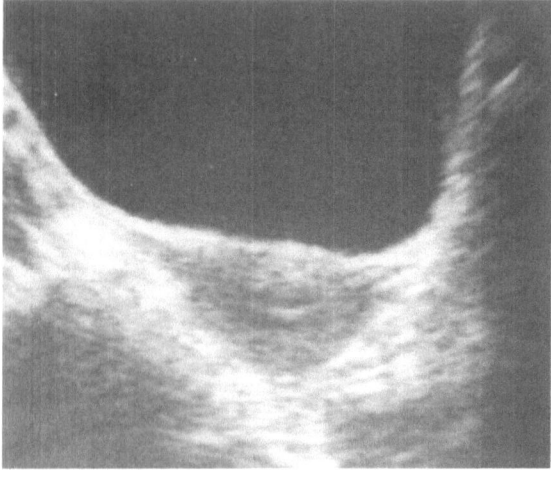

a

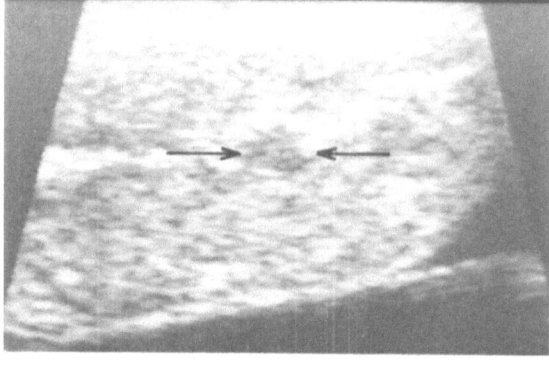

Figure 9.6. In vitro ultrasound examination of an early endometrial carcinoma. A small, irregular, hypoechoic mass (arrows) arises from the endometrial cavity. In vivo, only some irregularity of the endometrial cavity could be seen.

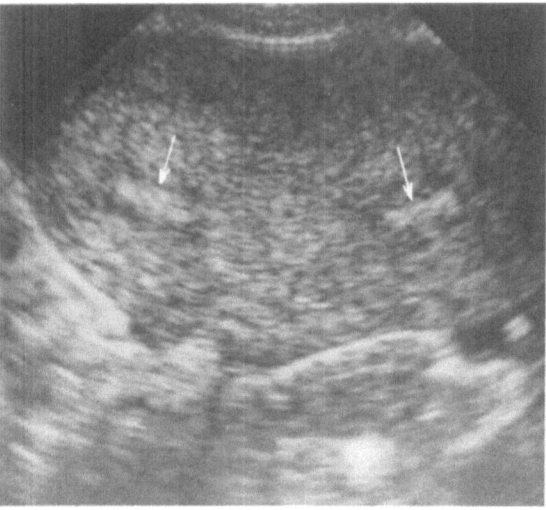

b

Figure 9.5. Arcuate uterus. (a) Transabdominal transverse scan of the fundus shows no abnormality. (b) Transvaginal transverse scan shows two endometrial cavities (arrows), indicating an arcuate uterus.

discrete tumors are hypoechoic (Fig. 9.6). In the diagnosis of tumor extension, it is not yet clear whether sonography, magnetic resonance imaging, or computed tomography is the most accurate.

Besides endometrial carcinoma, a variety of sonographic findings have been observed in postmenopausal patients, including echogenic polypoid masses; focal, irregular thickening of the endometrium; and fluid-filled collections. Further echopathologic correlation is needed

before the clinical significance of such findings can be established. Endometrial carcinoma can be sonographically mimicked by a marked, irregular, hyperplastic reaction in patients with breast carcinoma treated with antiestrogens (Figs. 9.7, 9.8).

Fibroids

Transvaginal sonography provides optimal demonstration of the myometrium. It delineates fibroids better than transabdominal sonography and detects lesions not found by the latter approach (Fig. 9.9); accurate localization of a fibroid relative to the myometrium and endometrium can be crucial when myomectomy is considered. Transvaginal sonography also readily differentiates a retroverted uterus from a fibroid, and extrauterine masses from subserosal fibroids. Finally, transvaginal sonography provides more information than does transabdominal examination on the texture of a fibroid, for example by showing areas of calcification or necrosis. In a series of 55 patients with fibroids, the lesions were better demonstrated transvaginally in 46 patients (84%), better seen transabdominally in 7 patients (13%), and equally well seen with the two techniques in 2 patients (3%) [12]. Transvaginal sonography is limited in this application by the insufficient sound penetration of high-frequency transducers, which precludes accurate delineation of large fibroids. Large lesions are measured by transabdominal sonography.

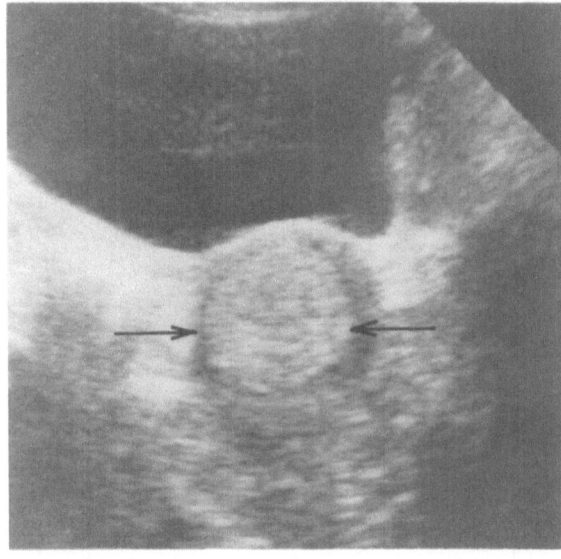

a

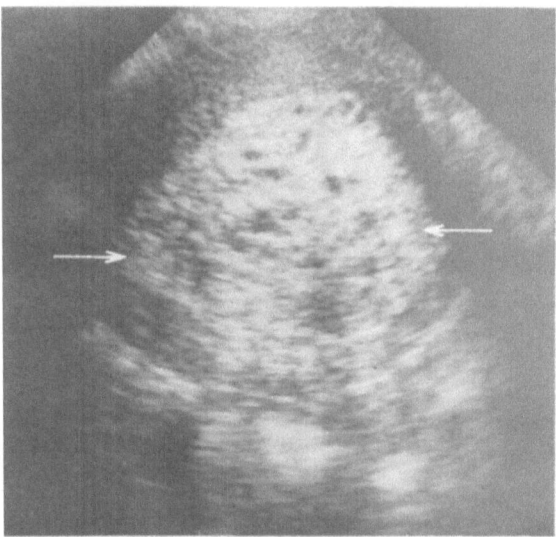

b

Figure 9.7. Endometrial hyperplasia in a patient receiving antiestrogen therapy for breast cancer. (a) Transabdominal transverse scan shows a large, hyperechoic mass in the center of the uterus (arrows). (b) Transvaginal transverse scan better shows the hyperplastic endometrium (arrows).

Cervical pathology

Nabothian cysts are common lesions of the cervix. These small, well-delineated retention cysts more frequently occur in the lower cervix and are more often depicted transvaginally than transabdominally.

Sonography can be used to stage cervical carcinoma. Clinical staging is inaccurate in 34%

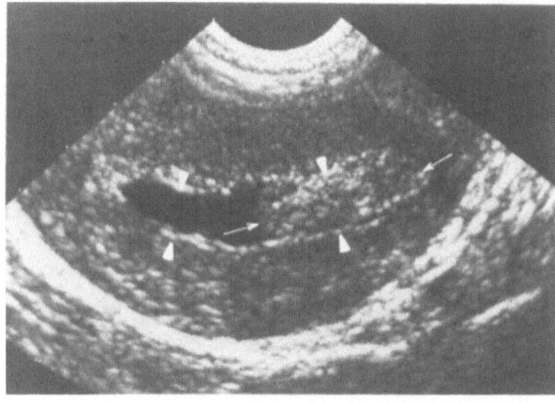

Figure 9.8. Endometrial polyp in a patient receiving antiestrogen therapy for breast cancer. Transvaginal sagittal scan of the uterus shows a large, fluid-filled, irregular endometrial cavity (arrowheads) containing an echogenic polyp (arrows).

to 39% of patients with stage IB cervical carcinoma (carcinoma confined to the cervix), whereas CT is accurate in only 50% of cases in the differentiation between stage IB and stage IIB lesions [19]. In this application, magnetic resonance imaging is a promising technique [20], and endosonography is expected to be accurate and more cost-effective. Transvaginal scans delineate the tumor and show its proximal extension, whereas transrectal sonography can demonstrate any infiltration into the vagina, parametrium, bladder, or rectum.

Fallopian tubes

The fallopian tubes are 10 to 12 cm long. They comprise interstitial (or intramural), isthmic, ampullar, and infundibular segments. The lumen varies from 1 mm in the uterine part to 8 or 9 mm in the ampulla and is filled with mucus. The tubes extend laterally to the posterolateral aspect of the ovaries, where they terminate with the fimbriae.

Normal ultrasound anatomy

Normal fallopian tubes have only rarely been visualized on transabdominal sonography [21], mainly because of the suboptimal spatial resolution of transabdominal transducers at depth. On

136

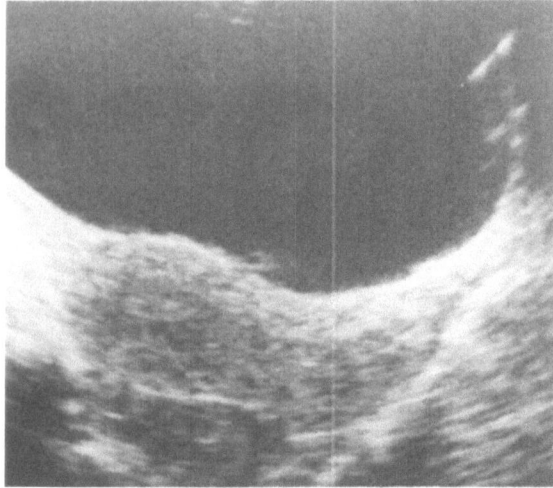

a

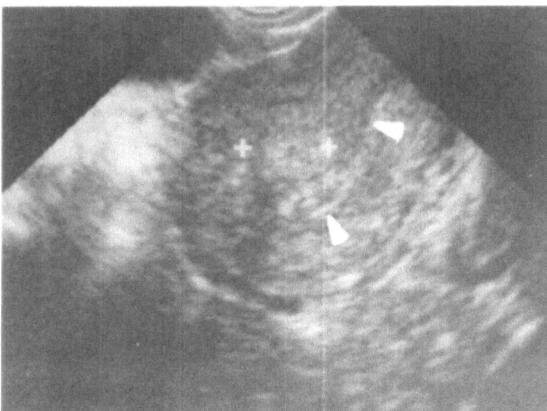

b

Figure 9.9. Uterine fibroid. (a) Transabdominal sagittal scan shows normal uterus. (b) Transvaginal sagittal scan of the uterine fundus. A small (2-cm) fibroid (markers) is seen to displace the endometrium posteriorly (arrowheads).

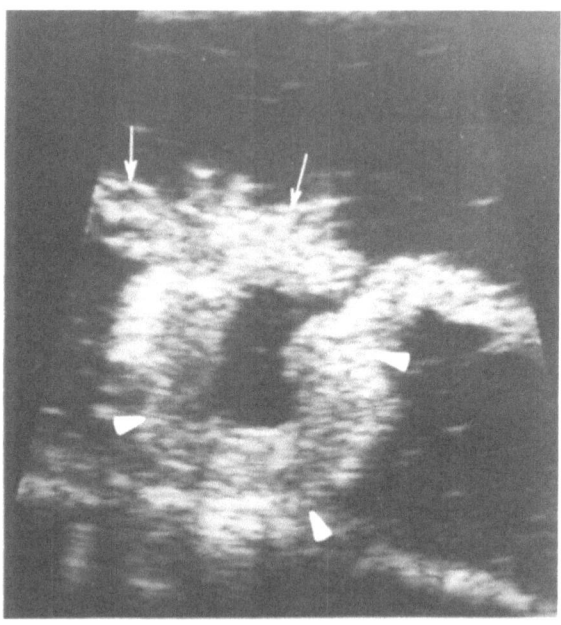

Figure 9.10. Normal fallopian tube. In vitro longitudinal scan of the tube (arrowheads). The arrows point to the fimbriae.

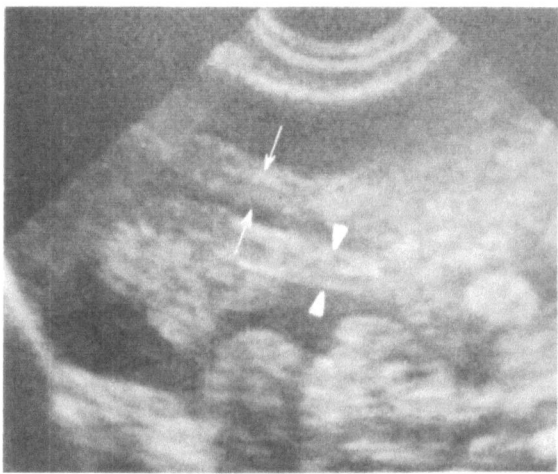

Figure 9.11. Normal fallopian tube in a patient with ascites. Oblique scan shows the right tube (arrows) and the utero-ovarian ligament (arrowheads). The two structures show a similar echogenicity.

in vitro study of surgical specimens, the normal fallopian tube appears as a well-defined, echogenic structure (Fig. 9.10). Limiting factors in the visualization of the tubes include their tortuous course, the absence of ultrasound contrast with the structures surrounding them, and the lesser maneuverability of endovaginal transducers.

Normal tubes have been demonstrated on transvaginal sonography in patients with fluid (of a minimal amount) in the pelvis (Fig. 9.11) [22]. They appear as tortuous structures whose echogenicity is similar to that of the uterus; normally, the lumen of the tube is collapsed and

not seen. In our experience, even in patients without fluid in the pelvis, a short proximal segment of the normal tube can routinely be demonstrated as an echogenic band 6 to 9 mm thick and 1 to 3 cm long (Fig. 9.12). There is sometimes a bright line in the center of the tube, which is thought to represent the endosalpingeal

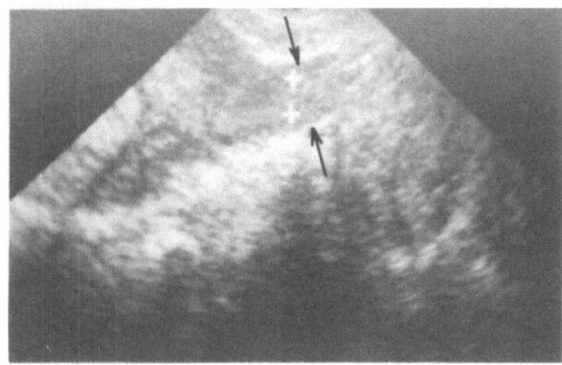

Figure 9.12. Transvaginal transverse scan shows a normal left tube (arrows).

interface. Fluid-filled tubular structures are often seen adjacent and parallel to the tube; these are believed to represent tubo-ovarian vessels. The major pitfall in fallopian tube visualization is the utero-ovarian ligament, which has a similar echo pattern. However, this ligament attaches to the uterus below the horn and joins the ovary at its medial aspect, whereas the tube attaches to the lateral aspect of the ovary (Fig. 9.11).

Pathologic findings

In *pelvic inflammatory disease* (PID), the tube may be thickened and, even without fluid in the lumen, become hypoechoic in relation to the uterus (Fig. 9.13). The fluid contained in the

lumen in *hydrosalpinx* enables easy demonstration of the tube. The presence of pus in *pyosalpinx* is usually associated with the finding of echogenic material in the fluid-distended tube. If fluid is present both inside and outside the tube, the thickness of the wall can be accurately measured. When the tube is significantly dilated, an elongated, cystic structure is seen in the adnexal region (Fig. 9.14). Hydrosalpinx is occasionally mistaken for an adnexal cystic mass on transabdominal views, but the characteristic pattern of a dilated tube is readily recognized transvaginally.

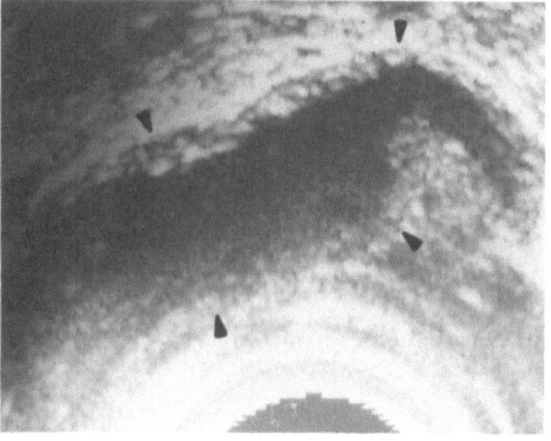

a

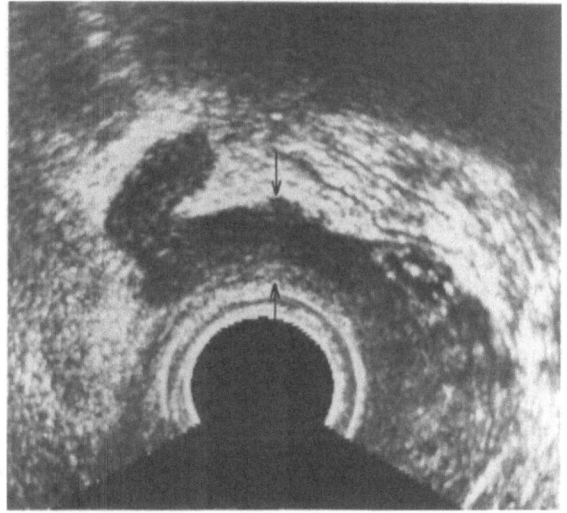

Figure 9.13. Pelvic inflammatory disease. Transvaginal scan shows the thickened tube (arrows). No fluid is present inside or outside the tube.

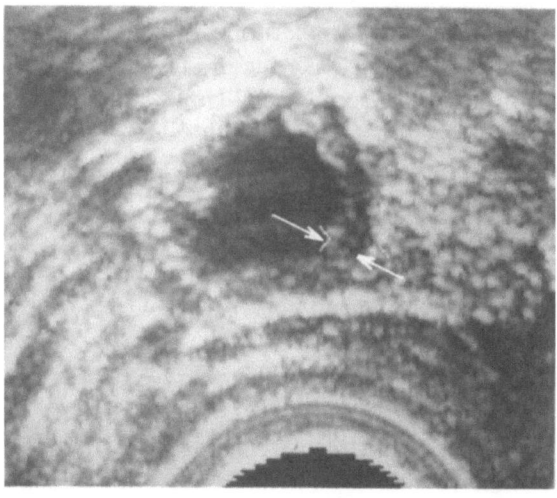

b

Figure 9.14. Hydrosalpinx. (a) Transvaginal longitudinal scan of the dilated tube (arrowheads). (b) Transvaginal transverse scan confirms the fluid-distended tube and shows the thickened, irregular wall (arrows).

A *tubo-ovarian abscess* appears sonographically as a complex adnexal mass, typically made up of a dilated, thickened tube surrounding an ill-defined ovary. Transvaginal sonography can distinguish between a tubal and a tubo-ovarian abscess (Fig. 9.15). It can also be used to evaluate the response of the abscess to antibiotic therapy and occasionally to direct diagnostic aspiration or drainage of the abscess. Tubal pregnancy is discussed below.

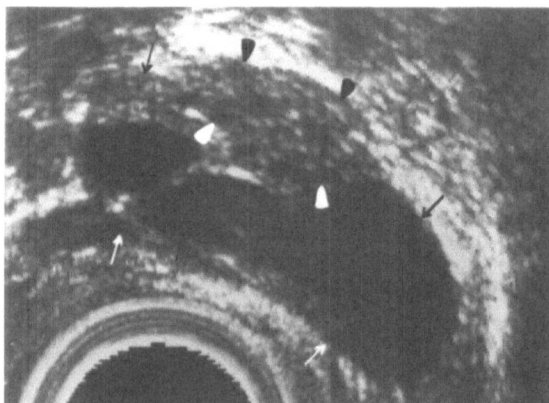

Figure 9.15. Tubal abscess. Transvaginal scan shows a significantly dilated tube (arrows). The ovary (arrowheads) is normal.

Ovaries

The ovaries are intraperitoneal, located lateral and slightly posterior to the uterus and adjacent to the internal iliac vessels. However, they are characterized by great mobility, even during the sonographic examination, and are sometimes found high in the pelvis or in the cul-de-sac. They are approximately $3 \times 2.5 \times 2$ cm in size.

Normal ultrasound anatomy

Ovarian size and echotexture vary considerably according to the patient's age, number of pregnancies, and menstrual phase. With high-resolution endovaginal transducers, the normal ovary in the reproductive years may show an interface between the hypoechoic cortex, where ovarian follicles are found, and the more echogenic medulla. The mature follicle has an average size of 2 cm and is readily demonstrated.

Immature or atretic follicles only a few millimeters in size may also be visualized. The formation of the corpus hemorrhagicum immediately after ovulation results in echoes in the follicle.

Accuracy of sonography in the visualization of ovaries

In the premenopausal patient, both ovaries can usually be identified on transabdominal sonography by the visualization of follicles. After menopause, ovaries decrease in size and cystic structures are less common, so that the rate of detection decreases. In a series of 30 healthy postmenopausal women examined transabdominally, Hall *et al.* [23] could see the ovaries in 68% of cases; our retrospective study of 105 routine pelvic ultrasound examinations in women over the age of 50 found that ovaries were identified in only 49% of the cases (Bret *et al.*, unpublished data). Transvaginal sonography is expected to increase the rate of visualization of normal ovaries; however, in our series of 201 pre- and postmenopausal patients undergoing transabdominal and transvaginal ultrasound examination during the same session, both approaches failed to demonstrate 28 and 26 ovaries, respectively [12]. Interestingly, those ovaries that were not detected transabdominally were not the same as those undetected transvaginally, confirming the two methods as complementary. Also, when the ovaries were identified by both techniques ($n = 305$), they were better seen on transvaginal scans in 70% (Fig. 9.16), better seen on transabdominal scans in 18%, and equally well seen by the two techniques in 12% of cases.

Volume measurement

It has often been suggested that the measurement of ovarian volume could be useful, especially in the postmenopausal woman, for detecting early ovarian cancer. With transabdominal scanning, the volume of the normal postmenopausal ovary has been reported at 1.2 to 4.3 cm^3 [23—26]. No significant difference was found between transvaginal and transabdominal scanning in a comparative study of normal ovarian volume measurement in either pre- or postmenopausal healthy women [24].

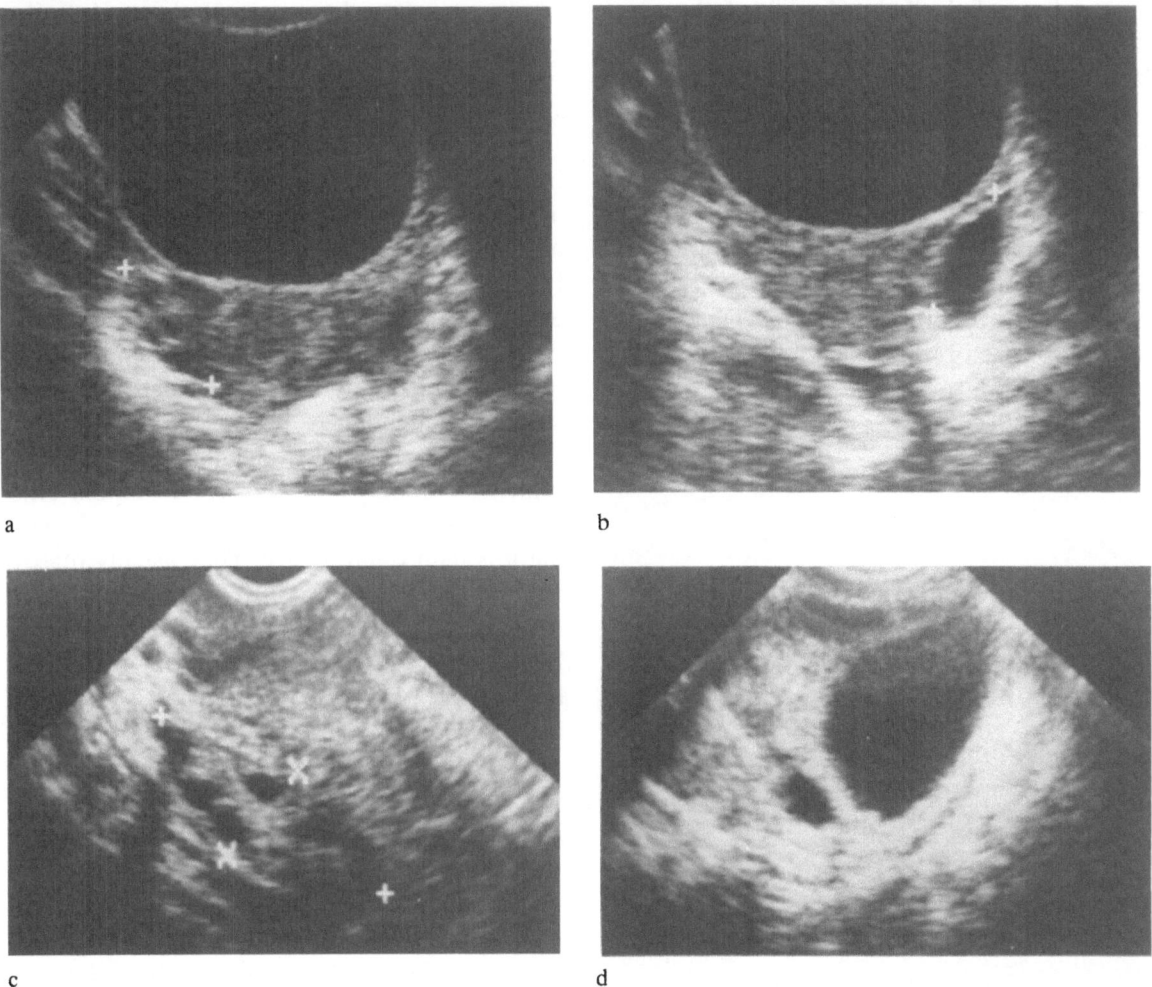

a   b

c   d

Figure 9.16. Normal ovaries. (a and b) Transabdominal transverse scans of the patient's right ovary and left ovary (markers), respectively. (c and d) Transvaginal scans better depict both ovaries. A dominant follicle is seen in the left ovary (d).

Monitoring follicle maturation
See Chapter 11.

Pathologic findings

Transvaginal sonography provides more detailed images of adnexal masses than transabdominal examination. In our above-mentioned series of 201 patients [12], 80 had adnexal masses. The transvaginal approach was found to be superior in depicting the mass in 79%, equal to transabdominal scanning in 15%, and inferior in 6%. Usually, a much clearer visualization allows better characterization of the lesion, although this does not always lead to a specific diagnosis.

The roles of transvaginal sonography in the evaluation of an adnexal mass are to determine the site of the origin and characterize the echotexture of the mass. When origin is ovarian, transvaginal scans usually show a rim of ovarian tissue at the periphery of the lesion. Endosonography can also readily confirm an exophytic or pedunculated subserous uterine fibroid by demonstrating continuity between the uterine muscle and the mass. Endosonography is limited in remote adnexal masses and large lesions that extend beyond the field of view of the transducer. In such cases, 5-MHz transducers should be used instead of 7.5-MHz transducers.

Ovarian polycystic disease
In most cases of ovarian polycystic disease, transabdominal imaging shows bilaterally enlarged ovaries with a grossly normal sonographic texture. Transvaginal sonography shows small, uniform cysts (each less than 1 cm) gathered at the periphery of the ovary (Fig. 9.17), and

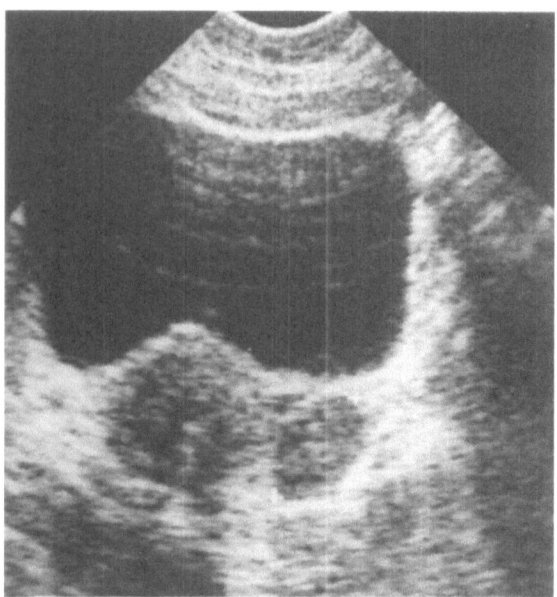

a

b

Figure 9.17. Polycystic ovarian disease. (a) Transabdominal transverse scan shows a normal-appearing left ovary (markers). (b) Transvaginal scan of the left ovary (markers) shows multiple cysts at the periphery of the ovary, each measuring less than 1 cm.

occasionally an echogenic central zone (see also Chapter 11).

Ovarian cysts
In cystic masses of the ovary, demonstration of internal echoes, wall proliferation, and septation is better achieved with transvaginal than transabdominal sonography. Differentiation between fluid-filled bowel loops and ovarian cysts is also easier on transvaginal scanning. Benign ovarian cysts include functional (follicle and corpus luteum) and proliferative cysts (dermoids, mucinous cystadenomas).

Follicle cysts result from failure of developing follicles to undergo atresia after ovulation. They appear sonographically as typical cysts measuring less than 6 cm in size. They usually regress without treatment. *Corpus luteum cysts* result from failure of the corpus luteum to regress. Blood degradation products from intracystic hemorrhage give rise to internal echoes and hence a complex sonographic pattern (Fig. 9.18). *Dermoid cysts* (Fig. 9.19) contain a thick sebaceous material, which creates a homogeneous, low-level echogenicity on transvaginal scans; these cysts may appear purely sonolucent on transabdominal scans performed at 3.5 MHz. Hair collections or teeth appear as highly echogenic, floating material. Rarely, a dermoid cyst is multilocular. *Cystadenomas* have a cystic appearance; they may be unilocular or multilocular, with very variable septation patterns.

Benign solid ovarian tumors
Benign solid ovarian tumors are rare. Chief among them are fibromas, which show a wide spectrum of sonographic features, from hypoechoic to highly echoic masses, occasionally associated with acoustic shadowing.

Ovarian carcinoma
Most ovarian carcinomas sonographically present as multilocular masses with papillary excrescences (Fig. 9.20). However, they can also appear as solid masses or unilocular cysts. In the presence of a complex ovarian mass, the sonographic detection of fluid and nodules in the cul-de-sac virtually establishes the diagnosis of malignancy.

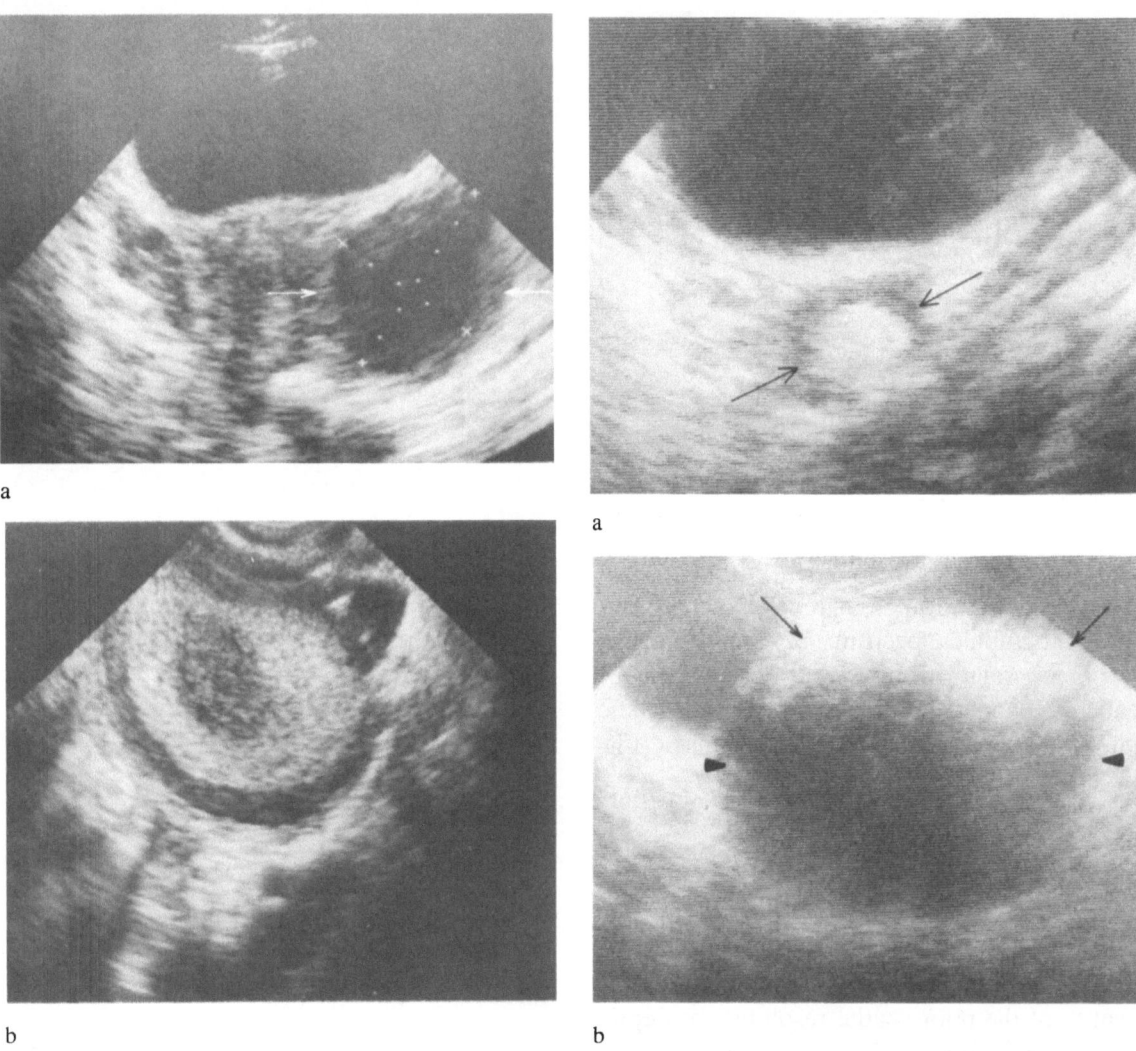

Figure 9.18. Corpus luteum cyst. (a) Transabdominal transverse scan shows a left cystic adnexal mass with thick walls
(arrows). (b) Transvaginal scan of the mass demonstrates an
echogenic area within the lesion, representing hemorrhagic
material.

Figure 9.19. Dermoid cyst. (a) Transabdominal scan shows
a mass with internal echogenic material (arrows). (b)
Transvaginal scan shows a cystic structure (arrowheads).
Hyperechoic intracystic material (arrows) close to the transducer is responsible for acoustic shadowing.

The silent progression of ovarian tumors to
large, palpable pelvic masses is well known.
Efforts should be aimed at early detection, and
transvaginal sonography has recently been contemplated as a screening modality for enlarged
ovaries in postmenopausal women. Transabdominal scanning has already been used in this
application. In each of two studies that com-
prised 1084 patients [26] and 805 patients [27],
respectively, only one ovarian carcinoma was
detected. In an evaluation of adnexal masses in
postmenopausal patients, only 1 of 32 lesions

less than 5 cm in diameter was found to be
malignant [28]. The diagnostic value (and cost-
effectiveness) of transvaginal sonography in this
application needs further evaluation. Prospective studies are under way [29].

Endometriosis

Besides the ovaries, endometriotic implants can
involve the fallopian tubes, cul-de-sac, serosal
surface of the uterus, and bowel. Bleeding in
endometriomas at the time of menstruation
results in the formation of loculated blood

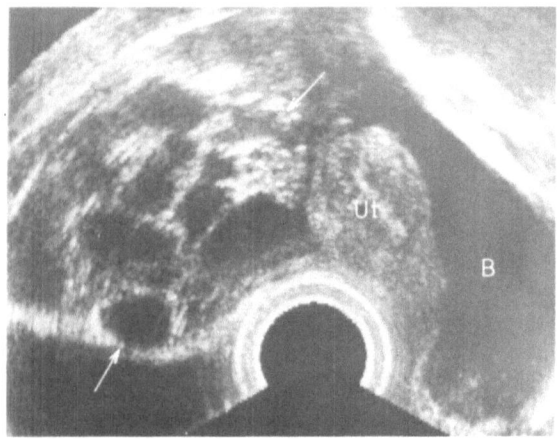

Figure 9.20. Ovarian carcinoma. Transvaginal scan shows a large, multicystic adnexal mass (arrows) with intracystic proliferation. B = bladder; Ut = uterus.

collections: the endometrial, or 'chocolate', cysts. The sonographic spectrum of ovarian endometriomas ranges from a well- defined, homogeneous, hypoechoic mass to a nonspecific complex, nonhomogeneous adnexal mass (Fig. 9.21) (see also Chapter 11).

Cul-de-sac

Fluid collections in the cul-de-sac may be mistaken for solid masses on suprapubic scans because of the poor spatial resolution at depth. Transvaginal sonography has proved to be extremely accurate in the detection of free fluid in the cul-de-sac and differentiating that fluid from fluid-filled bowel loops. The minimal amount (4 to 8 mL) of purely anechoic fluid often seen on transvaginal scans performed after ovulation arises from the follicular rupture. However, not infrequently, a somewhat lesser amount of fluid can also be detected before ovulation.

The presence of free fluid in the cul-de-sac is a crucial finding in patients with ovarian cancer, PID, or ectopic pregnancy. Echogenic fluid representing pus is also better characterized on transvaginal scans.

Transvaginal sonography has also proved accurate in differentiating solid masses in the cul-de-sac (e.g., metastatic implants versus uterine masses) [30].

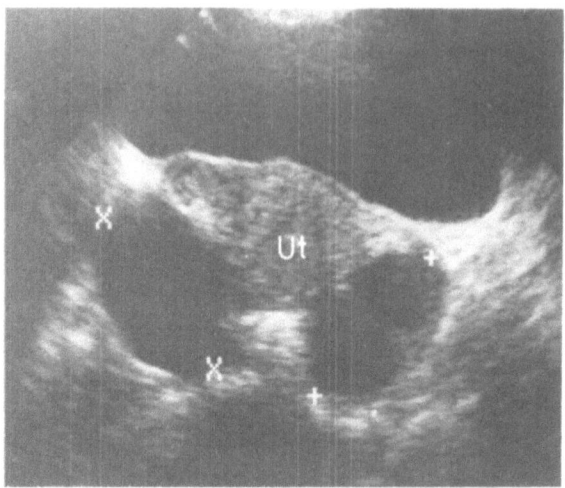

a

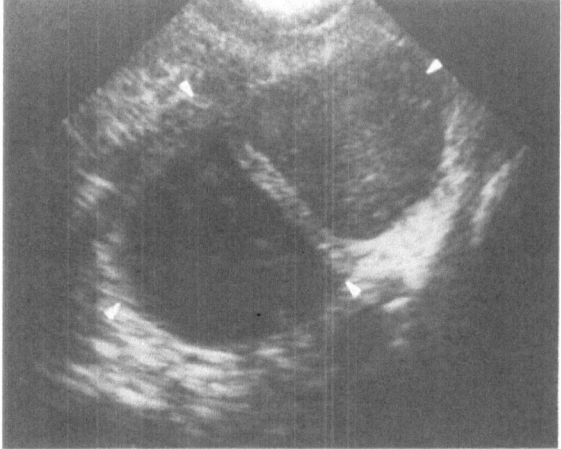

b

Figure 9.21. Endometriomas. (a) Transabdominal transverse scan shows two cystic adnexal masses (markers). Ut = uterus. (b) Transvaginal scan of the left adnexal mass (arrowheads) demonstrates internal echoes, a thick wall, and septation.

Ectopic pregnancy

Because of its polymorphism, extrauterine pregnancy is one of the most difficult sonographic diagnoses. However, this diagnosis is one of the best applications of transvaginal sonography. Transvaginal sonography is instrumental in visualizing adnexal abnormalities or in early confirmation of an intrauterine pregnancy.

The demonstration of intrauterine pregnancy virtually excludes coexisting ectopic pregnancy (except for patients treated for infertility).

Transvaginal sonography identifies normal intrauterine pregnancy 5—7 days earlier than transabdominal sonography. This is crucial in the management of patients with bleeding, pain, and a positive serum beta-human chorionic gonadotropin (HCG) test.

Although the only definitive sign of an ectopic pregnancy is the visualization of a live embryo outside the uterine cavity, the demonstration of an ectopic gestational sac or hematosalpinx is considered fairly specific to this diagnosis. The ectopic gestational sac is seen as a small cystic structure with thick, echogenic walls (ring-like structure). Transvaginal sonography demonstrates its outline and contents better than transabdominal ultrasound. A live or dead embryo, a yolk sac, or (occasionally) echogenic fluid can be seen within the sac (Fig. 9.22). If the embryo is alive, the sac is rounded and has well-delineated, smooth contours; if the embryo is dead, the contours are irregular and ill defined. Transvaginal Doppler study may show a low-resistance

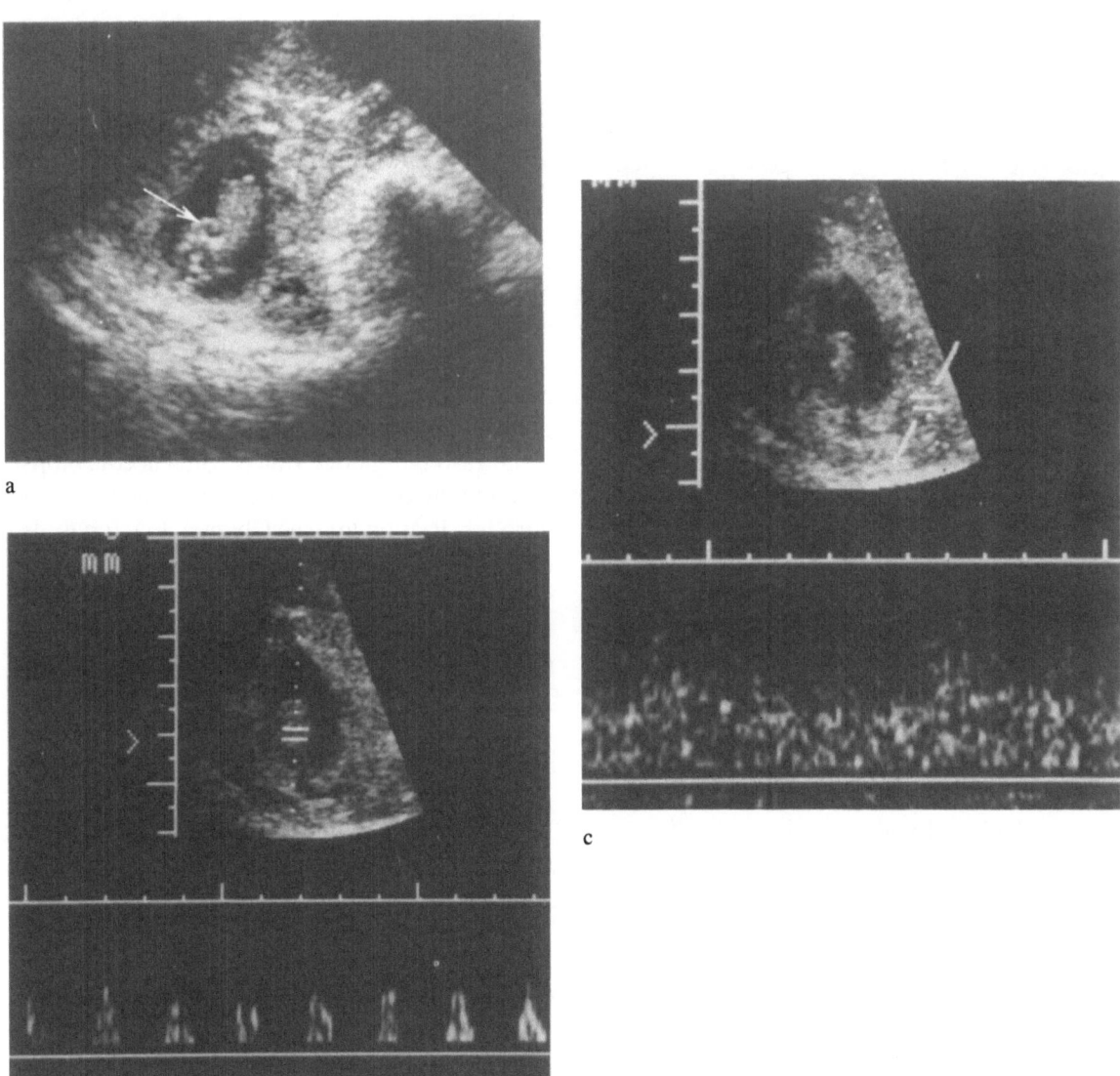

Figure 9.22. Ectopic pregnancy. (a) Transvaginal scan shows an extrauterine gestational sac containing an embryo (arrow). (b) Transvaginal duplex Doppler examination confirms embryonic heart activity. (c) Transvaginal duplex Doppler examination of the trophoblastic region demonstrates low-resistance flow signals.

flow signal in the trophoblastic reaction around the sac (Fig. 9.22c). Hematosalpinx is seen as a relatively echogenic tubular structure in the adnexal region (Fig. 9.23).

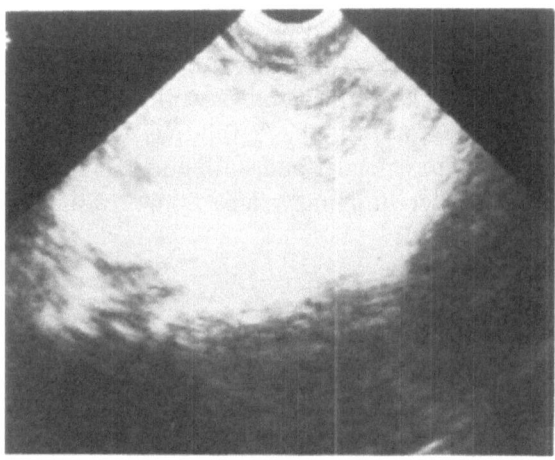

Figure 9.23. Ectopic pregnancy. Transvaginal scan shows an echogenic, elongated mass, which represents hematosalpinx.

Indirect signs of ectopic pregnancy are the presence of a complex adnexal mass, an endometrial reaction (pseudogestational sac), and free fluid in the cul-de-sac. Although transvaginal sonography better demonstrates small amounts of fluid in the cul-de-sac, the limited field of view of the intracavitary transducer can hamper the evaluation of large intraperitoneal fluid collections. Ruptured ectopic pregnancies usually present as complex pelvic masses in which no sac or embryo can be identified.

In a review of 18 cases of proved ectopic pregnancy examined with transvaginal sonography, we found no case in which transvaginal sonography was totally negative, and diagnosis based on the presence of either an ectopic gestational sac (with or without an embryo), or hematosalpinx was achieved in 13 (72%) of the cases. It should be noted that with growing experience, specific diagnosis of ectopic pregnancy was made in 11 (92%) of the last 12 patients of this series [31]. The exact location of the pregnancy in relation to the various segments of the tube or to the ovary was accurately determined whenever a gestational sac was demonstrated.

The superiority of transvaginal sonography over transabdominal examination in the early

diagnosis of ectopic pregnancy has been documented by Nyberg *et al.* [8], who found that transvaginal examination was more informative in 60% of their patients. Most authors recommend that transvaginal sonography be performed whenever ectopic gestation is suspected and transabdominal study fails to demonstrate a viable intrauterine pregnancy [8, 29, 31].

Transvaginal biopsy

Although transvaginal sonography is more accurate than transabdominal imaging, it does not always provide a specific diagnosis of pelvic masses. Transvaginal needle biopsy might prove useful in this setting. However, pelvic masses in the female patient present a special situation: most of them are benign, even in postmenopausal women, and fine-needle aspiration biopsy of benign masses is associated with a high rate of nondiagnostic results. Also, the risk of malignant seeding in the peritoneal cavity, especially in cases of cystic masses, has not yet been completely ruled out.

Ultrasound-guided transvaginal needle biopsy was initially described to aspirate oocytes for in vitro fertilization [6] (see Chapter 11). It has also been described for cephalocentesis in a case of severe fetal hydrocephaly [32]. Only recently has this technique been used in the evaluation of gynecologic masses [33, 34].

Transabdominal sonographic guidance

Transabdominal (suprapubic) sonography can be used for the continuous monitoring of transvaginal biopsy. With the patient in the lithotomy position, a speculum is inserted in the vagina. The vaginal fornices are antiseptically prepared. The needle is then introduced under continuous transabdominal real-time guidance. This freehand technique gives the operator flexibility in directing and repositioning the needle during the biopsy.

Transvaginal sonographic guidance

Transvaginal biopsy can be more accurately performed under transvaginal than under transabdominal sonographic guidance. A needle guide that attaches to the transducer is required (Fig. 9.24). Because of the length of the guide, 25—35-cm-long needles must be used.

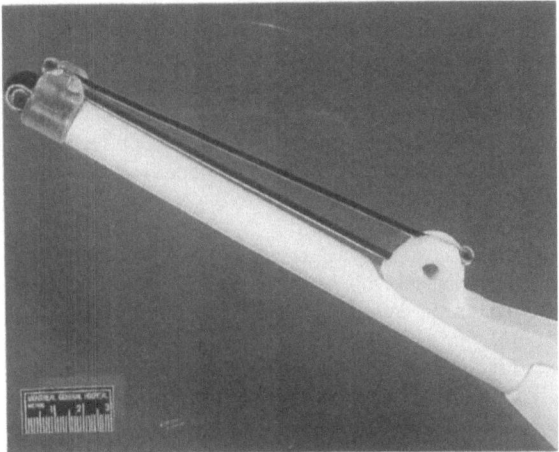

Figure 9.24. Biopsy needle guide mounted on an endovaginal transducer.

After the biopsy guide has been mounted on the probe and the combination inserted in the vagina, the lesion to be sampled is localized in the coronal and sagittal planes. The transducer is positioned in such a way that the electronic dotted line indicating the planned needle track crosses the lesion. The distance from the outer end of the guide to the lesion is then measured, and the needle is introduced in the guide to that distance. The needle is visualized on the video monitor as soon as it enters the ultrasonic field of view (Fig. 9.25). It appears as a bright line, sometimes associated with comet-tail artifacts. When the lesion is reached, the biopsy or drainage is performed.

Indications

Indications for transvaginal biopsy other than oocyte retrieval are listed in Table 9.4. A recurrent mass in the pelvis after total hysterectomy and bilateral salpingo-oophorectomy for cancer can be sampled by fine-needle aspiration under transvaginal ultrasound guidance. If the biopsy is positive for malignancy, the patient can be treated immediately and is spared second-look laparotomy. When a mass is unchanged after treatment for PID, aspiration should be performed to rule out another cause of pelvic

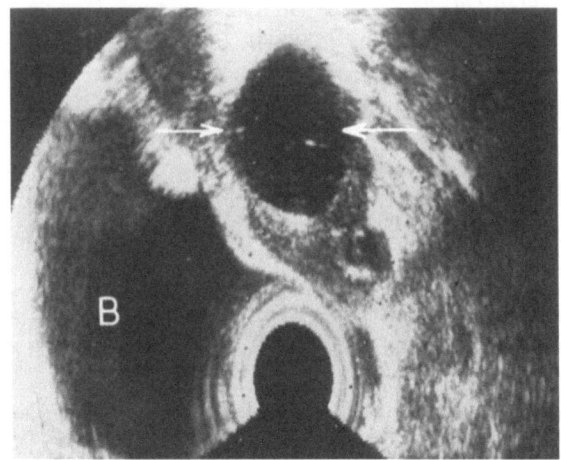

a

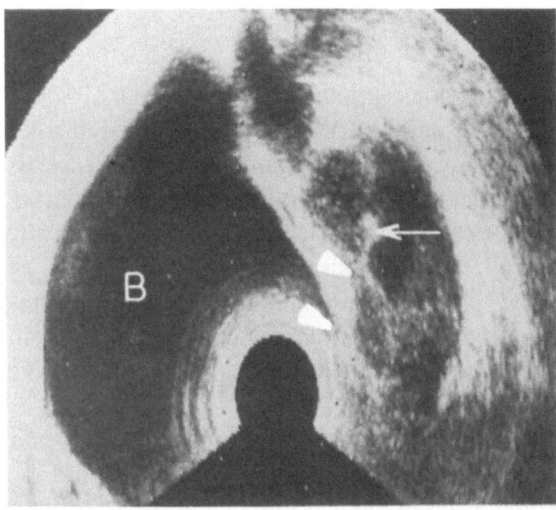

b

Figure 9.25. Ovarian remnant syndrome. Transvaginal aspiration biopsy performed under transvaginal sonographic guidance. (a) Transvaginal scan shows a cystic mass (arrows) with low-level echoes, surrounded by remnant ovarian tissue. (b) Transvaginal scan obtained during transvaginal fine-needle aspiration shows the needle (arrowheads) with a bright tip (arrow). B = bladder.

mass. The indication for biopsy of a newly diagnosed pelvic mass, particularly if cystic, is still controversial.

Ultrasound-guided transvaginal aspiration could be used as a therapeutic procedure in patients with acute symptoms from a hemorrhagic corpus luteum or follicular cyst, the risk of malignancy in either type of lesion being extremely low. Transvaginal drainage of a pelvic abscess can be performed under transabdominal [35] or transvaginal sonographic guidance.

Table 9.4. Indications for ultrasound-guided transvaginal biopsy (excluding oocyte retrieval).

Diagnostic
- Recurrent pelvic mass after treatment for ovarian or other pelvic malignancy
- No change of sonographic appearance of pelvic inflammatory disease after treatment
- Solid pelvic mass of unknown origin
- Cystic ovarian mass (controversial)

Therapeutic
- Symptomatic hemorrhagic corpus luteum or follicle cyst
- Pelvic abscess drainage

Conclusion

In gynecologic applications, transvaginal sonography usually provides more detailed images than transabdominal examination. As regards the clinical impact of this additional information, it has been shown that transvaginal sonography altered the diagnosis in approximately 30% of cases, provided better images than transabdominal scans but similar clinical information in about 50% of patients and was noncontributive in 20% of patients [12].

Because of its high resolution, low cost, and simplicity, transvaginal sonography should be widely used in clinical practice as an adjunct to transabdominal examination, which it cannot totally replace at present.

References

1. Kratochwil A.: Ultraschalldiagnostik in der Gynäkologie. Gynakologe, 1976, 9, 166—180.
2. Popp L. W., Lueken R. P., Müller-Holve W., Lindemann H. J.: Gynäkologische Endosonographie: erste Erfahrungen. Ultraschall Med., 1983, 4, 92—97.
3. Morimoto N., Noda Y., Takai I., Yamada I., Tojo S.: Ultrasonographic observation of ovarian follicular development via vaginal route. Nippon Sanka Fujinka Gakkai Zasshi, 1983, 35, 151—158.
4. Schwimer S. R., Lebovic J.: Transvaginal pelvic ultrasonography. J. Ultrasound Med., 1984, 3, 381—383.
5. Meldrum D. R., Chetkowski R. J., Steingold K. A., Randle D.: Transvaginal ultrasound scanning of ovarian follicles. Fertil. Steril., 1984, 42, 803—805.
6. Dellenbach P., Nisand I., Moreau L., *et al.*: Transvaginal, sonographically controlled ovarian follicle puncture for egg retrieval (letter). Lancet, 1984, 1, 1467.
7. Pennell R. G., Baltarowich O. H., Kurtz A. B., *et al.*: Complicated first trimester pregnancies: Evaluation with endovaginal US versus transabdominal technique. Radiology, 1987, 165, 79—83.
8. Nyberg D. A., Mack L. A., Jeffrey R. B. Jr., Laing F. C.: Endovaginal sonographic evaluation of ectopic pregnancy. A prospective study. AJR, 1987, 149, 1181—1186.
9. Mendelson E. B., Bohm-Velez M., Joseph N., Neiman H. L.: Gynecologic imaging: Comparison of transabdominal and transvaginal sonography. Radiology, 1988, 166, 321—324.
10. McSweeney M. B., Baber R. J., Kossoff G., Gill R. W.: Transvaginal Doppler assessment of blood flow to the ovaries in infertile patients. Presented at the 88th Meeting of the American Roentgen Ray Society, San Francisco, May 8—13, 1988.
11. Schwimer S. R., Rothman C. M., Lebovic J., Oye D. M.: The effect of ultrasound coupling gels on sperm motility in vitro. Fertil. Steril., 1984, 42, 946—947.
12. Bret P. M., De Stempel J., Atri M., Illescas F. F., Aldis A.: Transvaginal ultrasound in gynecology (excluding infertility). Presented at the 88th Meeting of the American Roentgen Ray Society, San Francisco, May 8—13, 1988.
13. Duffield S., Picker R.: Ultrasonic evaluation of the uterus in the normal menstrual cycle. Med. Ultrasound, 1981, 5, 70—74.
14. Pupols A., Wilson S.: Ultrasonographic interpretation of physiologic changes in the female pelvis. J. Can. Assoc. Radiol., 1984, 35, 34—39.
15. Fleischer A. C., Kalemeris G. C., Entman S. S.: Sonographic depiction of the endometrium during normal cycles. Ultrasound Med. Biol., 1986, 12, 271—277.
16. Forrest T. S., Elyaderani M. K., Muilenburg M. I., Bewtra C., Kable W. T., Sullivan P.: Cyclic endometrial changes: US assessment with histologic correlation. Radiology, 1988, 167, 233—237.
17. Fleischer A. C., Mendelson E. B., Bohm-Velez M. Entman S.S.: Transvaginal and transabdominal sonography of the endometrium. Semin. Ultrasound CT MR, 1988, 9, 81—101.
18. Mendelson E. B., Bohm-Velez M., Joseph N., Neiman H. L.: Endometrial abnormalities: Evaluation with transvaginal sonography. AJR, 1988, 150, 139—142.
19. Walsh J. W., Goplerud D. R.: Prospective comparison between clinical and CT staging in primary cervical carcinoma. AJR, 1981, 137, 997—1003.
20. Rubens D., Thornbury J. R., Angel C., *et al.*: Stage IB cervical carcinoma: Comparison of clinical, MR, and pathologic staging. AJR, 1988, 150, 135—138.
21. Hall D. A.: Sonographic appearance of the normal ovary, of polycystic ovary disease, and of functional ovarian cysts. Semin. Ultrasound, 1983, 4, 149—165.
22. Timor-Tritsch I. E., Rottem S.: Transvaginal ultrasonographic study of the fallopian tube. Obstet. Gynecol., 1987, 70, 424—428.

23. Hall D. A., McCarthy K. A., Kopans D. B.: Sonographic visualization of the normal postmenopausal ovary. J. Ultrasound Med., 1986, 5, 9—11.

24. Granberg S., Wikland M.: Comparison between endovaginal and transabdominal transducers for measuring ovarian volume. J. Ultrasound Med., 1987, 6, 649—653.

25. Campbell S., Goessens L., Goswamy R. K., Whitehead M.: Real-time ultrasonography for determination of ovarian morphology and volume. A possible early screening test for ovarian cancer? Lancet, 1982, 1, 425—426.

26. Goswamy R. K., Campbell S., Whitehead M. I.: Screening for ovarian cancer. Clin. Obstet. Gynaecol., 1983, 10, 621—643.

27. Andolf E., Svalenius E., Astedt B.: Ultrasonography for early detection of ovarian carcinoma. Br. J. Obstet. Gynaecol., 1986, 93, 1286—1289.

28. Rulin M. C., Preston A. L.: Adnexal masses in postmenopausal women. Obstet. Gynecol., 1987, 70, 578—581.

29. Mendelson E. B., Bohm-Velez M., Neiman H. L., Russo J.: Transvaginal sonography in gynecologic imaging. Semin. Ultrasound CT MR, 1988, 9, 102—121.

30. Lande I. M., Hill M. C., Cosco F. E., Kator N. N.: Adnexal and cul-de-sac abnormalities: Transvaginal sonography. Radiology, 1988, 166, 325—332.

31. Atri M., De Stempel J., Bret P. M., Illescas F. F., Aldis A., Gillett P.: Accuracy of transvaginal ultrasound for detection of ectopic pregnancy. Presented at the 51st Meeting of the Canadian Association of Radiologists, Edmonton, June 12—16, 1988.

32. Chayen B., Rifkin M. D.: Cephalocentesis. Guidance with an endovaginal probe and endovaginal needle placement. J. Ultrasound Med., 1987, 6, 221—223.

33. Schwimer S. R., Marik J., Lebovic J.: Percutaneous ovarian cyst aspiration using continuous transvaginal ultrasonographic monitoring. J. Ultrasound Med., 1985, 4, 259—260.

34. Bret P. M., Atri M., Illescas F. F., Seymour R. J., De Stempel J.: US-guided transvaginal biopsies in pelvic masses: Preliminary experience. Presented at the 88th Meeting of the American Roentgen Ray Society, San Francisco, May 8—13, 1988.

35. Nosher J. L., Winchman H. K., Needell G. S.: Transvaginal pelvic abscess drainage with US guidance. Radiology, 1987, 165, 872—873.

10. Transvaginal sonography in obstetrics

Transvaginal sonography with the use of small, high-frequency transducers has proved particularly beneficial in the evaluation of first-trimester pregnancy.

Instrumentation and technique of examination

The end-firing sector probes have proved the best option in transvaginal scanning, although electronic linear-array probes have also been used. The sector probes are either mechanically activated, oscillating or rotating single-transducer probes or electronic, sector phased-array or curved-array probes. Electronic scanning systems provide dynamic electronic focusing and a high frame rate (20 to 30 images per second), the latter allowing visualization of the early vascular features of pregnancy.

Endovaginal probes are available with 5–7.5-MHz transducers. The outer diameter of the probe is about 15 mm, and the scanhead is usually rounded for adequate contact with the vaginal mucosa. The endovaginal probe can be sterilized between patients by immersion in an antiseptic solution (Cidex). A single-use latex protective device, such as a surgical glove, condom, or specially designed commercial covering sheath, is filled with standard coupling gel and placed over the transducer. A liberal amount of gel is applied to the external surface of the probe just before its vaginal insertion.

The major limitations of endovaginal scanning are its small field of view and limited sound beam penetration, both of which diminish the technique's usefulness for evaluating pregnancy after the first trimester. Transvaginal sonography is extremely well tolerated by patients, most of whom prefer this procedure to the discomfort of the overdistended bladder required in transabdominal imaging (see also Chapter 9).

Several particular points must be borne in mind when transvaginal examination is performed:

1. The procedure must first be explained to the patient. Ultrasound is known as a non-invasive imaging technique; in transvaginal sonography, physical and psychological boundaries must be overcome. The examination might not be well tolerated by the uninformed patient.
2. Since the probe is inside the body, the orientation of the transducer must be noted with precision for interpretation of the images displayed on the video monitor. Endocavitary images are usually displayed with the endocavitary probe at the top of the image.
3. As a consequence of the reduced field of view, the images displayed on the screen are apparently magnified.
4. Gain settings must be adjusted to compensate for the attenuation of the beam associated with high-frequency transducers.
5. The endovaginal probe must be handled gently and the deformation of the vagina must remain painless.

The indications for transvaginal sonography in obstetrics are listed in Table 10.1

Bruno D. Fornage (ed.), *Endosonography*, pp. 149–156.
© 1989 *Kluwer Academic Publishers*.

Table 10.1. Indications for transvaginal sonography in first-trimester pregnancy.

- Limited transabdominal study of the pelvis (including obese patients and insufficient bladder distension)
- Early detection and precise dating of intrauterine pregnancy
- Suspicion of ectopic pregnancy
- First-trimester bleeding
- Absence of embryonic vital signs on transabdominal scans

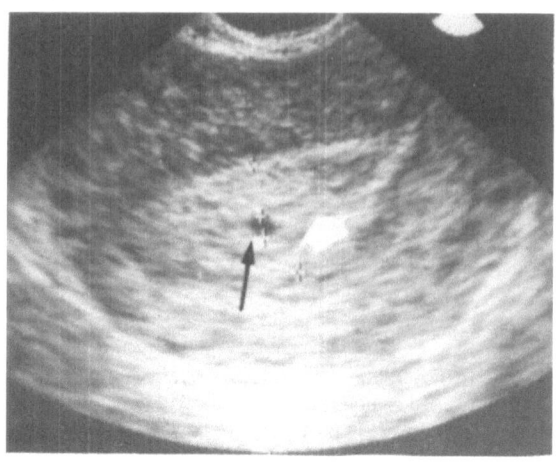

Figure 10.1. Four-week, 1-day pregnancy. Transverse transvaginal scan of the uterine fundus obtained using a 5-MHz sector probe shows a 3.2-mm gestational sac (black arrow), which is eccentric to the endometrial echoes (white arrow).

Normal first-trimester pregnancy

Intrauterine pregnancy has been diagnosed as early as 4 weeks and 2 days amenorrhea on the basis of the visualization of the echogenic chorionic ring and central, anechoic cavity (as small as 2—3 mm) [1]. It is now commonly accepted that an intrauterine gestational sac can be detected on high-frequency transvaginal sonography between 4 and 5 menstrual weeks (Figs. 10.1—10.3). The early gestational sac is characterized by its location in the endometrium, off the uterine cavity, which allows differentiation from a pseudogestational sac in the case of an ectopic pregnancy or uterine bleeding. At 5 menstrual weeks, the gestational sac is about 1 cm in diameter and appears as a rounded, echo-free area surrounded by an echogenic ring, the chorion, which comprises the extraembryonic mesenchyma, chorionic villi, and lacunae [2]. Transvaginal sonography has proved reliable in detecting normal intrauterine pregnancy when the sac size is more than 4 mm or when the serum beta-human chorionic gonadotropin (HCG) level exceeds 1000 IU/L. It typically detects intrauterine gestation 1 week earlier than transabdominal sonography.

Cavity of the gestational sac

The yolk sac, amniotic cavity, embryo, and umbilical cord are visualized at between 5 and 6 menstrual weeks.

Yolk sac

The yolk sac is the first structure to be seen in

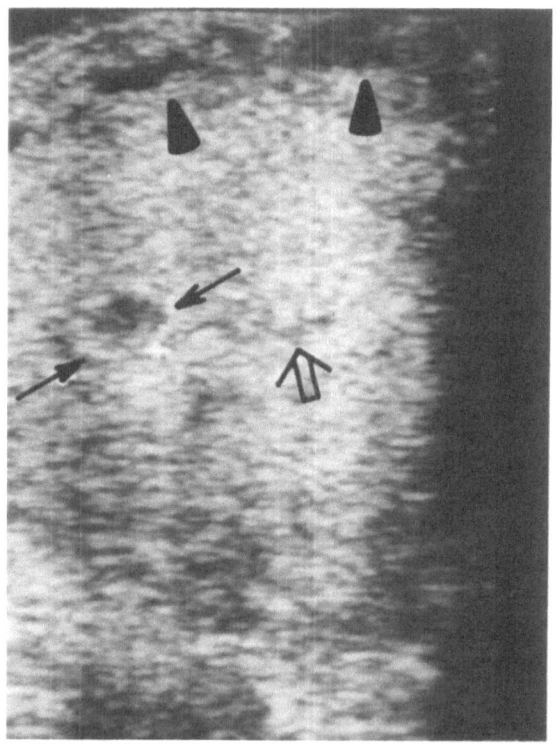

Figure 10.2. Gestational sac in a 4-week, 3-day pregnancy. Transvaginal scan obtained using a linear-array probe shows the sac surrounded by an echogenic ring (arrows). The open arrow points to the uterine cavity. Note the subserous uterine vessels (arrowheads).

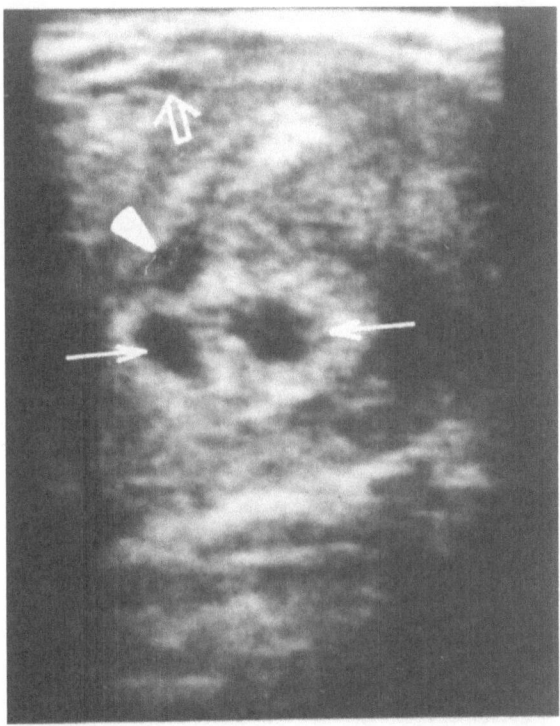

Figure 10.3. Transvaginal scan of a twin pregnancy at 5 menstrual weeks shows the two gestational sacs (arrows) located off the uterine cavity (arrowhead), in the endometrium. The open arrow points to subserous uterine vessels.

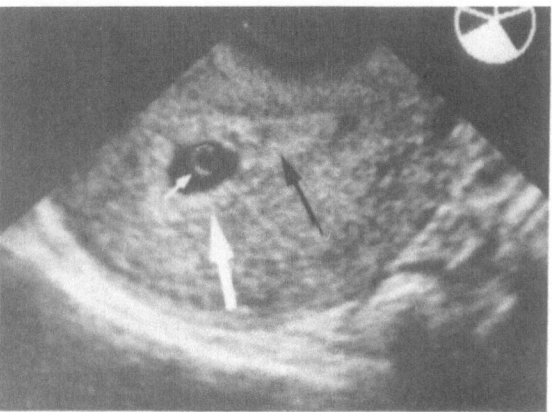

Figure 10.4. Early pregnancy. Transverse transvaginal scan of the uterine fundus obtained using a 7.5-MHz sector probe at 5 menstrual weeks shows the gestational sac (white arrow), yolk sac (small white arrow), and endometrium (black arrow).

the gestational sac, appearing at 5 menstrual weeks. It is spherical in shape, its diameter unchanged at about 4 mm until 10 menstrual weeks (Figs. 10.4, 10.5), when it blends into the gestational sac upon the collapse of the extraembryonic coelom. The stalk of the yolk sac is of variable length, so that the yolk sac is not a reliable landmark for the implantation site and the area of future placental development. This variation is also to be considered when sampling chorionic villi.

Amniotic cavity

At 6 weeks, the amniotic cavity is separated from the extraembryonic coelom by the thin, faintly echogenic amniotic membrane, eccentric in relation to the gestational sac. The membrane is best demonstrated when it lies perpendicular to the beam (Fig. 10.6). The amniotic cavity progressively occupies the gestational sac, filling it at 10 to 12 menstrual weeks.

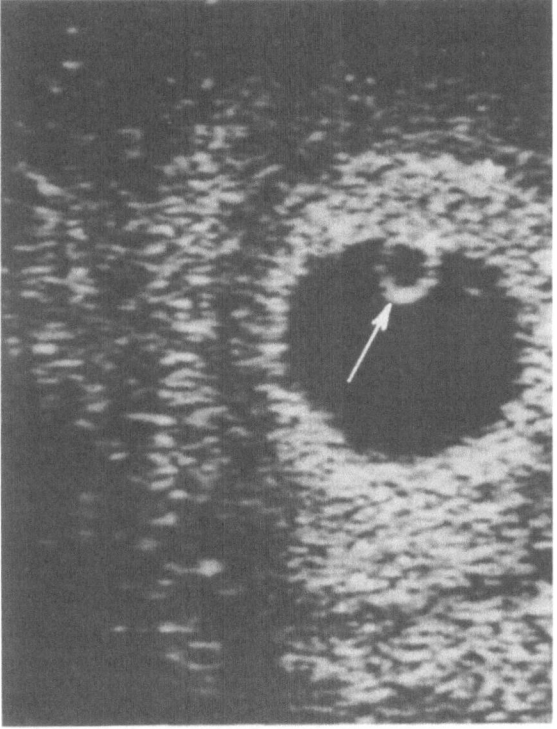

Figure 10.5. Early pregnancy. Transvaginal scan shows the yolk sac (arrow) in the extraembryonic coelom. The yolk sac is approximately 4 mm in diameter.

Embryo

A few days after the detection of the yolk sac, the embryonic pole is seen. At 5 menstrual weeks, the embryo is 3 mm in size. Embryos as small as 2 mm have been detected adjacent to

152

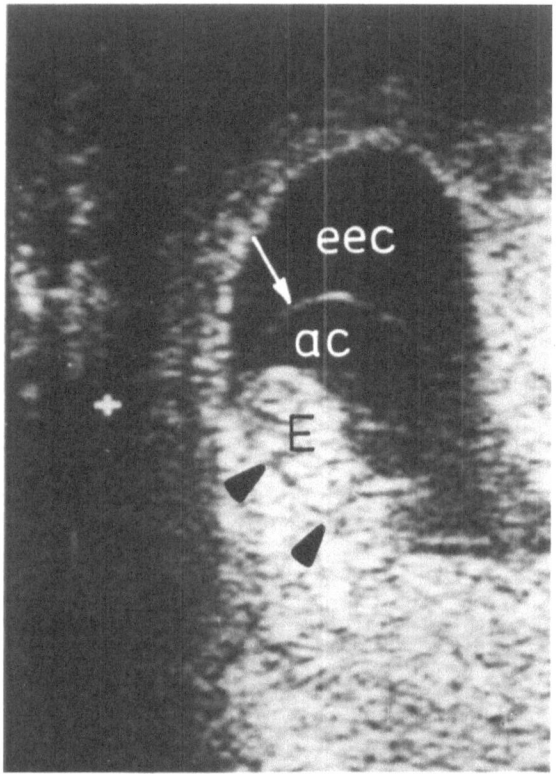

Figure 10.6. Early pregnancy. Transvaginal scan of the gestational sac shows the amniotic membrane (arrow), which separates the extraembryonic coelom from the amniotic cavity. It is eccentric to the gestational sac. Arrowheads point to the decidua basalis. ac = amniotic cavity; E = embryo; eec = extraembryonic coelom.

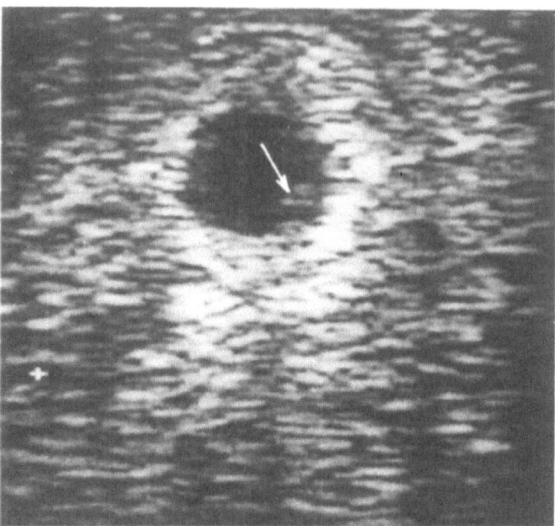

Figure 10.7. Early pregnancy. Transvaginal scan at 5 menstrual weeks shows a 1-cm gestational sac with some embryonic echoes (arrow) adjacent to the wall.

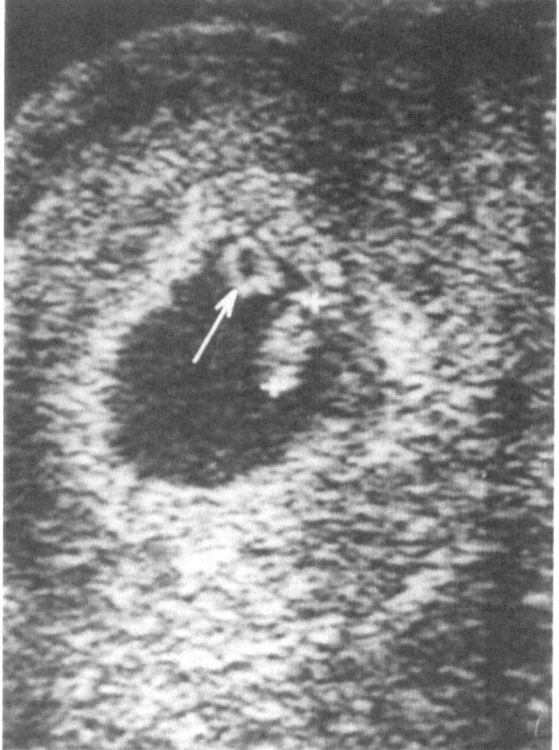

Figure 10.8. Transvaginal scan shows an 8-mm embryo (calipers), distinct from the yolk sac (arrow).

the yolk sac with transvaginal sonography [3, 4]. Sometimes the embryo cannot be clearly differentiated from the wall of the gestational sac (Fig. 10.7). However, such a situation is usually clarified within a few days (Fig. 10.8). Crown-rump length is the most reliable measurement in dating first-trimester pregnancy. Transvaginal ultrasound has proved more accurate than transabdominal scanning in this measurement because it avoids such errors as inclusion of the yolk sac or failure to identify the longest diameter of the embryo [5]. The visualization of embryonic cardiac activity is the definitive criterion for a viable pregnancy. Early cardiac activity is visualized at 5 1/2 menstrual weeks on transvaginal examination. At this stage of development, the heart is made of a simple tube, which later elongates and bends on itself. The heart activity is a peristaltic type of contraction;

the heart rate is close to 140 beats/min. These findings are similar to those described by Loeber *et al.* in guinea pig embryos [6]. Cardiac activity is synchronized between 7 and 8 weeks.

Transvaginal sonography provides an impressive depiction of the anatomy of the developing embryo during the first trimester.

Umbilical cord

The umbilical cord is seen on average after 6 gestational weeks (Fig. 10.9). Its appearance allows localization of the insertion zone of the gestational sac (decidua basalis). This localization may be crucial in evaluating patients with threatened abortion. In the first trimester, the cord appears large in relation to the embryo.

Trophoblastic zone

The trophoblastic zone, which is the area of nutritional exchange, completely surrounds the early gestational sac (Fig. 10.10). The increased echogenicity of this area is related to the high number of interfaces created by the numerous chorionic villi. At an early stage, a 'double-sac' sign can be seen peripheral to a portion of the gestational sac fluid. This finding is thought to represent the decidua parietalis (or vera) surrounding the decidua capsularis.

The chorionic ring is about 3 to 4 mm thick all around the gestational sac until about 7

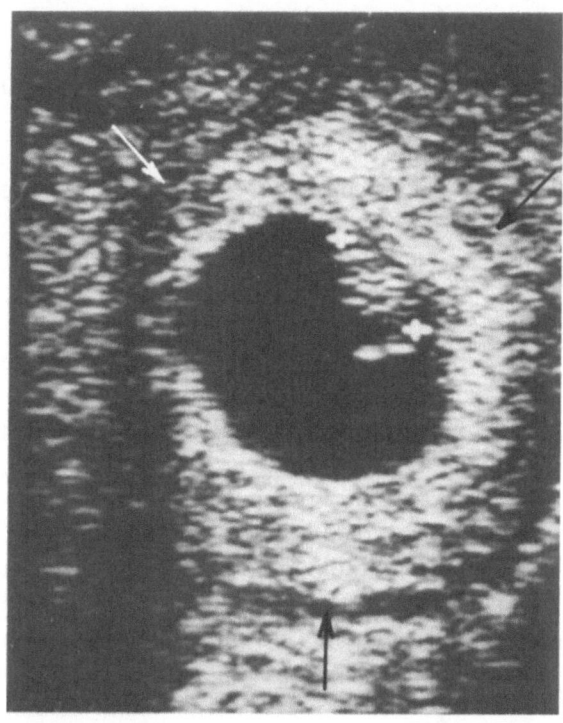

Figure 10.10. Transvaginal scan of a 10-mm embryo (calipers). The gestational sac is entirely surrounded by the chorion (arrows).

menstrual weeks. Then, within a period of 2 weeks, its thickness will be tripled. Endosonography can differentiate between the chorion laeve and the chorion frondosum because of their different thicknesses. On the side of the decidua capsularis, the chorion laeve, or smooth chorion, develops to a minimal extent; in comparison, the chorion frondosum, which faces the decidua basalis, increases further in thickness and will become the placenta.

Some kind of pulsatile activity can be detected within the chorion after 7 menstrual weeks. This pattern appears as a subtle flickering of some areas in phase with the fetal cardiac pulsations. After 11 menstrual weeks, some hypoechoic, lacunar areas with slow-moving echoes can also be visualized in the chorion frondosum.

Uterus

Early pregnancy is associated with a relatively hypoechoic uterus. This finding is better demonstrated by transvaginal than by standard transabdominal sonography.

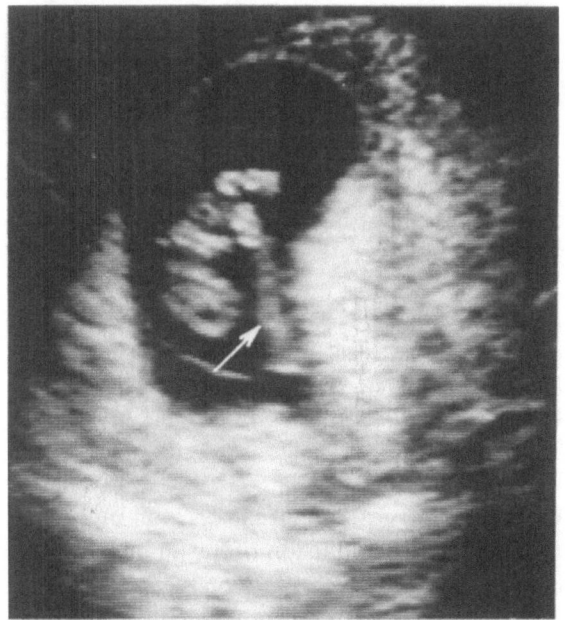

Figure 10.9. Nine-week pregnancy. Transvaginal scan shows the umbilical cord (arrow).

154

After 5 menstrual weeks, vessels are visualized in the external part of the myometrium (Figs. 10.2, 10.3). The diameter of each is about 5 mm. Numerous smaller vessels are also detected at some distance from the chorionic ring (Fig. 10.11). When electronic transducers are used, these vessels show some internal moving echoes, accounted for by blood flow. Over time, the vessels increase in size and approach the decidua basalis (Fig. 10.12). However, no invasion of the area of the future placenta by these maternal vessels can be demonstrated.

The intervillous space is nonvascularized during the first trimester, which has been confirmed at chorionoscopy by the direct observation of villi floating in a clear, watery liquid free of maternal blood [7—9]. After the first trimester, the maternal vessels communicate with the intervillous space and blood circulation develops.

Abnormal first-trimester pregnancy

Vaginal bleeding in the first trimester is a symptom of abnormal pregnancy. It may be related to subchorionic bleeding, an incomplete (missed) or complete abortion, or a blighted ovum.

Subchorionic hematoma

Normally, the chorionic ring is in intimate contact with the decidua basalis and myometrium. With transvaginal scanning, a small crescent-shaped, virtually anechoic area can be visualized between the chorion and the uterus (Fig. 10.13). This finding is fairly common and may be associated with bleeding and pain, or there may be no symptoms. Although it has been suggested that this hypoechoic crescent represents the decidua parietalis or even fluid in the uterine cavity [10], the anechoic fluid collection is thought more likely to represent a hematoma [11, 12]. The lesion was probably previously misdiagnosed as a vanishing twin gestational sac [13—16]. Since this fluid collection is always located outside the chorionic sac, it is readily differentiated from the clearly visualized two

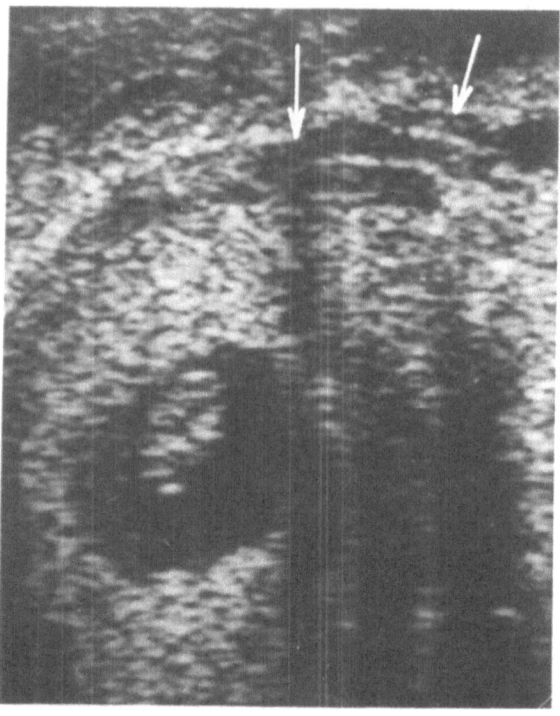

Figure 10.11. Transvaginal scan shows intramyometrial vessels (arrows) around the chorionic ring.

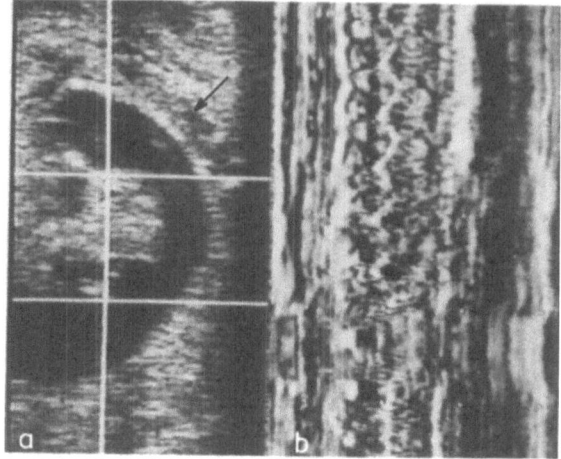

Figure 10.12. Transvaginal scan of an 11-week pregnancy. (a) The sac wall is thin at the level of the chorion laeve. Maternal vessels are seen adjacent to the wall of the gestational sac (arrow). (b) M-mode representation of fetal cardiac activity.

cavities of the gestational sac or, later in the first trimester, from nonfusion of the amnion and the chorion. It may be the size of a gestational sac and usually persists for several weeks with a constant size. The pregnancy will continue normally in about 60% to 70% of cases.

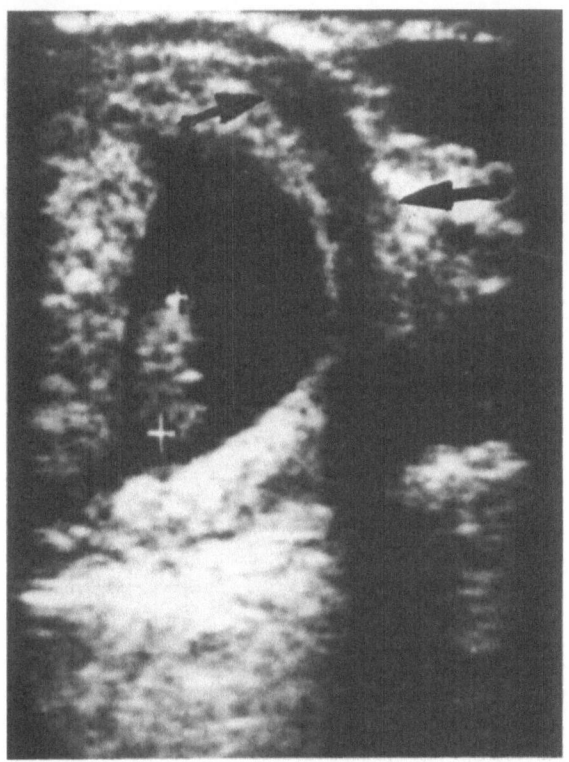

Figure 10.13. Transvaginal scan performed at 8 menstrual weeks shows a 15-mm embryo and partial hemorrhagic detachment of the sac. The hematoma (arrows) is opposite the site of insertion of the gestational sac, in the area of the decidua capsularis.

Abortions

It has been shown that transabdominal sonography detects arrest of development before the spontaneous abortion occurs [17]. Transvaginal scanning is the examination of choice in threatened abortion, particularly when no vital sign can be detected on transabdominal scans.

After a complete spontaneous abortion, an 'empty' uterus is usually seen. In missed abortion, a nonviable pregnancy that has not yet been evacuated, the nonviability is confirmed by the absence of embryonic cardiac activity. A missed abortion usually presents with intrauterine retention of embryonic and trophoblastic debris.

In recently interrupted pregnancies, the gestational sac is visualized with a grossly normal appearance. The amount of fluid is either normal or slightly increased. However, the chorion shows subtle dynamic changes. Echoes in

motion can be depicted in the chorion at the site of implantation. These echoes may move slowly and diffusely, or whirl and suggest vessels emptying into a large fluid collection, similar to the circulation in the intervillous space. Occasionally, a communication between a peritrophoblastic vessel and the trophoblast can be visualized with a typical jet phenomenon confirming the wide opening of the vessel in the intervillous space. These findings are thought to be associated with an early-stage embryonic demise prior to the onset of clinical symptoms, at a time when the gestational sac and embryo are still apparently normal.

A *blighted ovum* is defined as anembryonic gestation. There is no embryo, amniotic cavity, or yolk sac, the cavity of the gestational sac being entirely made of coelom. Sonographically, a blighted ovum appears as a gestational sac larger than 20—25 mm that is totally empty, as opposed to missed abortion. The outline of the sac is in many cases irregular.

Size-date discrepancy is confirmed by transvaginal sonography in early pregnancy failure.

Ectopic pregnancy

See Chapter 9.

Miscellaneous

In molar pregnancy, transvaginal scanning demonstrates the vesicles more clearly than transabdominal scanning.

In pregnancy coexisting with an intrauterine contraceptive device (IUD), the relationships of both are accurately demonstrated on transvaginal scans.

Certain pathologic conditions commonly encountered in evaluation of pregnancy (or infertility), including uterine malformations, synechiae, scars after hysterotomy, and fibroids (Fig. 10.14), are accurately assessed with transvaginal sonography (see also Chapter 11).

Second- and third-trimester pregnancy

Because of its restricted field of view, transvaginal

156

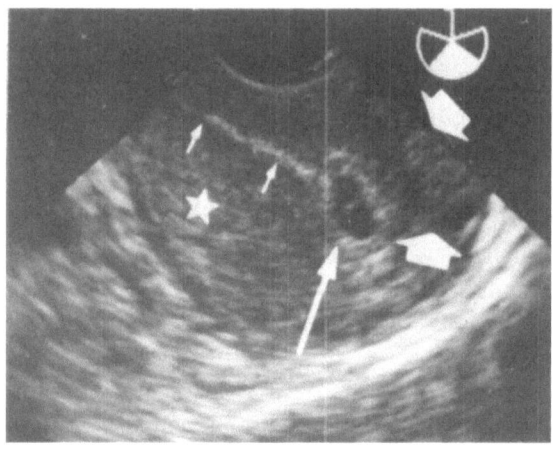

Figure 10.14. Leiomyomas and pregnancy. Longitudinally oriented transvaginal scan at 5 menstrual weeks shows a gestational sac (long arrow) clearly demarcated from the uterine cavity (short arrows). Two intramural myomas are also visualized (star and large arrows).

scanning during the second and third trimesters is limited to the evaluation of the cervix and lower part of uterus, with special reference to the relation between a low inserted placenta and the internal os.

References

1. De Crespigny L. Ch., Cooper D., McKenna M.: Early detection of intrauterine pregnancy with ultrasound. J. Ultrasound Med., 1988, 7, 7—10.
2. Schaaps J. P., Lambotte R.: Ultrasonic observation of pregnancy during the first trimester using a vaginal approach. In: Fraccaro M., Simoni G., Brambati B. (eds). First trimester fetal diagnosis. Berlin, Springer-Verlag, 1985, 78—91.
3. Baltarowich O. H., Kurtz A., Pennell R. G., *et al.*: Normal detailed embryonic anatomy with endovaginal sonography (abstract). Radiology, 1987, 165 (P), 158.
4. Timor-Tritsch I. E., Rottem S.: Transvaginal sonography. New York, Elsevier, 1988.
5. Lyons E., Levi C., Lindsay D.: Discrepancies in CRL measurements done endovaginally and transvesically. Presented at the 32nd Meeting of the American Institute of Ultrasound in Medicine, New Orleans, October 6—9, 1987.
6. Loeber C., Goldberg S. J., Hendrix M. J. C., Sahn D. J.: Dynamic mammalian cardiogenesis investigated by high-resolution ultrasound in guinea pigs. Circulation, 1983, 68, 841—845.
7. Gustavii B.: First-trimester chromosomal analysis of chorionic villi obtained by direct vision technique. Lancet, 1983, 2, 507—508.
8. Gustavii B., Chester M. A., Edvall H., *et al.*: First-trimester diagnosis on chorionic villi obtained by direct vision technique. Hum. Genet., 1984, 65, 373—376.
9. Nordenskjold F., Gustavii B.: Direct-vision chorionic villi biopsy for prenatal diagnosis in the first trimester. J. Reprod. Med., 1984, 29, 572—574.
10. Cadkin A. V., McAlpin J.: The decidua-chorionic sac: A reliable sonographic indicator of intrauterine pregnancy prior to detection of a fetal pole. J. Ultrasound Med., 1984, 3, 539—548.
11. Schaaps J. P., Thoumsin H. J.: Vaginal ultrasonography of early pregnancies. Presented at the Annual Meeting of the Society of Perinatal Obstetricians, San Antonio, 1986.
12. Hustin J., Schaaps J. P.: Echocardiographic and anatomic studies of the maternotrophoblastic border during the first trimester of pregnancy. Am. J. Obstet. Gynecol., 1987, 157, 162—168.
13. Levi S.: Ultrasonic assessment of the high rate of human multiple pregnancy in the first trimester. J. Clin. Ultrasound, 1976, 4, 3—5.
14. Robinson H. P.: The diagnosis of early pregnancy failure by sonar. Br. J. Obstet. Gynaecol., 1975, 82, 849—857.
15. Robinson H. P., Caines J. S.: Sonar evidence of early pregnancy failure in patients with twin conceptions. Br. J. Obstet. Gynaecol., 1977, 84, 22—25.
16. Kurjak A., Lantin V.: Ultrasound diagnosis of fetal abnormalities in multiple pregnancy. Acta Obstet. Gynecol. Scand., 1979, 58, 153—161.
17. Szabo J., Szemere G.: Optimal timing of chorionic biopsy and its application in the second trimester of pregnancy. In: Fraccaro M., Simoni G., Brambati B. (eds). First trimester fetal diagnosis. Berlin, Springer-Verlag, 1984, 65—68.

11. Transvaginal sonography in infertility

NABIL F. MAKLAD

The development of endovaginal ultrasound probes and their subsequent improvement and refinement over the past few years have extended the role of sonography in the diagnosis and management of female infertility. Transvaginal ultrasound provides a convenient and efficient method of evaluating the female reproductive system and has greatly expanded our understanding of reproductive physiology.

Evaluation of the pelvis in the infertile female

Transvaginal sonography affords detailed visualization of the uterus and adnexa. Transvaginal 'screening' ultrasound is increasingly being performed as part of the workup of infertility.

Uterus

A variety of uterine conditions are associated with infertility, including congenital malformations, fibroids, and endometrial abnormalities. Recent comparisons between transabdominal and transvaginal sonography have demonstrated the superiority of the latter technique in imaging the myometrium and endometrium [1] and in detecting fibroids.

Congenital malformations

Although congenital uterine anomalies occur in fewer than 0.5% of women, their incidence in infertile women has been reported to be as high as 9% [2—4]. Hysterosalpingography (HSG) is the primary imaging modality in the evaluation of congenital uterine malformations. The anomalies that result from the total or partial nonre-

sorption of the sagittal uterine septum — namely, uterus septus and subseptus, respectively — are the congenital malformations most frequently associated with infertility [5]. The external uterine contour is normal in both uterus septus and subseptus, while a bilobed fundal configuration is characteristic of bicornuate uterus. As HSG cannot demonstrate the external uterine morphology, transabdominal ultrasound has been utilized with some success in diagnosing a septate uterus, and in distinguishing between this anomaly and bicornuate uterus [6—8]. However, an intrauterine septum is often difficult to demonstrate on transabdominal sonography, and an artifactual bilobed appearance of the uterus sometimes results from overdistension of the urinary bladder. The use of transvaginal ultrasound in the diagnosis of various congenital uterine anomalies is still being evaluated. Preliminary results indicate that transvaginal sonography is superior in outlining the uterine cavity and in delineating subtle differences in the external uterine contour (Fig. 11.1). The proximity of the high-frequency endovaginal transducer to the uterus and the ability to image in various planes contribute to a more accurate demonstration of uterine morphology. In addition, the improved soft tissue textural imaging by transvaginal ultrasound enables the differentiation of the fibrous septum seen in septate uteri from the myometrial tissue that separates the two uterine cavities in bicornuate uteri (Fig. 11.2).

After uterus septus and uterus subseptus, the uterine anomaly most commonly associated with infertility is unicornuate uterus. This malformation results from the unilateral arrest of müllerian

Bruno D. Fornage (ed.), *Endosonography*, pp. 157—177.
© 1989 *Kluwer Academic Publishers*.

158

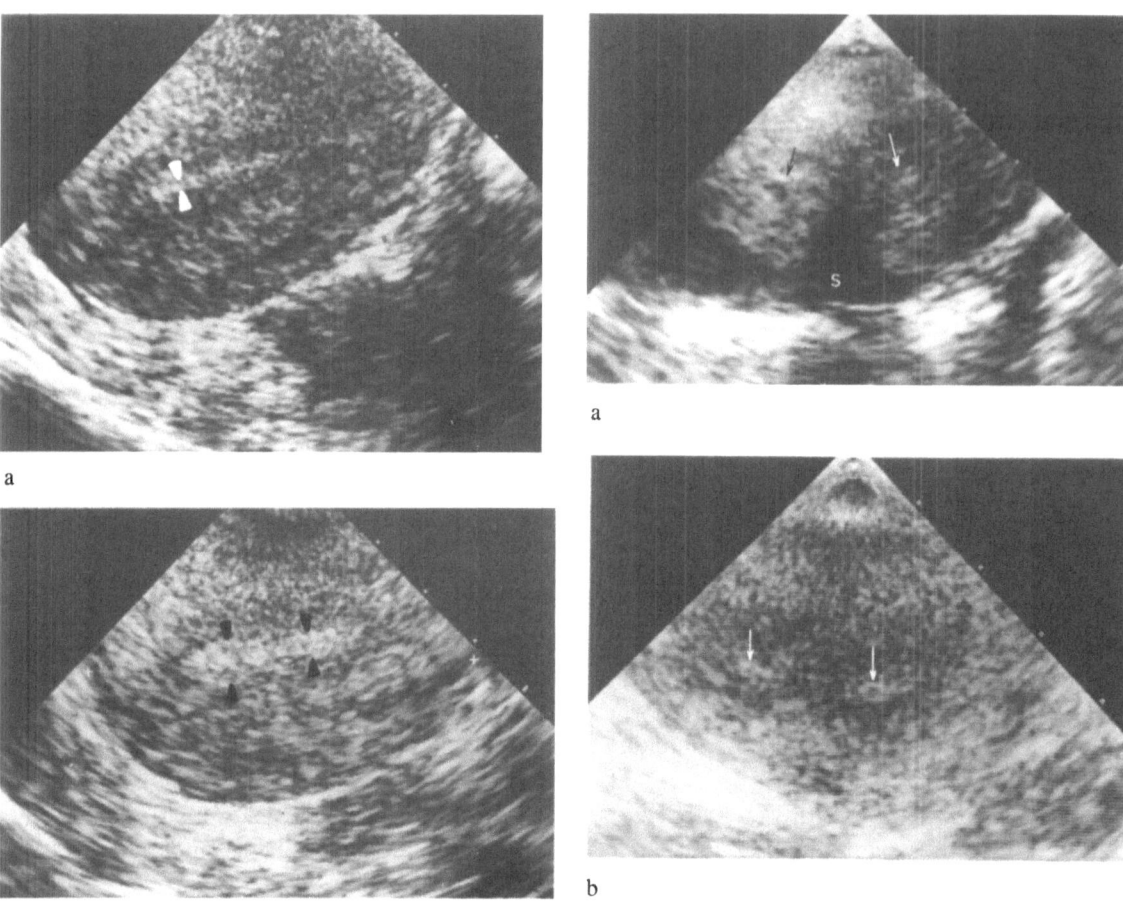

a

b

Figure 11.1. Normal uterus. Sagittal (a) and coronal (b) transvaginal scans. The echogenic endometrium (arrowheads) is surrounded by the hypoechoic inner myometrium. The external uterine contour is well delineated.

a

b

Figure 11.2. Uterine malformations. Transvaginal coronal scans. (a) Septate uterus. The fibrous septum (S) separating the two uterine cavities (arrows) is hypoechoic. (b) Bicornuate uterus. The two echogenic endometria (arrows) are separated by myometrium.

duct development. Fedele and co-workers investigated the usefulness of transabdominal ultrasound in diagnosing the various subclasses of unicornuate uterus [9]. They reported a high sensitivity and specificity for diagnosis of a rudimentary horn and for demonstration of a cavity in such a horn. Transvaginal ultrasound, still under investigation in this setting, may prove helpful in the diagnosis of unicornuate uterus and its various types, because of the excellent depiction of the endometrium and the external uterine contour.

Uterine hypoplasia, especially in women exposed to diethylstilbestrol (DES) in utero, is associated with infertility, endometriosis, ectopic pregnancy, and repeated pregnancy loss. A T-shaped uterine configuration is sometimes seen in DES-exposed women [10]. Transvaginal ultrasound is well suited for the diagnosis of this condition, since the organ's volume and shape, as well as the shape of the uterine cavity, are accurately demonstrated (Fig. 11.3). It is conceivable that transvaginal sonography will be utilized as a screening procedure for uterine hypoplasia in women at high risk for this anomaly, such as those exposed to DES in utero [11].

Fibroids

Fibroids are rarely a solitary cause of infertility, and the mechanisms by which these tumors interfere with gestational capacity are still unclear [12]. Some of the mechanisms suggested are (a) distortion of the uterine cavity, causing

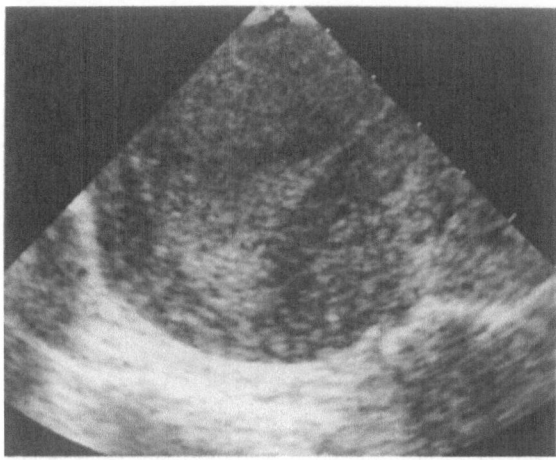

a

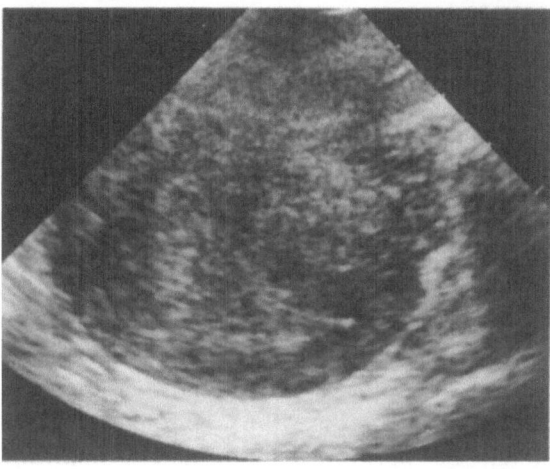

b

Figure 11.3. Uterus in patient exposed to DES in utero. Sagittal (a) and coronal (b) scans demonstrate the characteristic T-shaped uterine contour and cavity.

mechanical compromise and increasing the distance required for sperm transport; (b) obstruction of the uterotubal junction, interfering with uterotubal transport [13]; (c) alteration of the blood flow to the endometrium by submucous myomas, leading to compromise of vessels required for endometrial proliferation; (d) irritation of the myometrium by degenerating intramural and submucous fibroids, resulting in dynamic changes in uterine contractility [14]; and (e) alteration in uterine fluid volume and composition, impairing blastocyst implantation. It is estimated that 18% of infertile patients have fibroids that are at least partially responsible for failure to conceive [15].

The diagnostic tests used to determine the presence, number, and location of fibroids include HSG, hysteroscopy, and sonography. Transvaginal ultrasound is superior to transabdominal scanning in detecting and delineating fibroids. Of particular importance in the infertile female is the demonstration of small submucous fibroids impinging on the endometrium, which may interfere with implantation. These small tumors are rarely visible on transabdominal ultrasound, and hysteroscopy is often required for their accurate diagnosis and differentiation from endometrial polyps [16]. Transvaginal ultrasound allows the demonstration of very small fibromyomas and the accurate delineation of their relationship to the endometrium (Fig. 11.4). In addition, fibroids encroaching on the uterotubal junction can be identified by transvaginal ultrasound, because of the easy visualization of the region of the tubal ostia (Fig. 11.5).

The traditional treatment of fibroids in infertile patients in whom no other cause of infertility can be found after adequate evaluation is myomectomy, either via the abdominal route or by hysteroscopy. The results of myomectomy in properly selected infertility cases were reviewed by Buttram and Reiter, who found a 40% postoperative pregnancy rate in a review of 18 studies reporting on 1202 women [17]. Recent reports indicate that the administration of luteinizing hormone-releasing hormone (LHRH) agonists for several months is a valid alternative to myomectomy in premenopausal women with symptomatic fibroids [18]. Transvaginal sonography can be used for follow-up of fibroids during this nonsurgical therapy.

Endometrial abnormalities

The role of the endometrium in the process of implantation is well known. Less familiar is the function of the underlying inner myometrium in the process of blastocyst attachment and nidation. Both the endometrium and inner myometrium must be anatomically and functionally normal for successful implantation. With the advent of transvaginal scanning, a renewed interest has developed in evaluation of the endometrium-myometrium zone, particularly in its variation in width, volume, and texture under

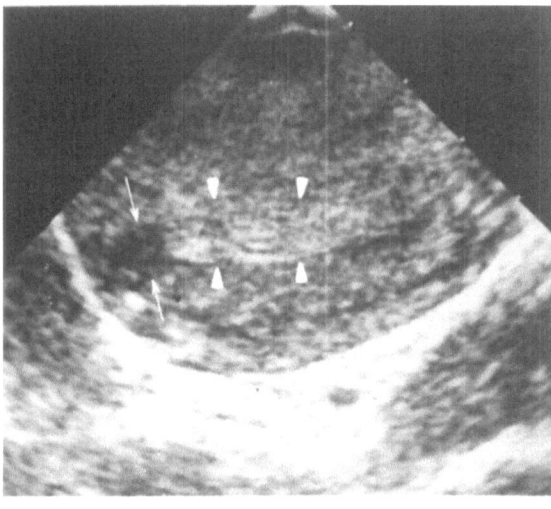

a

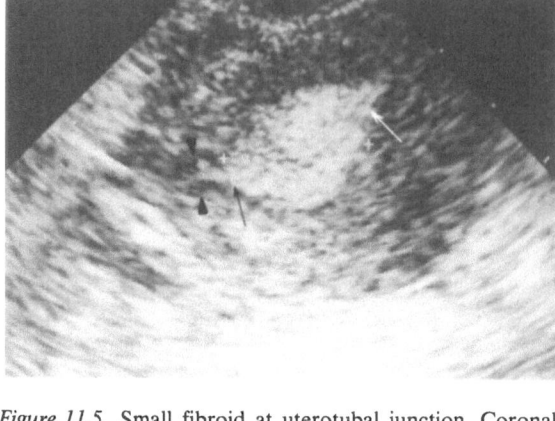

Figure 11.5. Small fibroid at uterotubal junction. Coronal transvaginal scan shows the regions of the tubal ostia (arrows), and a small, hypoechoic submucous fibroid (arrowheads) at the right uterotubal junction.

b

Figure 11.4. Submucous fibroid. (a) A small, hypoechoic submucous fibroid (arrows) is recognized by the subtle difference in echogenicity from the surrounding myometrium. Note the proximity of the fibroid to the echogenic endometrium (arrowheads). (b) The submucous fibroid (markers), which measures 9 mm, impinges on the echogenic endometrium (arrowheads).

the influence of the various medications utilized to induce ovulation in infertile patients.

The thickness of the normal endometrium in women of reproductive age varies with the menstrual cycle phase. During menses, the endometrium appears on transvaginal sonography as a thin central interface, 2 to 3 mm in thickness. In the proliferative phase, and under the influence of estrogen, the endometrial thickness is 4 to 6 mm. A progressive increase in thickness occurs in the periovulatory phase, with a maximum of 6 to 8 mm, and in the secretory phase, up to 8 to 12 mm.

Endometrial abnormalities encountered in infertile women include hyperplasia (most commonly seen in patients with polycystic ovaries), intrauterine synechiae (Asherman's syndrome), polyps, and inflammatory conditions (acute and chronic endometritis).

Endometrial hyperplasia can be diagnosed by transvaginal ultrasound when the thickness of the endometrium exceeds the normal limits for the cycle phase (Fig. 11.6). A follow-up scan should be performed immediately following cessation of menses in the next menstrual cycle to demonstrate persistent endometrial thickening. Confirmation is by endometrial biopsy, which is also useful in 'endometrial dating,' especially in patients suspected of luteal-phase deficiency [19, 20].

Intrauterine synechiae typically are associated with menstrual abnormalities and infertility. They are of traumatic or less commonly inflammatory origin and result in partial or complete obliteration of the endometrial cavity. The most common etiology is vigorous curettage after delivery or abortion. The diagnosis of Asherman's syndrome is suspected by history and confirmed by HSG and hysteroscopy, the latter technique having substantially altered the management of the condition. With the widespread use of transvaginal scanning, intrauterine synechiae are being detected with greater frequency and accuracy. The typical sonographic appearances are serpiginous echogenic endometrial

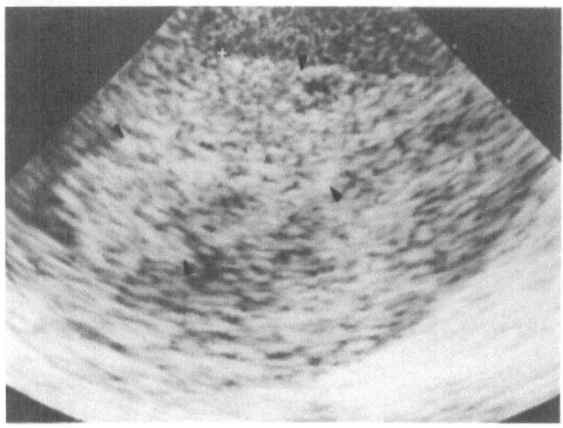

Figure 11.6. Endometrial hyperplasia. The markedly thickened endometrium (arrowheads) measures 23 mm on this sagittal scan of the uterus made during the secretory phase (normal thickness of endometrium, 8 to 12 mm).

irregularities and multiple cystic or hypoechoic areas within the endometrium (Fig. 11.7). The importance of diagnosing this condition in infertile women can be appreciated when the results of hysteroscopic lysis of the adhesions are reviewed: pregnancy rates as high as 70% to 80% have been reported [21].

Endometrial polyps appear as single or multiple hypoechoic lesions within a thickened endometrium, as nonhomogeneous echogenic material filling the uterine cavity, or as multiple echogenic foci [22]. Transvaginal scanning has improved the accuracy of diagnosing polyps and differentiating them from submucous fibroids (Fig. 11.8).

Endometritis, whether acute or chronic, shows thickened and/or irregular endometrium on transvaginal ultrasound. Associated tubal and ovarian inflammatory masses can be easily demonstrated (Fig. 11.9).

Ovaries

Monitoring of ovarian activity by sonography during ovulation induction is currently an essential part of all regimens of ovarian stimulation. Three conditions affecting the ovaries and known to be associated with varying degrees of infertility are the polycystic ovary, endometriosis, and the luteinized unruptured follicle syndrome (LUFS).

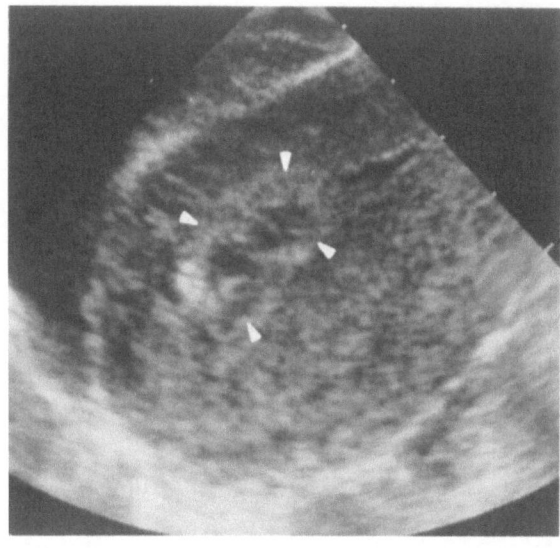

a

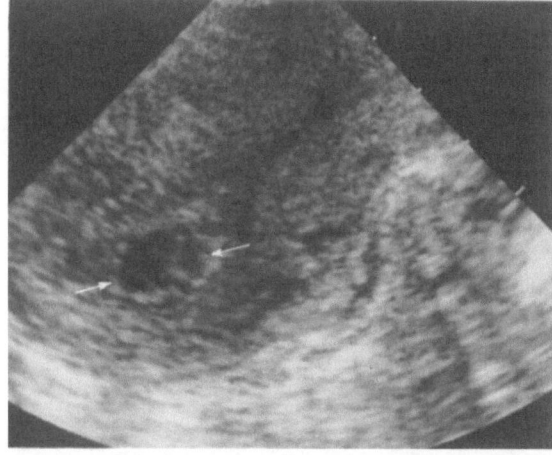

b

Figure 11.7. Intrauterine synechiae. (a) Sagittal scan of the uterus demonstrates thick echogenic strands surrounding multiple hypoechoic areas within the endometrium (arrowheads). (b) Serpiginous echogenic endometrial irregularities are associated with two cystic areas (arrows).

Polycystic ovarian disease
The association of enlarged polycystic ovaries with oligomenorrhea or amenorrhea, hirsutism, obesity, and infertility was first described by Stein and Leventhal in 1935 [23]. The incidence of polycystic ovaries has been reported at 1.4%, with the majority of affected women having ovulatory failure (89%) and infertility (74%) [24]. Ovarian enlargement two to five times greater than normal is found in 70% to 85% of patients with polycystic ovaries (normal range

162

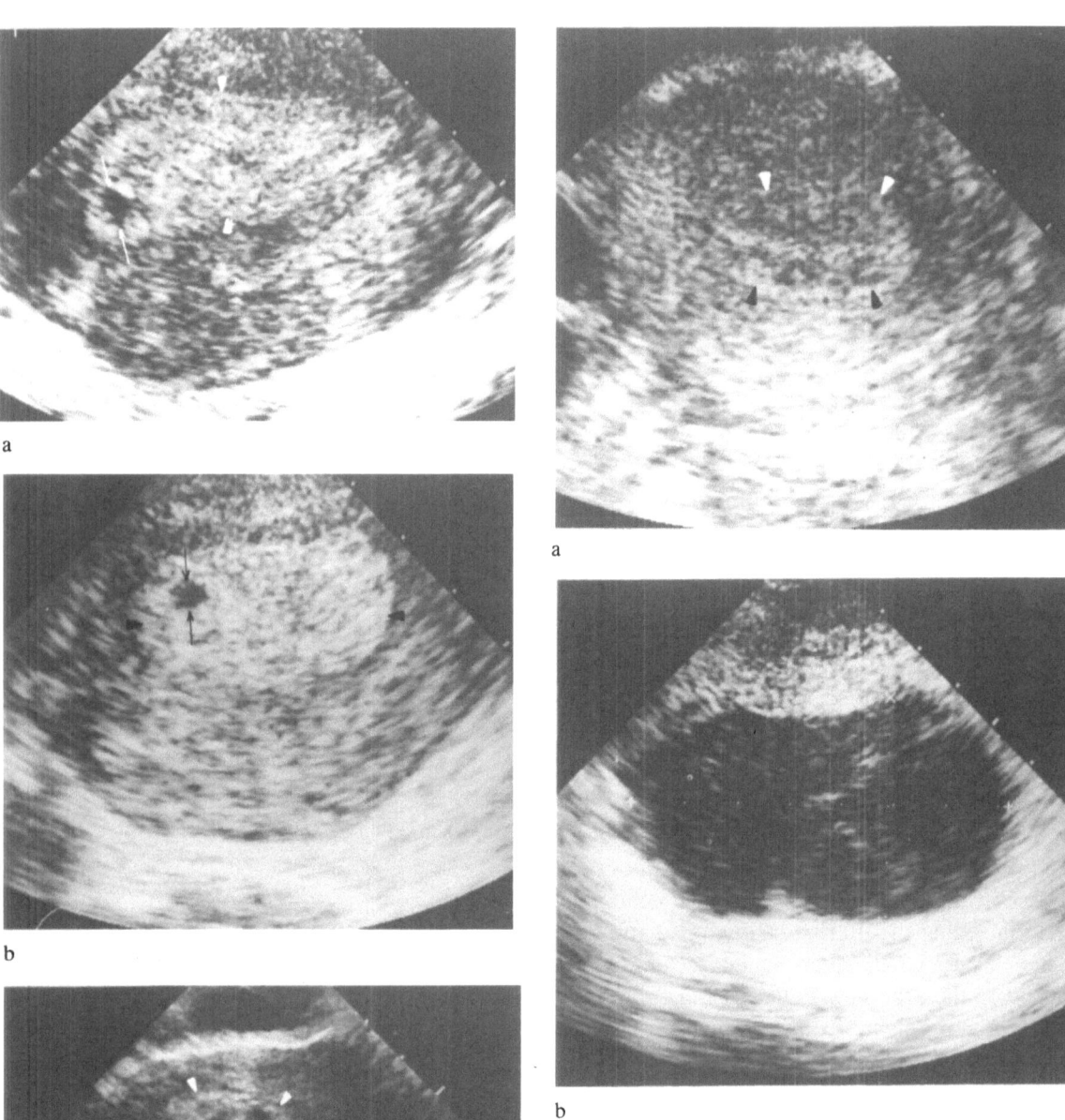

Figure 11.8. Endometrial polyps. Sagittal (a) and coronal (b) scans show a single hypoechoic endometrial polyp (arrows) within the markedly thickened hyperechoic endometrium (arrowheads). (c) Multiple hypoechoic endometrial polyps and multiple echogenic foci are seen within the hyperplastic endometrium (arrowheads) in a different patient.

Figure 11.9. Endometritis and tubo-ovarian inflammatory mass. (a) Coronal scan of the uterus shows a thickened, irregular, nonhomogeneous endometrium (arrowheads) due to endometritis. (b) Oblique scan of the adnexa in the same patient demonstrates a complex tubo-ovarian inflammatory mass.

in the reproductive years, 6—14 cm³). The enlarged ovaries are easily demonstrated on both transabdominal and transvaginal scanning, are spherical and contain numerous small cysts (Fig. 11.10). The presence of multiple 2—4-mm cysts associated with increased ovarian stroma is considered diagnostic (Fig. 11.11). Another, less common sonographic appearance is the hypo-

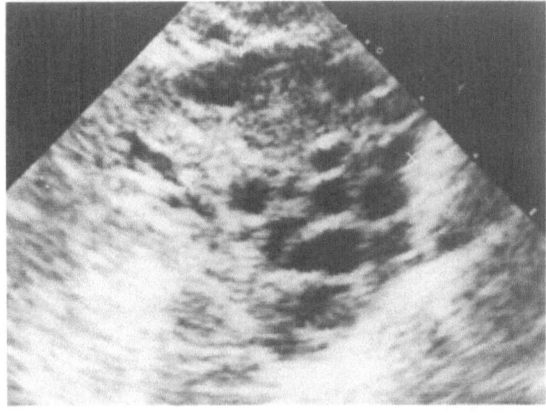

a

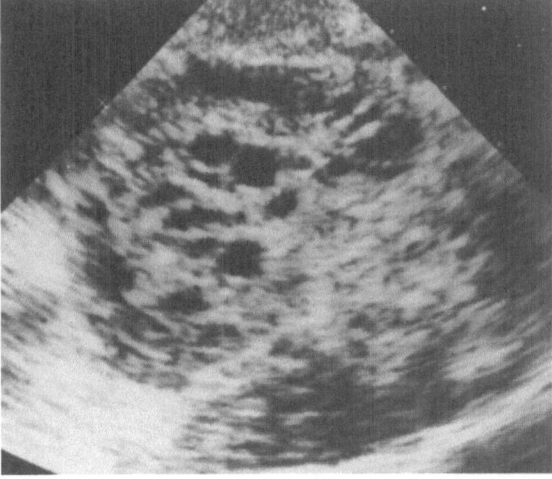

b

Figure 11.10. Polycystic ovaries. Transvaginal transverse scans of the right (a) and left (b) ovaries show enlargement, with numerous small cysts (2 to 5 mm) throughout the ovarian stroma.

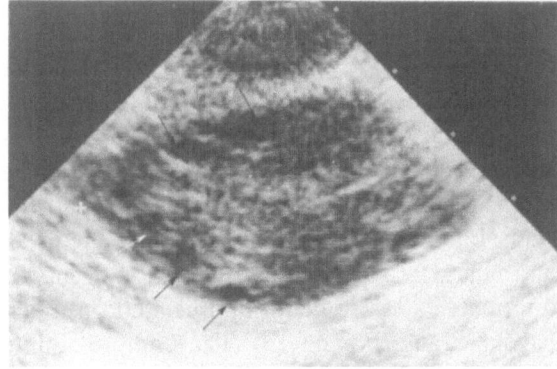

Figure 11.11. Polycystic ovary. Transvaginal scan shows an enlarged ovary with multiple small cysts (arrows) and increased ovarian stroma.

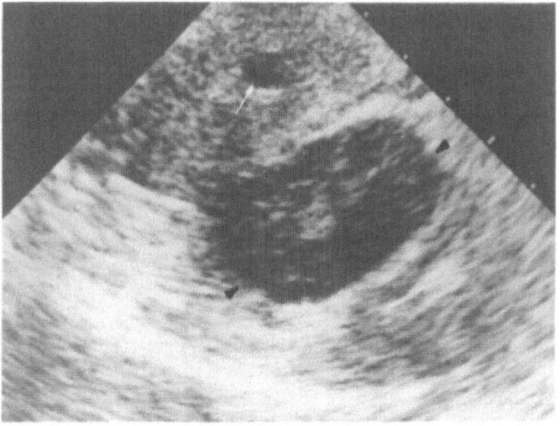

Figure 11.12. Polycystic ovary. Transverse scan shows a hypoechoic ovary without identifiable cysts (arrowheads). Note a small cyst (arrow) in the cervix uteri.

echoic ovary without identifiable cysts (Fig. 11.12). Because of the unopposed estrogenic milieu that occurs in many cases, and as mentioned above, endometrial hyperplasia, seen as endometrial thickening, is a common associated finding in patients with polycystic ovaries.

Endometriosis
Endometriosis, defined as the presence in various heterotopic locations of tissue that resembles endometrium, is apparently increasing in prevalence. The true incidence of the condition is unknown; it has been found at laparoscopy in 30% to 50% of infertile patients [25, 26]. Clinical manifestations include pelvic pain,

dysmenorrhea, and infertility. Pelvic examination often reveals tender nodularity along the uterosacral ligaments, posterior uterine surface, and cul-de-sac. The diagnosis is confirmed by direct visualization, during laparoscopy or laparotomy, of friable red tissue, 'powder burn' lesions, and bluish cysts.

Infertility occurs in 30% to 40% of women with endometriosis [27] and is 20 times more likely to occur in affected women than in controls [28]. Ovarian involvement, whether by implants on the surface or deposits within the organ, cannot be diagnosed by current ultrasound techniques. However, it is possible that in the near future the resolution of endovaginal probes will be enough improved to allow visual-

164

ization of these tiny endometrial deposits. Endometriomas, or 'chocolate' cysts, which result from bleeding into endometriosis deposits, are easily diagnosed by ultrasound. These loculated blood collections characteristically show debris of even echogenicity within a cystic lesion, more often demonstrated by transvaginal than by transabdominal sonography. The thickened wall and characteristic layering of the homogeneous internal echoes are better appreciated on transvaginal scans (Fig. 11.13). The compressibility of endometriomas, a well-known feature on laparoscopic examination, is also demonstrable on transvaginal ultrasound (Fig. 11.14). Transvaginal aspiration of endometriomas, for diagnostic and therapeutic purposes, is under investigation (Maklad, unpublished data).

Luteinized unruptured follicle syndrome
Luteinized unruptured follicle syndrome (LUFS)

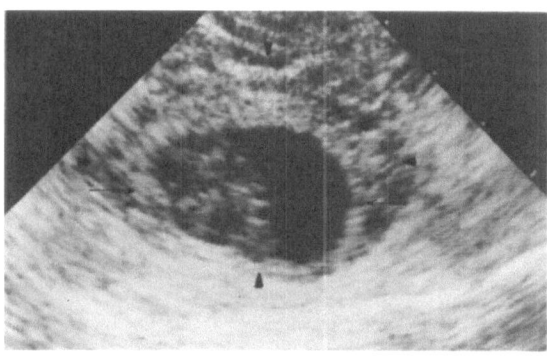

a

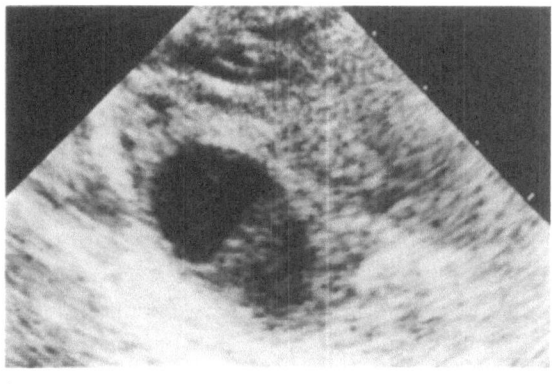

b

Figure 11.13. Ovarian endometrioma. (a) Longitudinal transvaginal scan of the adnexa demonstrates a thick-walled endometrioma (arrows) within the ovary (arrowheads). (b) Layering of the echogenic debris is seen when the patient is turned on her side.

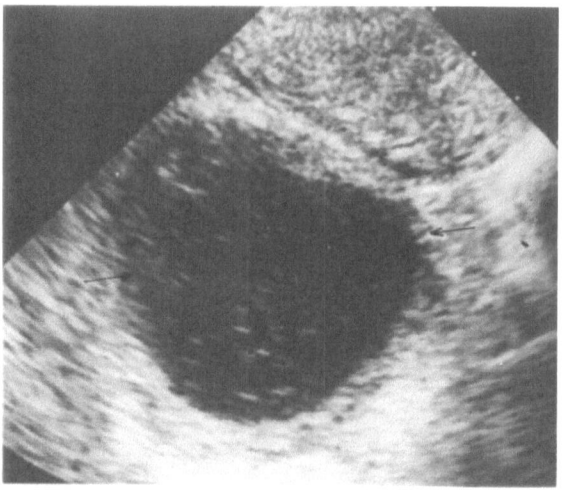

a

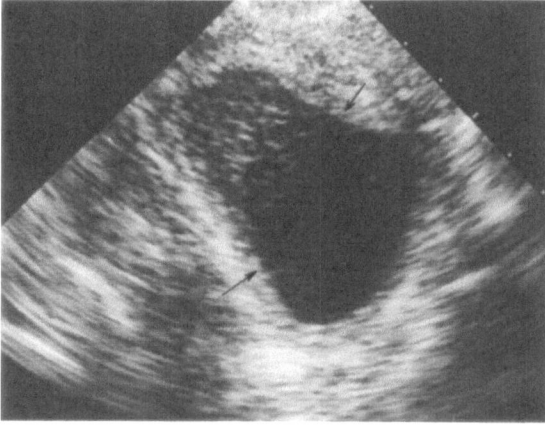

b

Figure 11.14. Compressibility of endometrioma. (a) Transverse scan of an endometrioma (arrows) showing homogeneous echogenic debris. (b) Change in shape of the endometrioma (arrows) from pressure by the transvaginal probe denotes its compressibility.

has recently received considerable attention, especially in patients with endometriosis, as a possible cause of infertility [29]. The syndrome is defined as failure of mechanical release of an ovum from a mature follicle at the presumed time of ovulation in spite of biochemical evidence of ovulation, such as rising serum progesterone levels, elevation of body temperature, and midcycle surge of luteinizing hormone (LH). The diagnosis of LUFS has been reported at laparoscopy when no postovulatory stigma of ovulation could be detected [30]. Difficulties associated with laparoscopic diagnosis of LUFS include limited accessibility to the ovary in some cases, suboptimal timing of the procedure referable to the midcycle LH surge, and lack of knowledge about how long an ovulatory stigma persists following ovulation. For these and possibly other reasons, some stigmas are not seen at laparoscopy, and serial sonography appears to be a superior diagnostic test [31]. The incidence of LUFS diagnosed by ultrasound criteria has been reported as 9% to 13% [32]. On serial sonography in patients with this condition, a persistent follicular cyst is seen, while the signs suggestive of ovulation, such as thickening of the follicular cyst wall, collapse of the follicle, and appearance of free fluid in the cul-de-sac, are absent. The role of transvaginal ultrasound in the diagnosis of this condition is evolving, with a possible role for duplex Doppler study of the ovary as discussed below.

Fallopian tubes

A patent tube, free of disease or adhesions, is essential for ovum pickup, sperm transport, fertilization, and embryo transport. Tubal obstruction, whether proximal or distal, and phimotic tubal ostia are readily demonstrable on HSG and laparoscopy. Fluid-filled dilated tubes can be detected by both transabdominal and transvaginal sonography. The fluid within the tube is usually echofree, as in hydrosalpinx (Fig. 11.15); in pyosalpinx, the fluid is uniformly echogenic (Fig. 11.16), or it is heterogeneous with hyperechoic strands and clumps due to organization (Fig. 11.17). While these appearances may suggest an etiology for the tubal disease, the lack of specificity limits the role of sonography to outlining the size and extent of the lesion. Transvaginal aspiration performed utilizing needles attached to the ultrasound probe for diagnostic or therapeutic purposes is being evaluated [33].

The presence of free pelvic fluid facilitates the delineation of pelvic organs by ultrasound. The importance of this fluid in demonstrating the normal or diseased tube by transvaginal ultrasound has recently been emphasized by Timor-Tritsch and Rottem [34]. By scanning patients on a midcycle day (increased pelvic fluid) in the lithotomy position with reverse Trendelenburg (to pool fluid into the pelvis), these investigators

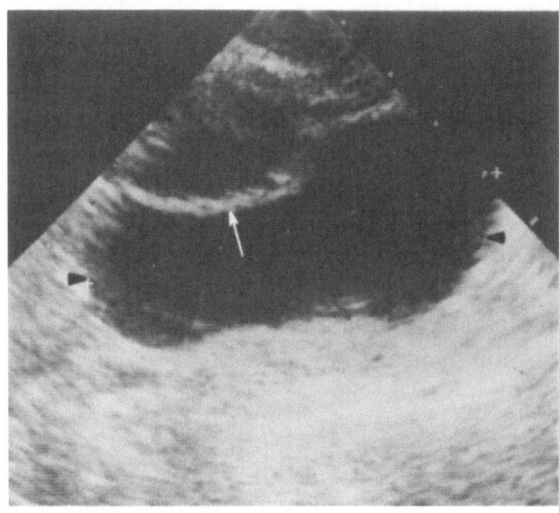

Figure 11.15. Hydrosalpinx. Transvaginal coronal view of the adnexa shows echo-free fluid filling the fallopian tube (arrowheads). The echogenic septum (arrow) represents a folding of the distended tube.

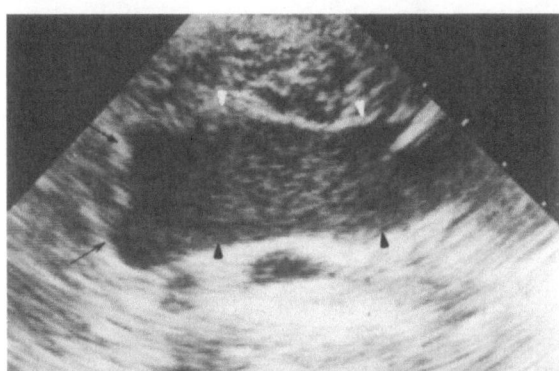

Figure 11.16. Pyosalpinx. Uniformly echogenic fluid fills the dilated fallopian tube (arrowheads). The fimbrial end of the tube is well depicted (arrows).

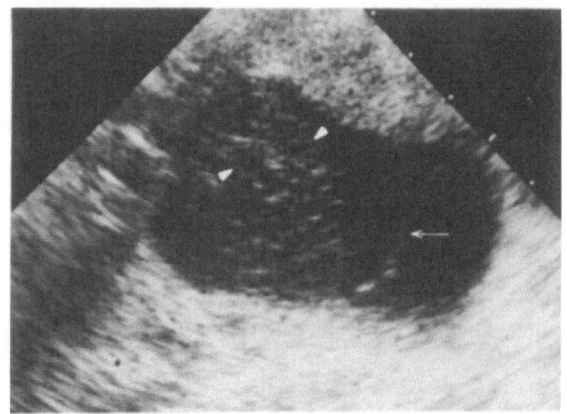

Figure 11.17. Pyosalpinx. Heterogeneous fluid with strands (arrow) and echogenic clumps (arrowheads), which result from organization, are demonstrated within the dilated fallopian tube.

demonstrated the normal tube as a tortuous echogenic structure of varying width (Fig. 11.18). Various pathologic conditions affecting the tubes were better evaluated using this technique.

Monitoring of ovulation-induction cycle

The ability to induce ovulation by chemical or hormonal means in anovulatory women was

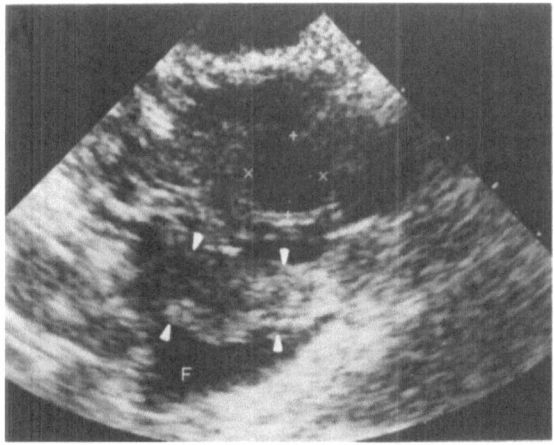

a

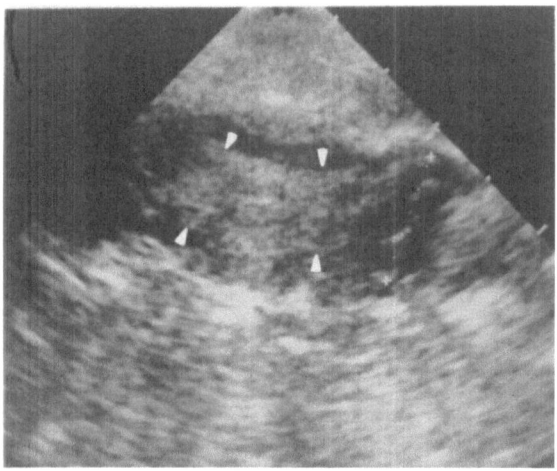

b

Figure 11.18. Fallopian tube. (a) The fallopian tube is outlined by fluid (F) in the pelvis. The echogenic structure (arrowheads) is seen to increase in thickness toward the fimbrial end. An ovarian follicle is also demonstrated (calipers). (b) The fimbrial end of the tube contains a small amount of fluid (calipers). The ampullary portion of the tube (arrowheads), which is 1 cm in thickness, is well seen due to the surrounding fluid.

introduced in the late 1950s. The availability of clomiphene citrate (Clomid, Merrell Dow) and gonadotropins afforded an effective means of ovulation induction and fostered many therapeutic techniques for assisted reproduction, such as in vitro fertilization and embryo transfer (IVF-ET) and gamete intrafallopian transfer (GIFT). Recently, new agents for follicular recruitment have been added, most notably gonadotropin-releasing hormone (Gn-RH). The advent of various ovulation induction regimens meant that effective methods for monitoring ovulation cycles were not only desirable but in many cases essential to gauge the success of treatment and to avoid such potential complications as ovarian hyperstimulation syndrome (OHS) and multiple pregnancy. Currently, ultrasound imaging of the pelvis, alone or in combination with serum estradiol (E2) determination, is the method of choice in monitoring stimulated as well as natural cycles. Accurately establishing the time of ovulation is essential for all techniques of assisted reproduction.

Various therapeutic regimens are used for ovarian stimulation with the following agents, used alone or in combination.

1. Clomiphene citrate stimulates endogenous secretion of gonadotropins from the pituitary gland.
2. Human menopausal gonadotropin (HMG) is obtained by purification of urine of menopausal women. The menotropins, as these are frequently called, are usually administered as equal parts of FSH and LH. This preparation is marketed as Pergonal (Serono Laboratories). Purified FSH (containing less than 0.1% LH) is available as Metrodin (Serono Laboratories).
3. Gonadotropin-releasing hormone is effective in inducing ovulation in anovulatory hypothalamic, hypogonadotropic women.
4. Human chorionic gonadotropin (HCG) is used to simulate the LH surge in the periovulatory period, to stimulate ovulation and luteinization. When to administer HCG to trigger ovulation is decided by sonographic criteria and results of hormonal assays.

Monitoring of ovulation

Ultrasound imaging of the ovaries is an established and effective method for tracking follicular development in natural and stimulated cycles [35—39]. Although estrogen levels can indicate the onset of ovarian response and can predict the likelihood of ovarian hyperstimulation, they cannot indicate follicle number, growth, or maturation, and a high E2 level can occur in the presence of one mature follicle or several immature ones. Sonography is used to:

1. demonstrate ovarian follicular formation,
2. determine the number and size of follicles,
3. track follicular growth, normally a 2—3-mm increase in mean diameter per day,
4. depict morphologic changes associated with the presence of mature ova,
5. detect premature luteinization of follicles during ovarian stimulation, and
6. predict the likelihood of development of OHS and the risk of multiple pregnancy.

The introduction of endovaginal ultrasound probes, with the demonstration of their superiority in imaging the ovaries, has made transvaginal sonography the technique of choice in monitoring ovulation induction [40].

Monitoring of cycles, usually by daily ultrasound studies, is begun once ovarian response has been established (from day 8 to day 10 of the cycle depending on the protocol of stimulation). The identified ovarian follicles are numbered and measured (Fig. 11.19). The size of each follicle is determined daily either by measurement of the largest diameter obtainable in the sagittal and coronal planes [41] or by averaging the three greatest dimensions. To facilitate reproducible measurements and to best follow follicular growth, it is preferable that the same operator perform the daily scans. Follicular size is used as an indicator of maturity. Follicles should be within the range of 17 to 25 mm mean diameter for ovulation. Consequently, the timing of the ovulation dose of HCG in stimulated cycles is dependent on follicle size; ovulation will occur within 48 hours of the HCG administration. It is generally accepted that the leading follicle (or follicles) should attain a diameter of

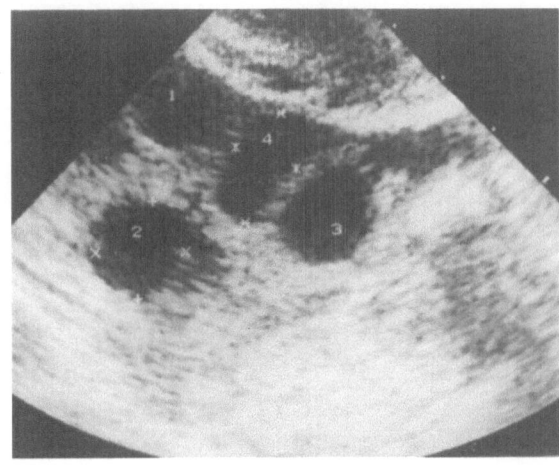

a

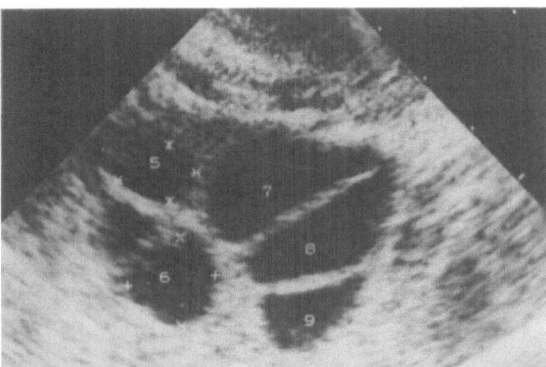

b

Figure 11.19. Stimulated ovary. Two coronal views of a stimulated ovary — inferior (a) and superior (b) — demonstrate multiple follicles. Each follicle has been numbered to facilitate monitoring of growth by daily ultrasound examination. Measurement of follicle dimensions is shown by various cursors.

at least 16 to 18 mm before the ovulating dose of HCG is given [42, 43].

In addition to determining size, transvaginal sonography can demonstrate subtle changes in the follicle that are associated with maturity, namely, thickening and crenation of the wall, the appearance of fine intrafollicular echoes and linear strands (presumed to represent cellular debris and clumping of granulosa cells), and the development of an echogenic focus within the follicle (thought to represent the cumulus oophorus) (Fig. 11.20). A recent study of 40 patients confirmed that the presence of these follicular changes was associated with a higher

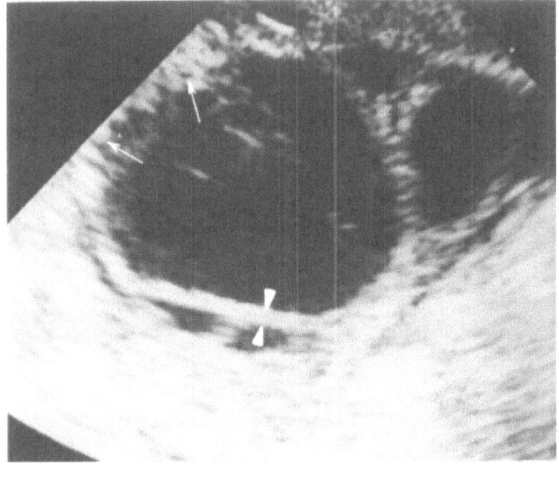

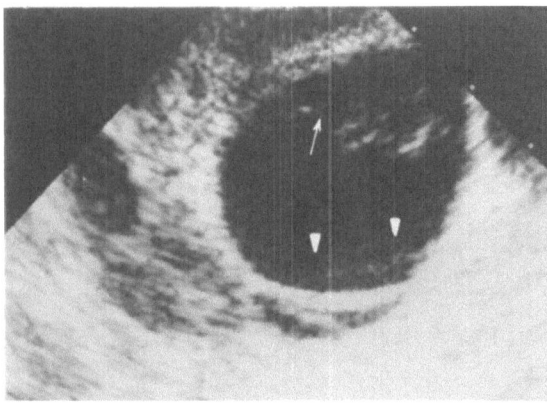

Figure 11.20. Sonographic signs of follicular maturity. (a) In the larger follicle, thickening (arrowheads) and crenation (arrows) of the wall indicate maturity. The smaller follicle is immature by sonographic criteria. (b) Mature follicle. The fine intrafollicular echoes (arrowheads) and the linear strands (arrow) are presumed to represent cellular debris and clumping of granulosa cells. (c) The echogenic focus (arrow) within the large ovarian follicle is thought to represent the cumulus oophorus, indicating maturity. Note the fine intrafollicular echoes (arrowheads).

rate of fertilization [44]. These sonographic findings are also useful in diagnosing premature follicular luteinization: Hamori *et al.* recently demonstrated premature luteinization in 21 of 271 patients [45]; implantation was not achieved in any of the 21 patients, and the authors recommend cancellation of the treatment cycle (to save effort and expense) in the presence of such findings.

The combined use of sonographic follicular monitoring and the hormonal profile (serial serum E2 determinations) is helpful in predicting OHS. This potentially severe complication of ovulation induction is a function of the circulating level of estrogens at the time of ovulation. Patients with serum E2 levels in excess of 2000 pg/mL are at high risk of developing OHS if they are given the ovulating dose of HCG. OHS is classified as mild, moderate, or severe [46]. Mild OHS occurs in about 25% of ovulation induction cycles that utilize HMG. It is associated with pelvic pain and discomfort and ovarian enlargement up to 5 cm. In moderate OHS, the ovaries measure up to 10 cm, and a weight gain of 5 kg or more occurs, often accompanied by nausea and vomiting. The development of ascites, pleural effusion, electrolyte imbalance, and/or marked ovarian enlargement (greater than 10 cm) constitutes severe OHS. The clinical manifestations of OHS are evident 5 to 7 days following the administration of HCG. The value of ovarian sonography in predicting OHS has been emphasized in several recent reports [47—49]. It was found that patients with OHS had significantly more follicles at the time of HCG administration than patients without OHS. Mild OHS was characterized by the presence of eight to nine follicles, two thirds of which were of intermediate size (9 to 15 mm), whereas in moderate and severe OHS, 95% of preovulatory follicles were less than 16 mm and over half of these were less than 9 mm in diameter.

Monitoring of endometrial changes

That the endometrium is well demonstrated on sonography has prompted many investigators to monitor its size and morphologic changes during stimulated cycles [50]. Such monitoring has been greatly facilitated by transvaginal ultrasound, with which endometrial thickness and growth are easily determined (Fig. 11.21). Initial efforts to correlate endometrial thickness and the probability of conception were disappointing, mainly because the studies were performed during the late proliferative (preovulatory) phase. Some reports indicate that sonographic measurement of the endometrium in the secretory phase may be helpful in predicting which patients are likely to conceive [51—54]. An endometrial thickness greater than 13 mm 11 days after follicular aspiration was associated with the greatest likelihood of conception. Other

authors have suggested estimation of endometrial volume as a more accurate measurement [55]. Endometrial volume is obtained by the product of the transverse dimension, the anteroposterior dimension at the level of the tubal ostia, and the length from the fundus to the internal os on long-axis views (Fig. 11.22). Smith *et al.*, in a study of stimulated cycles in IVF-ET, have described four distinct sonographic patterns of preovulatory endometrium [56]. Reflectivity and endometrial echotexture were used to grade the endometrial response into least

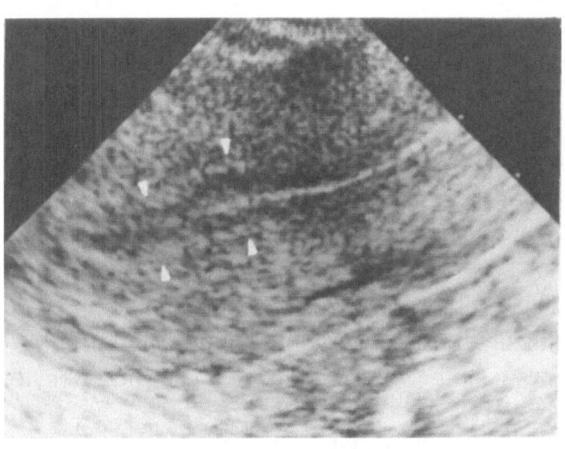

a

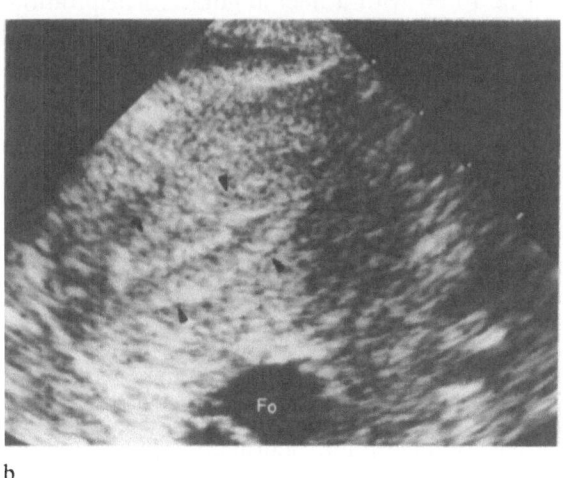

b

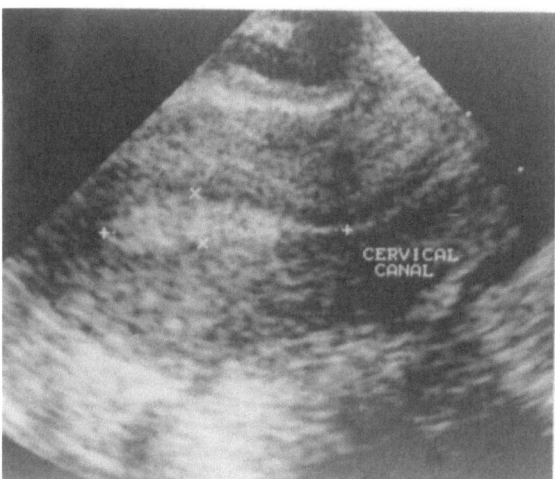

a

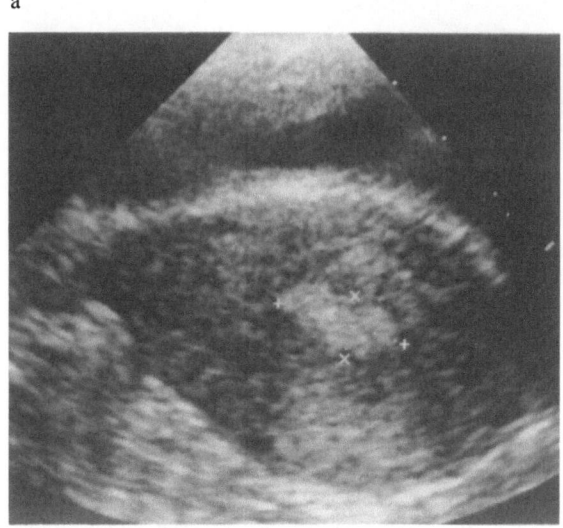

b

Figure 11.21. Endometrial changes during stimulated cycles. (a) Transvaginal sagittal scan of the uterus in the early proliferative phase shows hypoechoic endometrium and faintly echogenic interfaces (arrowheads). (b) Sagittal scan of the same uterus in the periovulatory phase. The endometrial thickness has increased, and the interfaces are more echogenic (arrowheads). Note a follicle (Fo) in the stimulated ovary.

Figure 11.22. Endometrial volume estimation. Sagittal (a) and coronal (b) scans of the uterus. Cursors delineate the endometrium. The endometrial volume is obtained by the product of the long (from fundus to internal os, the 'cervical canal' length being excluded), transverse, and anteroposterior greatest dimensions.

170

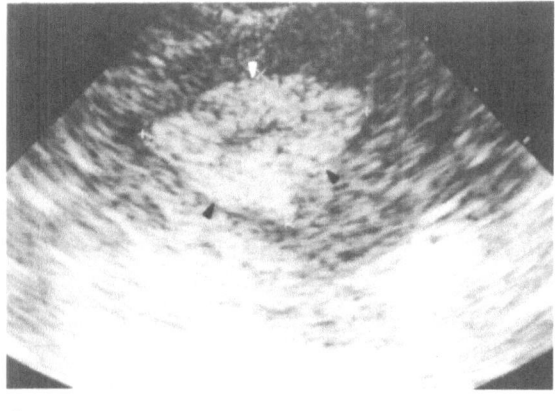

a

b

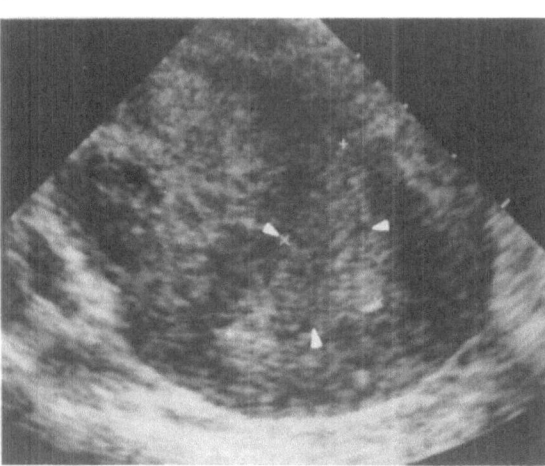

c

Figure 11.23. Endometrial response and likelihood of conception. Coronal scans of the uterus during the secretory phase in three different patients. (a) The endometrium (arrowheads) is markedly echogenic compared with surrounding myometrium. This is considered the most favorable response of the endometrium and is associated with the greatest likelihood of conception. (b) Less favorable response is indicated by only minimal increase in echogenicity of the endometrium (arrowheads). (c) The endometrium is isoechoic (arrowheads). This is less likely to be associated with conception.

favorable for conception (anechoic with a prominent midline echo), most favorable (hyperechoic endometrium, as compared with myometrium), and two intermediate grades (Fig. 11.23). These authors recommend the use of endometrial changes as an adjunct to hormonal assays, as a worthwhile parameter that adds greater flexibility to the management of treatment cycles.

Follicular aspiration guided by transvaginal sonography

Laparoscopy was originally the only method for follicular aspiration for oocyte recovery [57]. Alternative methods, such as transvesical needle aspiration using a transabdominal or a transurethral approach under ultrasound guidance, were subsequently developed to overcome the problems of inaccessible ovaries on laparoscopy [58—61]. Transvaginal aspiration followed, first under transabdominal ultrasound control [62], and later under transvaginal sonographic guidance [63]. Transvaginal follicular aspiration utilizing transvaginal ultrasound guidance has now become the method of choice for oocyte recovery.

Almost all available endovaginal transducers can be fitted with a needle guide for aspiration (Fig. 11.24). The puncturing needle is passed through the needle guide, and its expected path is indicated on the video monitor. Various needles from different suppliers are in use; most are 30 cm in length and have an inner diameter of 1.0 mm (17 gauge). The tip of the needle must be very sharp to puncture the ovary and follicles. Shallow grooves scored at the surface of the needle tip facilitate its sonographic visualization by increasing its ultrasound reflectivity (Fig. 11.25). Some operators prefer manual aspiration of the punctured follicles using a 5- or 10-mL syringe; others prefer suction units connected by means of a tubing system.

Technique

All patients receive premedication 45 minutes to 1 hour before the transvaginal follicular aspiration. Some patients require more sedation than others, although very few if any will need general

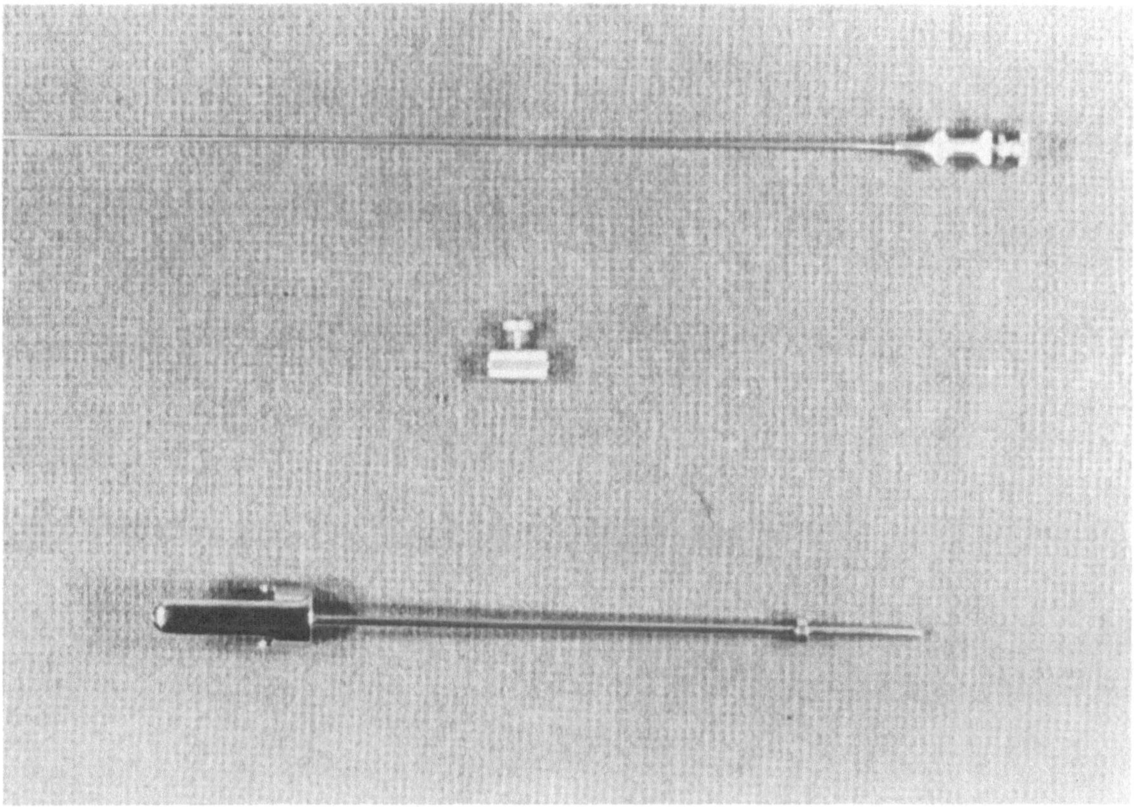

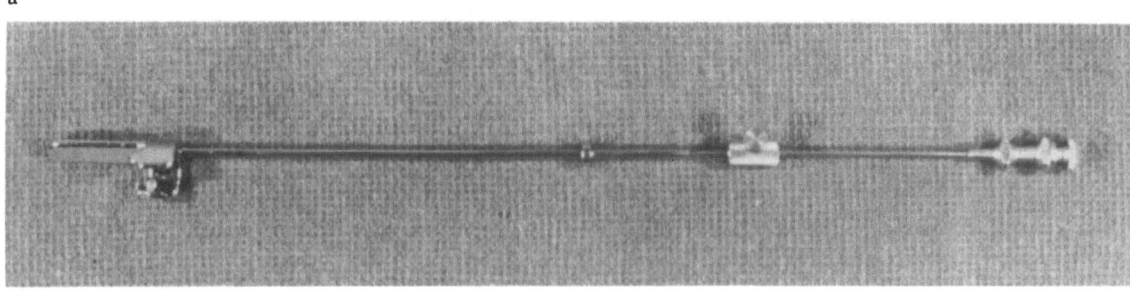

Figure 11.24. Needle guide and puncturing needle for follicular aspiration. (a) The needle guide (bottom) fits onto the transvaginal transducer. The puncturing needle (top) is 30 cm in length. The stopper (center) is used to prevent the needle tip from protruding beyond the guide during intravaginal insertion. (b) View of the needle guide, needle, and stopper assembled to fit on the transvaginal transducer.

anesthesia. The urinary bladder is emptied and the patient placed in the lithotomy position. The vagina is cleansed with sterile saline solution or with culture medium. The endovaginal transducer (covered with a latex condom), needle guide and puncturing needle (which is not protruding beyond the guide) are introduced into the vagina. The ovaries are carefully imaged to determine the number and size of the follicles and to plan the optimal approach for puncture. The follicle to be aspirated is aligned with the electronic puncture line (Fig. 11.26), and the needle is advanced through the vaginal wall. Once the follicle has been punctured, the needle tip is visualized within it as a strong specular reflection (Fig. 11.26). All the follicular fluid is aspirated, and on the video monitor the follicle is seen to collapse (Fig. 11.27). The follicular fluid is examined (by qualified members of the embryo laboratory) for the presence of granulosa

172

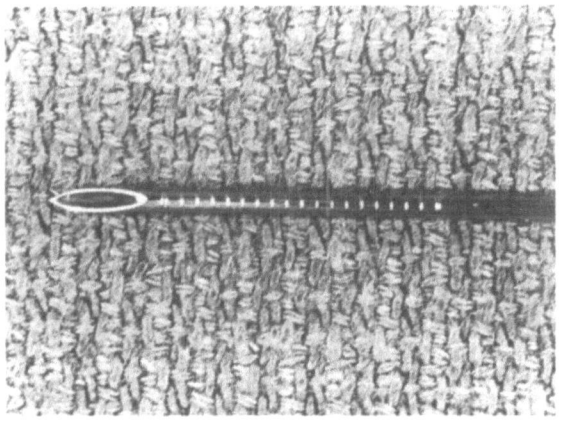

a

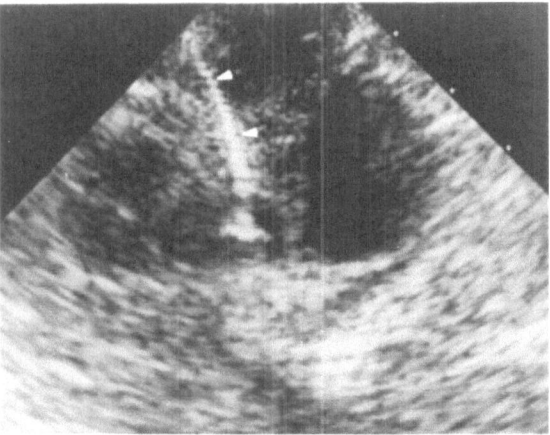

b

Figure 11.25. (a) Magnified view of the puncturing needle shows the shallow grooves scored at the surface of its tip to enhance sonographic visualization. (b) Sonogram obtained during transvaginal follicular aspiration demonstrates the enhanced visualization of the needle that results from the grooves (arrowheads).

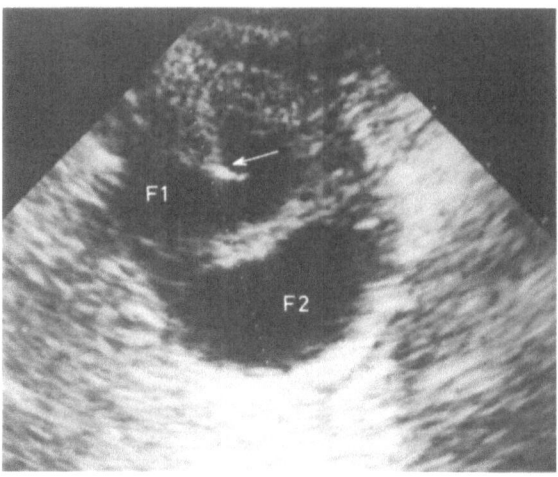

Figure 11.26. Transvaginal ultrasound-guided follicular aspiration. The follicle to be aspirated (F1) is aligned with the electronic puncture line (dotted line). The tip of the needle within the follicle is seen as a strong specular reflector (arrow). The second follicle (F2) can be aspirated by advancing the needle under sonographic monitoring, without need for reorientation of the needle.

cells and the oocyte. With the needle tip still within the follicle, one or more flushes are performed as necessary utilizing culture medium fluid. The process of flushing and reaspirating is monitored by continuous real-time scanning (Fig. 11.27).

Once an oocyte has been recovered from a punctured follicle, or alternatively a set number of flushes has been completed, the whole procedure is repeated for the next follicle. In many cases, a number of follicles can be aspirated without withdrawing the needle. However, it is essential to avoid excessive transducer manipulation with the needle protruded to prevent

inadvertent rupture of adjacent follicles and ovarian injury.

Complications of transvaginal aspiration are rare and can be managed without operative intervention. These include (a) excessive vaginal bleeding at the puncture site, usually responsive to a vaginal pack; (b) pelvic hematoma, which can be monitored by repeat ultrasound examination until its resolution; and (c) ovarian or pelvic abscess.

The most significant advantage of transvaginal follicular aspiration under transvaginal ultrasound guidance is the avoidance of general anesthesia and its risks and expense. Many centers now perform oocyte recovery under transvaginal ultrasound guidance as an outpatient procedure. Other advantages of this method are avoidance of a full urinary bladder, ease of performance, and the higher rates of oocyte retrieval reported by many [64, 65].

Role of transvaginal sonography in assisted reproduction

Now that endovaginal probes are both widely available and used, the use of transvaginal

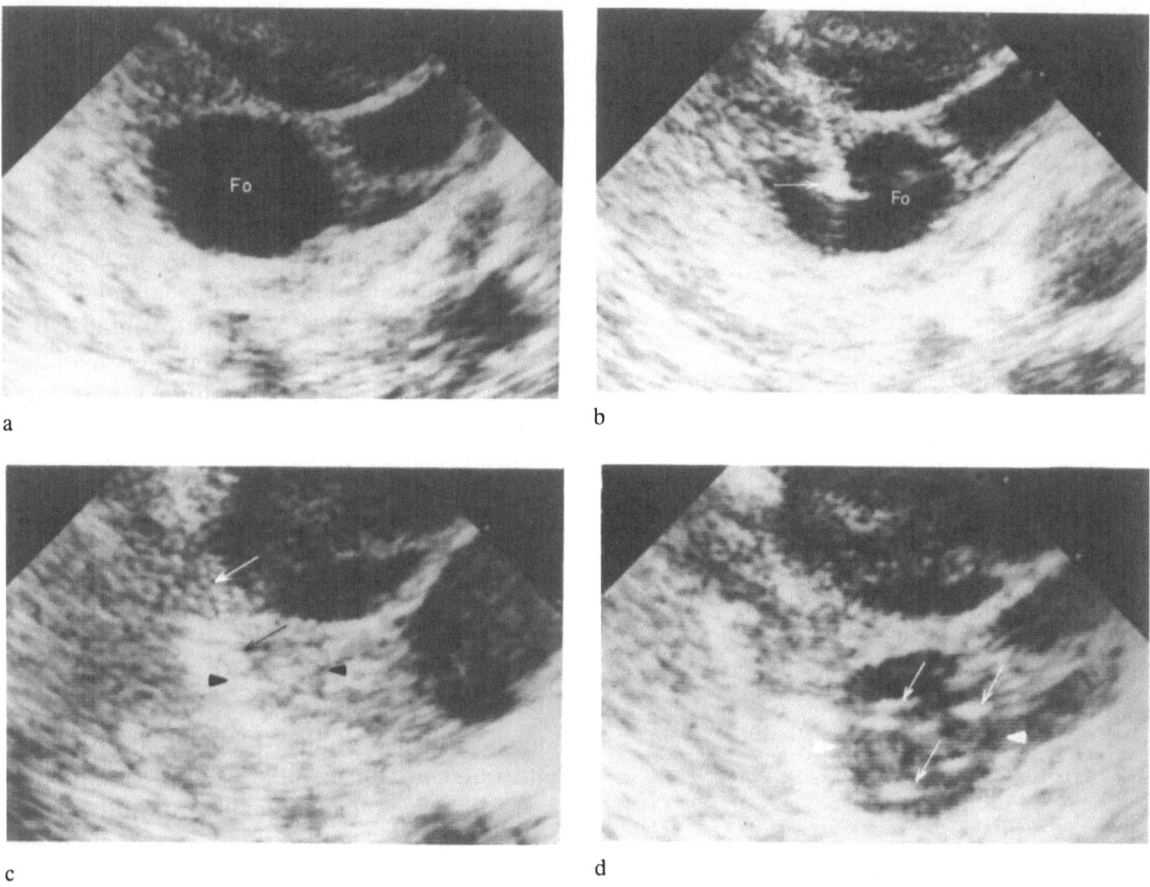

Figure 11.27. Aspiration and flushing of follicle. (a) Transvaginal scan of the follicle (Fo) to be aspirated. (b) The follicle (Fo) has been punctured and is being aspirated. Note the decrease in size compared with (a). The needle tip is seen as a specular reflector (arrow) within the follicle. (c) Collapse of the follicle occurs when all the follicular fluid has been aspirated. The collapsed follicle (arrowheads) and the needle path (arrows) are barely discernible. (d) Culture medium fluid has been introduced into the follicle during the process of flushing. The follicle (arrowheads) is distended and contains swirling echoes (arrows), which represent microbubbles in the flushing fluid.

ultrasound has been explored in many aspects of assisted reproduction, including embryo transfer (ET), gamete intrafallopian transfer (GIFT), zygote intrafallopian transfer (ZIFT), pronuclear-stage tubal transfer (PROST), and fallopian embryo transfer (FET).

Embryo transfer

Following fertilization and cleavage of recovered oocytes, the embryo (or embryos) is transferred into the uterine cavity, usually within 48 hours of follicular aspiration. The procedure is performed by 'loading' the embryo(s) into a sterile transfer catheter in a very small amount of culture medium (30 to 50 µL) and threading this

catheter through a metallic endocervical guide. Theoretically, the ideal site of embryo transfer is 1 to 2 cm from the cephalad aspect of the endometrial cavity. Transabdominal ultrasound has been used to guide the tip of the transfer catheter to the ideal location within the endometrial cavity, and it has occasionally demonstrated kinks in the catheter [66]. Transvaginal ultrasound-directed embryo transfer is being evaluated for a role in routine transfer following IVF. Both the metallic endocervical guide and the transfer catheter can be visualized by transvaginal ultrasound (Fig. 11.28). Surgical embryo transfer by perurethral or transvaginal techniques utilizing ultrasound guidance has been found to be useful in patients in whom

174

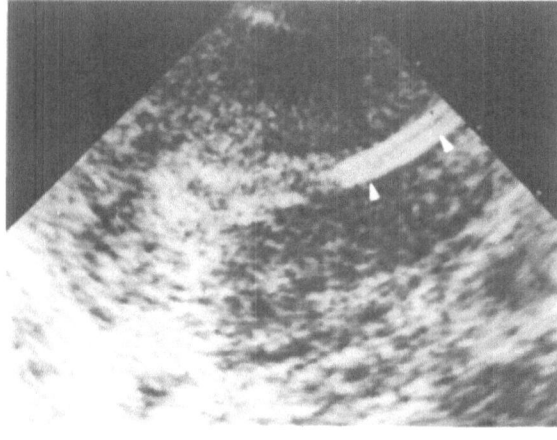

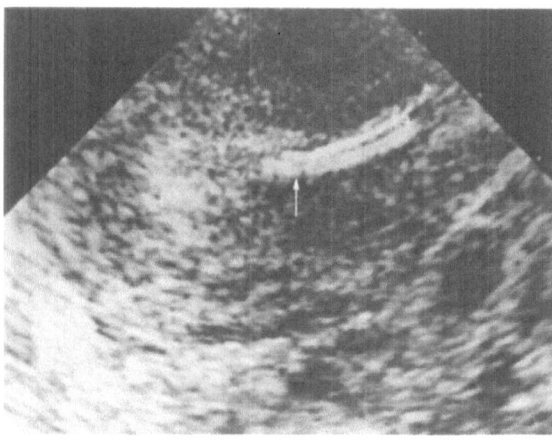

Figure 11.28. Transvaginal ultrasound-directed embryo transfer. (a) Sagittal scan of the uterus shows the endocervical guide (arrowheads) in place. (b) The embryo transfer catheter (arrow) has been inserted into the uterine cavity through the endocervical guide.

nonsurgical cervical transfer is difficult because of stenosis or spasm of the cervix [67].

Gamete intrafallopian transfer

GIFT has gained popularity in recent years as an alternative to IVF-ET. Oocyte recovery was initially performed at laparoscopy or minilaparotomy with the patient under general anesthesia [68]. The recovered oocytes (usually two) and prepared sperm (approximately 500,000 sperm, in 50 µL of buffered medium) are transferred into the fallopian tube via a catheter introduced through the fimbriated end. The technique

obviously requires at least one anatomically normal and patent fallopian tube. Because the gametes are placed in the fallopian tube, fertilization occurs in its normal site (with natural surrounding fluids and temperature) and development of the embryo and its entry into the uterus proceed at a normal pace. The recent development of transvaginal ultrasound-guided endocervical cannulation of the fallopian tube [69] has fostered attempts at performing GIFT solely by transvaginal ultrasound, thus avoiding laparoscopy. A similar technique is currently being evaluated for intrafallopian transfer of fertilized oocytes at various stages under transvaginal sonographic guidance in such procedures as ZIFT [70], PROST [71], and FET [72].

Transvaginal Doppler study

Studies of blood flow to the ovaries and corpus luteum utilizing duplex Doppler transvaginal ultrasound are being investigated for possible use in assessing the functional status of the ovary prior to conception, and in predicting the likelihood of pregnancy following assisted reproduction.

The Doppler waveform obtained from the ovary in the proliferative phase is characteristic of high-impedance flow, with a reduced diastolic component and a high resistance index (Fig. 11.29). In the luteal phase, duplex Doppler studies of the corpus luteum have been found to provide information about the likelihood of pregnancy. In those patients destined to achieve a pregnancy, Porter *et al.* found that the mean resistance index of the corpus luteum flow was significantly lower than in patients who did not become pregnant [73]. No patient with a resistance index greater than 0.5 became pregnant in the Porter series. Kossoff and McSweeney compared the resistance index of the corpus luteum flow at 3 and 10 days following embryo transfer in 55 patients [74]. The mean resistance index decreased from 0.47 to 0.45 in patients with subsequent pregnancy, whereas it increased from 0.82 to 0.98 in the patients who did not become pregnant. A resistance index greater

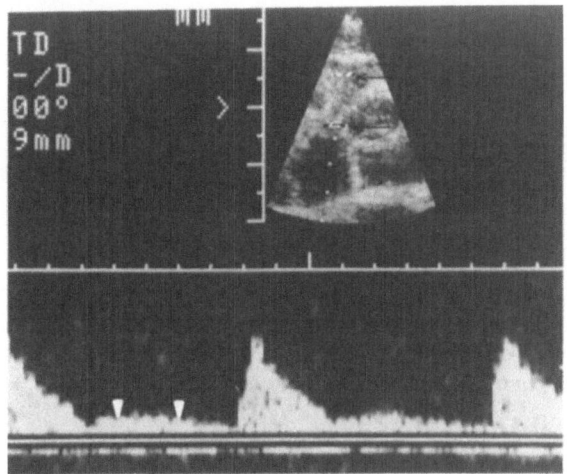

Figure 11.29. Transvaginal duplex Doppler of the ovary. The magnified transvaginal scan of the ovary (top) confirms that the Doppler sample gate between cursors (arrows) is within ovarian tissue. The Doppler waveform (bottom) is characteristic of high-impedance flow, with a reduced diastolic component (arrowheads).

than 0.55 was associated with a poor chance for pregnancy in this latter series.

The addition of color flow Doppler imaging to transvaginal scanning is expected to facilitate the evaluation of blood flow to the ovaries, corpus luteum, and endometrium.

Summary

Transvaginal ultrasound plays a pivotal role in the evaluation and management of the infertile female. It has gained widespread acceptance in monitoring ovarian and endometrial response in stimulated cycles and is the method of choice in oocyte retrieval. Transvaginal sonography is gradually replacing laparoscopy in many procedures of assisted reproduction, including GIFT, ZIFT, and PROST. New methods for managing infertility are being developed, based on the experience gained through the use of transvaginal sonography. Transvaginal duplex and color flow Doppler will undoubtedly enhance our understanding of the physiopathologic aspects of female infertility.

References

1. Mendelson E. B., Bohm-Velez M., Joseph N., Neiman H. L.: Gynecologic imaging: Comparison of transabdominal and transvaginal sonography. Radiology, 1988, 166, 321—324.
2. Woolf R. B., Allen W. M.: Concomitant malformations: The frequent simultaneous occurrence of congenital malformations of the reproductive and urinary tracts. Obstet. Gynecol., 1953, 2, 236—265.
3. Wiersma A. F., Peterson L. F., Justema E. J.: Uterine anomalies associated with unilateral renal agenesis. Obstet. Gynecol., 1976, 47, 654—657.
4. Zanetti E., Ferrari L. R., Rossi G.: Classification and radiographic features of uterine malformations. Br. J. Radiol., 1976, 51, 161—170.
5. Buttram V. C. Jr., Gibbons W. E.: Müllerian anomalies: A proposed classification. An analysis of 144 cases. Fertil. Steril., 1979, 32, 40—46.
6. McArdle C. R., Berezin A. F.: Ultrasound demonstration of uterus subseptus. J. Clin. Ultrasound, 1980, 8, 139—141.
7. Valdes C., Malini S., Malinak L. R.: Ultrasound evaluation of female genital tract anomalies: A review of 64 cases. Am. J. Obstet. Gynecol., 1984, 149, 285—292.
8. Randolph J. F. Jr., Ying Y. K., Maier D. B.: Comparison of real-time ultrasonography, hysterosalpingography, and laparoscopy/hysteroscopy in the evaluation of uterine abnormalities and tubal patency. Fertil. Steril., 1986, 46, 828— 832.
9. Fedele L., Dorta M., Vercellini P., Brioschi D., Candiani G. B.: Ultrasound in the diagnosis of subclasses of unicornuate uterus. Obstet. Gynecol., 1988, 71, 274—277.
10. Kaufman R. H., Binder G. L., Gray P. M. Jr., et al.: Upper genital tract changes associated with exposure in utero to diethylstilbestrol. Am. J. Obstet. Gynecol., 1977, 128, 51—59.
11. Mintz M. C., Grumbach K.: Imaging of congenital uterine anomalies. Semin. Ultrasound CT MR, 1988, 9, 167—174.
12. Buttram V. C. Jr., Reiter R. C.: Uterine leiomyomata: Etiology, symptomatology, and management. Fertil. Steril., 1981, 36, 433—445.
13. Wallach E. E.: The uterine factor in infertility. Fertil. Steril., 1972, 23, 138—158.
14. Malone L. H., Ingersoll F. M.: Myomectomy in infertility. In: Behrman S. J., Kistner R. W., (eds.). Progress in infertility, ed. 2. Boston, Little, Brown & Co., 1975.
15. Ranney B., Frederick I.: The occasional need for myomectomy. Obstet. Gynecol., 1979, 53, 437—441.
16. Hamou J.: Hystéroscopie et microcolpohystéroscopie: Atlas et traité. Palermo, Cofese, 1984.
17. Buttram V. C. Jr., Reiter R. C.: Surgical treatment of the infertile female. Baltimore, Williams & Wilkins, 1985.
18. Maheux R.: LH-RH agonists. How useful against uterine leiomyomas? Contemp. Ob/Gyn, 1986, 28, 66—77.

176

19. Balasch J., Vanrell J. A., Creus M., Marquez M., Gonzalez-Merlo J.: The endometrial biopsy for diagnosis of luteal phase deficiency. Fertil. Steril., 1985, 44, 699—701.
20. Witten B. I., Martin S. A.: The endometrial biopsy as a guide to the management of the luteal phase defect. Fertil. Steril., 1985, 44, 460—465.
21. March C. M., Israel R., March A. D.: Hysteroscopic management of intrauterine adhesions. Am. J. Obstet. Gynecol., 1978, 130, 653—657.
22. Fleischer A. C., Kalemeris G. C., Machin J. E., Entman S. S., James A. E. Jr.: Sonographic depiction of normal and abnormal endometrium with histopathologic correlation. J. Ultrasound Med., 1986, 5, 445—452.
23. Stein I. F., Leventhal M. L.: Amenorrhea associated with bilateral polycystic ovaries. Am. J. Obstet. Gynecol., 1935, 29, 181.
24. Raj S. G., Thompson I. E., Berger M. J., et al.: Clinical aspects of the polycystic ovary syndrome. Obstet. Gynecol., 1977, 49, 552—556.
25. Cohen M. R.: Laparoscopic diagnosis and pseudomenopause treatment of endometriosis with danazol. Clin. Obstet. Gynecol., 1980, 23, 901—915.
26. Williams T. J., Pratt J. H.: Endometriosis in 1,000 consecutive celiotomies: Incidence and management. Am. J. Obstet. Gynecol., 1977, 129, 245—250.
27. Kistner R. W.: Management of endometriosis in the infertile patient. Fertil. Steril., 1975, 26, 1151—1166.
28. Strathy J. T., Molgaard C. A., Coulam C. B., et al.: Endometriosis and infertility: A laparoscopic study of endometriosis among fertile and infertile women. Fertil. Steril., 1982, 38, 667—672.
29. Marik J., Hulka J.: Luteinized unruptured follicle syndrome: A subtle cause of infertility. Fertil. Steril., 1978, 29, 270—274.
30. Portuondo J. A., Agustin A., Herran C., et al.: The corpus luteum in infertile patients found during laparoscopy. Fertil. Steril., 1981, 36, 37—40.
31. Liukkonen S., Koskimies A. I., Tenhunen A., et al.: Diagnosis of luteinized unruptured follicle (LUF) syndrome by ultrasound. Fertil. Steril., 1984, 41, 26—30.
32. Graf M. J., Dunaif A.: Association of reproductive endocrine dysfunction with pelvic endometriosis. Semin. Reprod. Endocrinol., 1985, 3, 319—324.
33. Nosher J. L., Winchman, H. K., Needell G. S.: Transvaginal pelvic abscess drainage with US guidance. Radiology, 1987, 165, 872—873.
34. Timor-Tritsch I. E., Rottem S.: Transvaginal ultrasonographic study of the fallopian tube. Obstet. Gynecol., 1987, 70, 424—428.
35. Hackelöer B. J., Fleming R., Robinson H. P., et al.: Correlation of ultrasonic and endocrinologic assessment of human follicular development. Am. J. Obstet. Gynecol., 1979, 135, 122—128.
36. Maklad N. F.: Monitoring follicular development with ultrasound. In: Wolf D. P., Quigley M. M. (eds.). Human in vitro fertilization and embryo transfer. New York, Plenum Press, 1983.
37. Quigley M. M., Maklad N. F., Wolf D. P., et al.: Monitoring follicular development in IVF-ET program: Comparison of ultrasonic imaging and serum estradiol measurement. Fertil. Steril., 1983, 39, 416—420.
38. Ritchie W. G. M.: Ultrasound in the evaluation of normal and induced ovulation. Fertil. Steril., 1985, 43, 167—181.
39. Ritchie W. G. M.: Sonographic evaluation of normal and induced ovulation. Radiology, 1986, 161, 1—10.
40. Yee B., Barnes R. B., Vargyas J. M., Marss R. P.: Correlation of transabdominal and transvaginal measurements of follicle size and number with laparoscopic findings for in vitro fertilization. Fertil. Steril., 1987, 47, 828—832.
41. Fleischer A. C., Daniell J. F., Rodier J., et al.: Sonographic monitoring of ovarian follicular development. J. Clin. Ultrasound, 1981, 9, 275—280.
42. Marrs R. P., Vargyas J. M., March C. M.: Correlation of ultrasonic and endocrinologic measurements in human menopausal gonadotropin therapy. Am. J. Obstet. Gynecol., 1983, 145, 417—421.
43. Seibel M. M., McArdle C., Smith D., et al.: Ovulation induction in polycystic ovarian syndrome with urinary follicle-stimulating hormone or human menopausal gonadotropin. Fertil. Steril., 1985, 43, 703—708.
44. Smith B., Evans J., Simons E., Craft I.: The use of vaginal transducers in the detailed studies of periovulatory follicular and endometrial changes. Oral presentation, First World Congress on Vaginosonography in Gynecology, Washington, D.C., June 9—12, 1988.
45. Hamori M., Stuckensen J. A., Rumpf D., Kniewald T., Kniewald A., Kurz C. S.: Premature luteinization of follicles during ovarian stimulation for in vitro fertilization. Hum. Reprod., 1987, 2, 639—643.
46. Schwartz M., Jewelewicz R.: The use of gonadotropins for induction in ovulation. Fertil. Steril., 1981, 35, 3—12.
47. Painvain E., Barlese M. G., Mastrojanni F., et al.: Ultrasound evaluation of the ovarian hyperstimulation syndrome. Acta Eur. Fertil., 1987, 18, 39—43.
48. Blankstein J., Shalev J., Saadon T., et al.: Ovarian hyperstimulation syndrome: Prediction by number and size of preovulatory ovarian follicles. Fertil. Steril., 1987, 47, 597—602.
49. Nader S., Berkowitz A. S., Maklad N., Winkel C. A.: Ovarian hyperstimulation syndrome: Combined use of ultrasound and hormonal profile to identify the patient at low risk in an IVF/ET program. Infertility, 1988, 11, 157—165.
50. Fleischer A. C., Pittaway D. E., Beard L. A., et al.: Sonographic depiction of endometrial changes occurring with ovulation induction. J. Ultrasound Med., 1984, 3, 341—346.
51. Brandt T. D., Levy E. B., Grant T. H. et al.: Endometrial echo and its significance in female infertility. Radiology, 1985, 157, 225—229.
52. Glissant A., de Mouzon J., Frydman R.: Ultrasound study of the endometrium during in vitro fertilization cycles. Fertil. Steril., 1985, 44, 786—790.
53. Giorlandino C., Gleicher N., Nanni C., Vizzone A.,

Gentili P., Taramanni C.: The sonographic picture of endometrium in spontaneous and induced cycles. Fertil. Steril., 1987, 47, 508—511.

54. Rabinowitz R., Laufer N., Lewin A., *et al.*: The value of ultrasonographic endometrial measurement in the prediction of pregnancy following in vitro fertilization. Fertil. Steril., 1986, 45, 824—828.

55. Fleischer A. C., Mendelson E. B., Böhm-Velez M., Entman S. S.: Transvaginal and transabdominal sonography of the endometrium. Semin. Ultrasound CT MR, 1988, 9, 81—101.

56. Smith B., Porter R., Ahuga K., Craft I.: Ultrasonic assessment of endometrial changes in stimulated cycles in an in vitro fertilization and embryo transfer program. J. In Vitro Fert. Embryo Transfer, 1984, 1, 50—55.

57. Wood C., Leeton J. F., McTalbot J., *et al.*: Technique for collecting mature human oocytes for in vitro fertilisation. Br. J. Obstet. Gynaecol., 1981, 88, 756—760.

58. Lenz S., Lauritsen J. G.: Ultrasonically guided percutaneous aspiration of human follicles under local anesthesia: A new method of collecting oocytes for in vitro fertilization. Fertil. Steril., 1982, 38, 673—677.

59. Wikland M., Nilsson L., Hansson R., *et al.*: Collection of human oocytes by the use of sonography. Fertil. Steril., 1983, 39, 603—608.

60. Robertson R. D., Picker R. H., O'Neill C., Ferrier A. G., Saunders D. M.: An experience of laparoscopic and transvesical oocyte retrieval in an in vitro fertilization program. Fertil. Steril., 1986, 45, 88—92.

61. Parsons J., Riddle A., Booker M., *et al.*: Oocyte retrieval for in-vitro fertilisation by ultrasonically guided needle aspiration via the urethra. Lancet, 1985, 1, 1076—1077.

62. Dellenbach P., Nisand I., Moreau L., *et al.*: Transvaginal sonographically controlled follicle puncture for oocyte retrieval. Fertil. Steril., 1985, 44, 656—662.

63. Feichtinger W., Kemeter P.: Transvaginal sector scan sonography for needle-guided transvaginal follicle aspiration and other applications in gynecologic routine and research. Fertil. Steril., 1986, 45, 722—725.

64. Deutinger J., Reinthaller A., Csaicsich P., *et al.*: Follicular aspiration for in vitro fertilization: Sonographically guided transvaginal versus laparoscopic approach. Eur. J. Obstet. Gynecol. Reprod. Biol., 1987, 26, 127—133.

65. Baber R., Porter R., Picker R., Robertson R., Dawson E., Saunders D.: Transvaginal ultrasound directed oocyte collection for in vitro fertilization: Successes and complications. J. Ultrasound Med., 1988, 7, 377—379.

66. Leong M., Leung C., Tucker M., Wong C., Chan H.: Ultrasound-assisted embryo transfer. J. In Vitro Fert. Embryo Transfer, 1986, 3, 383—385.

67. Parsons J. H., Bolton V. N., Wilson L., Campbell S.: Pregnancies following in vitro fertilization and ultrasound-directed surgical embryo transfer by perurethral and transvaginal techniques. Fertil. Steril., 1987, 48, 691—693.

68. Asch R. H., Balmaceda J. P., Ellsworth L. R., Wong P. C.: Preliminary experiences with gamete intrafallopian transfer (GIFT). Fertil. Steril., 1986, 45, 366—371.

69. Jansen R. P. S., Anderson J. C.: Catheterisation of the fallopian tubes from the vagina. Lancet, 1987, 2, 309—310.

70. Devroey P., Braeckmans P., Smitz J., *et al.*: Pregnancy after translaparoscopic zygote intrafallopian transfer in a patient with sperm antibodies (letter). Lancet, 1986, 1, 1329.

71. Yovich J. L., Blackledge D. G., Richardson P. A., Matson P. L., Turner S. R., Draper R.: Pregnancies following pronuclear stage tubal transfer. Fertil. Steril., 1987, 48, 851— 857.

72. Jansen R. P. S., Anderson J. C., Sutherland P. D.: Clinical pregnancy after nonoperative embryo transfer to the fallopian tubes. Oral presentation, Society for Gynecologic Investigation, Baltimore, March 1988.

73. Porter R. N., Picker R. H., Robertson F. D., Saunders D. N.: The use of vaginal ultrasonography in an IVF program. Oral presentation, First World Congress on Vaginosonography in Gynecology, Washington, June 9—12, 1988.

74. Kossoff G., McSweeney M.: Obstetrical duplex Doppler. Oral presentation, 32nd Meeting of the American Institute for Ultrasound in Medicine, New Orleans, October 6—9, 1987.

Index of Subjects

SERIES IN RADIOLOGY

1. J. O. Op den Orth: *The Standard Biphasic-contrast Examination of the Stomach and Duodenum*. Method, Results, and Radiological Atlas. 1979   ISBN 90–247–2159–8
2. J. L. Sellink and R. E. Miller: *Radiology of the Small Bowel*. Modern Enteroclysis Technique and Atlas. 1982
                                                                                                                ISBN 90–247–2460–0
3. R. E. Miller and J. Skucas: *The Radiological Examination of the Colon*. Practical Diagnosis. 1983 ISBN 90–247–2666–2
4. S. Forgács: *Bones and Joints in Diabetes Mellitus*. 1982   ISBN 90–247–2395–7
5. Gy. Németh and H. Kuttig (eds.): *Isodose Atlas for Use in Radiotherapy*. 1981   ISBN 90–247–2476–7
6. J. Chermet: *Atlas of Phlebography of the Lower Limbs*. Including the Iliac Veins. 1982   ISBN 90–247–2525–9
7. B. K. Janevski: *Angiography of the Upper Extremity*. 1982   ISBN 90–247–2684–0
8. M. A. M. Feldberg: *Computed Tomography of the Retroperitoneum*. An Anatomical and Pathological Atlas with Emphasis on the Fascial Planes. 1983   ISBN 0–89838–573–3
9. L. E. H. Lampmann, S. A. Duursma and J. H. J. Ruys: *CT Densitometry in Osteoporosis*. The Impact on Management of the Patient. 1984   ISBN 0–89838–633–0
10. J. J. Broerse and T. J. Macvittie: *Response of Different Species to Total Body Irradiation*. 1984   ISBN 0–89838–678–0
11. C. L'Herminé: *Radiology of Liver Circulation*. 1985   ISBN 0–89838–715–9
12. G. Maatman: *High-resolution Computed Tomography of the Paranasal Sinuses, Pharynx and Related Regions*. Impact of CT Identification on Diagnosis and Patient Management. 1986   ISBN 0–89838–802–3
13. C. Plets, A. L. Baert, G. L. Nijs and G. Wilms: *Computer Tomographic Imaging and Anatomic Correlation of the Human Brain*. A Comparative Atlas of Thin CT-scan Sections and Correlated Neuro-anatomic Preparations. 1987
                                                                                                                ISBN 0–89838–811–2
14. J. Valk: *MRI of the Brain, Head, Neck and Spine*. A Teaching Atlas of Clinical Applications. 1987
                                                                                                                ISBN 0–89838–957–7
15. J. L. Sellink: *X-Ray Differential Diagnosis in Small Bowel Disease*. A Practical Approach. 1988 ISBN 0–89838–351–X
16. Th.H.M. Falke (ed.): *Essentials of Clinical MRI*. 1988   ISBN 0–89838–353–6
17. B. D. Fornage: *Endosonography*. 1989   ISBN 0–7923–0047–5
18. R. Chisin (ed.): *MRI/CT and Pathology in Head and Neck Tumors*. A Correlative Study. 1989   ISBN 0–7923–0227–3
19. G. Gozzetti, A. Mazziotti, L. Bolondi and L. Barbara (eds.): *Intraoperative Ultrasonography in Hepato-biliary and Pancreatic Surgery*. A Practical Guide. With Contributions by Y. Chapuis, J.-F. Gigot and P.-J. Kestens. 1989
                                                                                                                ISBN 0–7923–C 261–3
20. A. M. A. De Schepper and H. R. M. Degryse: *Magnetic Resonance Imaging of Bone and Soft Tissue Tumors an Their Mimics*. A Clinical Atlas. With Contributions by F. De Belder, L. van den Houwe, F. Ramon, P. Parizel   nd N. Buyssens. 1989   ISBN 0–7923–)343–1